Singapore's Health Care System
What 50 Years Have Achieved

Page 81

World Scientific Series on Singapore's 50 Years of Nation-Building

*The complete list of titles in the series can be found at
http://www.worldscientific.com/series/wss50ynb

SINGAPORE'S HEALTH CARE SYSTEM

What 50 Years Have Achieved

Editors

Lee Chien Earn

Changi General Hospital, Singapore

K. Satku

National University Health System, Singapore

World Scientific

NEW JERSEY · LONDON · SINGAPORE · BEIJING · SHANGHAI · HONG KONG · TAIPEI · CHENNAI · TOKYO

Published by

World Scientific Publishing Co. Pte. Ltd.
5 Toh Tuck Link, Singapore 596224
USA office: 27 Warren Street, Suite 401-402, Hackensack, NJ 07601
UK office: 57 Shelton Street, Covent Garden, London WC2H 9HE

Library of Congress Cataloging-in-Publication Data
Singapore's health care system : what 50 years have achieved / editors, Lee Chien Earn, K. Satku.
    p. ; cm. -- (World Scientific series on Singapore's 50 years of nation-building)
    Includes bibliographical references and index.
    ISBN 978-9814696043 (hardcover : alk. paper) -- ISBN 9814696048 (hardcover : alk. paper) --
    ISBN 978-9814696050 (pbk. : alk. paper) -- ISBN 9814696056 (pbk. : alk. paper)
    I. Lee, Chien Earn, editor. II. Satku, K. (Kandiah), editor. III. Series: World Scientific series on Singapore's
50 years of nation-building.
    [DNLM: 1. Delivery of Health Care--history--Singapore. 2. Health Resources--history--Singapore.
3. Health Services--history--Singapore. 4. History, 20th Century--Singapore. 5. History, 21st Century--
Singapore. W 84 JS6]
    RA395.S59
    362.1095957--dc23

                                  2015023642

British Library Cataloguing-in-Publication Data
A catalogue record for this book is available from the British Library.

Printed in Singapore

Preface

Singapore's healthcare system has come a long way within a relatively short period of 50 years. For example, 50 years ago the infant mortality rate (IMR) was 26 per thousand live births. Today, the IMR is 2. Similarly, life expectancy then was 64 years; today, it is 83. How did Singapore's healthcare system transform itself into one of the best in the world?

This book provides insights into the development of Singapore's healthcare system from the early days of fighting infections and providing supplemental nutrition for schoolchildren to today's management of lifestyle diseases and high-end tertiary care. A hallmark of the system is strong leadership and dedicated people that are prepared to learn from our own experiences while adapting best practices from around the world.

Our aim is not to be comprehensive, but to present key facets of our healthcare system with our various contributors sharing their perspectives in their own voice and style. We have thus taken the approach akin to that of a *Festschrift*, a term borrowed from German, which can be translated as celebratory publication or celebratory piece of writing. However, instead of honouring a person, this book is presented in honour of Singapore. In this regard, we would like to express our deepest appreciation to all who have willingly and expertly contributed to this book despite their busy schedules.

Even as we celebrate the achievements of the past 50 years, we recognise that our healthcare system is not without its challenges — not least those of an ageing population and an increasing market orientation. New challenges will also arise from time to time which require dynamic solutions. Our predecessors have laid a solid foundation that enables us to address these challenges from a stronger position compared with many other countries. Lastly, while the means may change, our goal remains the same — to help Singaporeans continue to "live well, live long, and with peace of mind."

Contents

1 The Transformation of the Health of Our People: An Overview

Lee Chien Earn* and K. Satku[†]

Singapore's healthcare system is recognised today as being one of the best in the world. The World Health Organisation ranked it 6th best among 191 countries in 2000, based on eight criteria;[1] Bloomberg declared Singapore as the healthiest country in the world in 2012, second among 51 countries in health efficiency in 2013 and first in 2014.[2] Indeed the statistics tell the story: the infant mortality rate in 2013 was 2 per thousand live births, maternal mortality was 0.025 per 1000 births and life expectancy was 82 years.[3] Per capita expenditure on healthcare in 2013 was US$2426.[4] In all these measures Singapore has, over many years, consistently ranked among the best in the world in terms of health outcomes and health efficiency.

Access to healthcare is assured, affordable, of good quality, and appropriate to need. The system remains viable because of a fiscal policy developed and refined over the last fifty years. The system can be improved, but in contrast to many developed countries, there is no looming crisis regarding sustainability.

The state of our health services today is contributed to by many factors. At the time of independence from Britain, Singapore was bequeathed a legacy of good health services and infrastructure. There was emphasis on developing preventive services and a network of curative services. Preventive services included public health services, maternal and child health (MCH) services, school health services and health education while curative services included outpatient dispensaries (OPDs) or primary care services, hospital services, and related supporting services such as pharmaceutical services and blood transfusion services. In the post-war years, the years leading up to independence of our nation, a ten-year building development

*Chief Executive Officer, Changi General Hospital, Singapore.
†Chairman, Health Sciences Authority, Singapore. Professor, Department of Orthopaedic Surgery, National University Health System, Singapore. Professor of Health Policy, Saw Swee Hock School of Public Health, National University of Singapore. Former Director of Medical Services (2004–2013), Ministry of Health, Singapore.

plan was drawn up, put into action in 1951, and completed in 1960.[5] Some of the buildings completed during this period included two operating theatre blocks (Surgery A and Surgery B), the Mistri Wing — for Paediatric care, and the School of Nursing, all at the General Hospital (later called the Outram Road General Hospital and now Singapore General Hospital); two new six storey blocks at Tan Tock Seng Hospital; and the Thomson Road Hospital, later known as Toa Payoh Hospital.[5]

The period immediately before and after independence was a time of great medical advances globally. New antibiotics and vaccines were discovered, as well as new drugs to control diseases such as leprosy, hypertension, and cancer. New technology resulted in better investigations such as the CT scan (computerised tomography) and MRI (magnetic resonance imaging) and new therapeutic procedures were developed, such as coronary artery by-pass grafting and later, coronary vessel stenting and joint replacement. Public health research revealed the effects of health-related behaviour such as smoking and its ill effects, and exercise and its benefits.

Singapore's healthcare professionals embraced the rapid progress happening in medical sciences globally. These advancements helped eradicate some illnesses like poliomyelitis and leprosy, prolong life by reducing premature death due to cancer and heart disease, and reduce years lived in disability by interventions such as cataract and joint replacement surgery, thereby improving quality of life.

However, the most significant factor in the progress of Singapore's health status was the Government's and the people's vision and commitment to the improvement of living conditions in general and of the health services in particular. Medical advances are, by themselves, useless unless there is access to them. Public health and other related developments were put in place as a result of good urban planning and a determination of the nation to succeed. The triumphs of public health that helped contain and eradicate the many infectious diseases that were rife in the early years of our nation were access to clean water, sanitation supplied to every household, health education, and accessible maternal and child healthcare. These were critical elements in the eradication of some of the more common causes of illnesses. In 1965, with independence and the economic success that followed, more healthcare infrastructure and manpower development took place. Ministry of Health's (MOH) per capita expenditure in 1965 was $38.[6] In 2013, Government Health Expenditure per person was estimated to be $1104.[4]

Health Services — The Early Years

There were a number of critical services already in place during the period of colonial rule which laid the foundations for further major developments and improvements in the health of our population. Prior to 1959, the environmental health services (including some personal health services) were run by the City Council Health Services and the Rural Board Health Services (Fig. 1.1). With self-government in

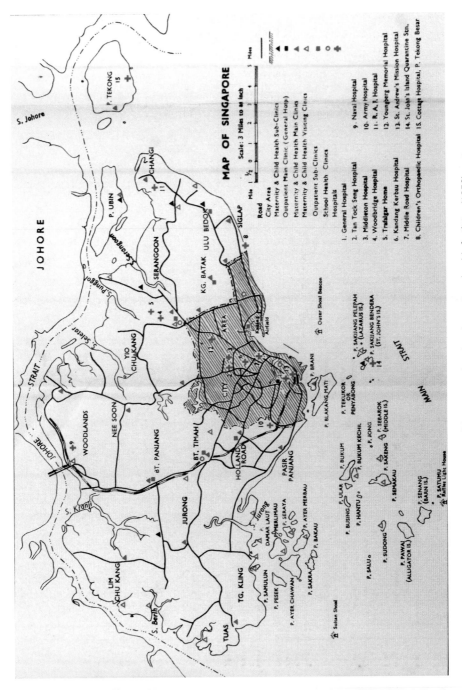

Fig. 1.1. Map of Singapore showing the various health facilities (1958).

1959, the Ministry of Health was reorganised. The functions of these two entities were brought under the Public Health Division (preventive services) of the Ministry of Health.[7]

The hospitals, including Middleton Hospital for infectious diseases, which were under the City Council, were included in the Hospitals Division (curative services) of the Ministry. Tan Tock Seng Hospital, which had been managed by a Committee of Management, was subjected to similar re-organisation and brought under the administration of the Hospitals Division of the Ministry.[7]

In 1965, the mid-year population was 1,864,900. There were 55,725 live births in 1965[6] giving a crude birth rate of 29.9/1000 population. This was a decline from the rate ten years earlier in 1955, which was 44.3/1000 population.

The infant mortality rate was 26/1000 live births, and the maternal mortality rate was 0.4/1000. Infectious diseases were common. Forty new cases of poliomyelitis, 230 cases of diphtheria, 278 cases of typhoid, 242 cases of leprosy and 201 cases of malaria were reported.[8] Life expectancy was 64 years.

There was an urgent need to improve both the preventive and curative services, and make them accessible to the citizens.

Preventive Health Services

School health services

School Health was one of the early preventive programmes. It was started in 1921.

The health status of our children in 1965 would be a fair reflection of the state of health of our population. There was a student population of 482,000 distributed across the 595 schools. A total of 150,000 were assessed by our School Health staff in 1965. About forty percent (40%) of students had varying degrees of dental caries. About 4% had skin conditions such as ringworm, eczema and scabies. 10 students were suspected to have leprosy. About 10% had defective vision. About 6 in 1000 or 0.6/100 had cardiac disease including acquired rheumatic heart disease, a condition in which heart valves malfunction after a bacterial infection. Worm infestation was present in about 6% of students. Despite a voluntary immunisation programme, 51 students were diagnosed with diphtheria, two (2) with poliomyelitis, and three (3) with whooping cough. Thirty-three thousand (33,000) undernourished children had to be put on a feeding scheme to help in their growth and development. Piped water was not available in about 10% of our schools on the main island. This was the state of the health of our school children when we gained independence.[6]

The immunisation programme was intensified through both the MCH services and schools; and soon diseases such as poliomyelitis, diphtheria and whooping cough became almost non-existent. The feeding scheme also contributed significantly to

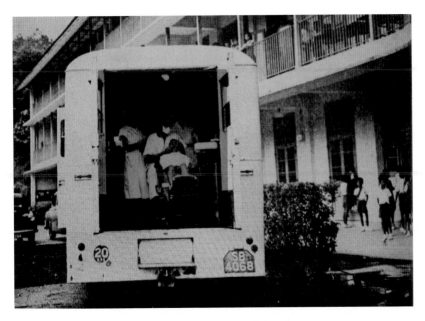

Fig. 1.2. Mobile dental clinic.

the improvement of health in the early years. A school dental service consisting of dental clinics in some primary schools and mobile dental clinics in others contributed to better dental hygiene (Fig. 1.2).

Improved sanitation across the island, and clean water supply through piped water including water from "stand pipes," contributed to the improvements to health of the school children and the general population. By the end of 1964, there were 2500 stand pipes distributed through the island[7] (Fig. 1.3).

School health services, including dental health services continues to be a major programme of the health services and has a one hundred percent reach to the children. The services at schools remain free.

Maternal and child health services

Another critical service that contributed to the rapid decline in infant mortality, maternal mortality and infectious diseases was the Maternal and Child Health services. Considered a preventive service, this service was also started during the colonial era and enhanced after independence.

In 1965, there was a network of clinics providing (i) main services (32 clinics); (ii) "kampong" (rural) midwives' services (10 clinics); and (iii) visiting centres (22 clinics).[6] Many mothers accessed antenatal services in the main clinics. The kampong midwives' services and visiting services reached out to mothers from the rural areas (Fig. 1.4).

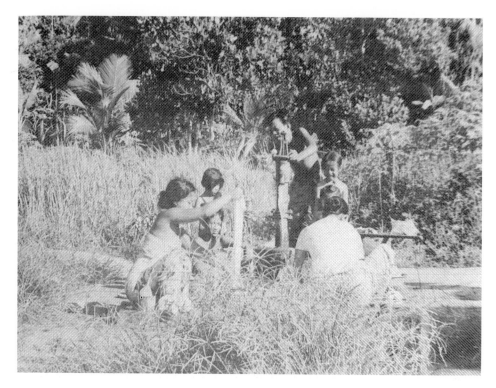

Fig. 1.3. Stand pipes that brought clean water to rural areas.

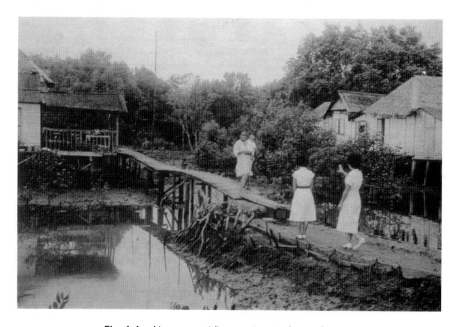

Fig. 1.4. Nurses providing services in the rural areas.

As a consequence, mothers had better care and an increasing number of deliveries took place in hospitals or under the supervision of midwives.

In 1965, 38,849 deliveries were done at the Kandang Kerbau Maternity Hospital (KKMH), about 12,000 deliveries were carried out by confinement midwives at the home and about 4000 deliveries were in private clinics or hospitals. Out of a total of 55,725 births that year, less than a thousand deliveries took place without trained medical care.[6]

The Child Health Service provided at these clinics included a comprehensive immunisation programme (smallpox, poliomyelitis and DPT (diphtheria, pertussis (whooping cough), and tetanus)) and advice to mothers on child care and treatment of minor ailments.

Training and Health Education Unit

The Training and Health Education Unit undertook a number of programmes, which included; (i) training healthcare workers so that they could provide better care to mothers at the Maternal and Child Health Clinics and uphold standards during public health inspection; (ii) public health campaigns such as a blood donation drive, a spring cleaning campaign, and an anti-leprosy campaign. The anti-leprosy campaign lasted a full year with an educational exhibit staged at the community centres. The exhibition included talks, film shows and screening clinics.

Following the publication of a White Paper on family planning and the recommendations of a review committee in 1965, the functions of the Singapore Family Planning Association were transferred to a newly constituted board, the Singapore Family Planning and Population Board. This Board was to function from within the Ministry supported by both the Maternal and Child Health branch and the Training and Health Education branch. The Board set targets to control birth rate and began operations in 1966, following the passage of a Bill establishing the Singapore Family Planning and Population Board on 31st December 1965.[6]

Public Health Services

A host of public health services were provided by the Ministry in 1965. These included Environmental Health (general hygiene and sanitation, including public cleanliness, food hygiene, the control of the sale of food and drugs, and mosquito control), Quarantine and Epidemiology (control of infectious diseases through surveillance of international traffic and local infectious disease occurrence), Markets and Hawkers (licensing and control of hawkers and markets), Public Health Engineering, and management of cemeteries and crematoria. The Public Health Division also worked with the Ministry of National Development to provide clean water through a network of piped water services, ensuring sanitary conditions in food manufacturing factories such as ice cream factories, and to provide appropriate disposal of refuse and night soil.

Many health issues arose with the rapid urbanisation and industrialisation of the country. The problems that were encountered included pollution of soil, water, food, air, and an increase in insect vectors such as mosquitoes and flies. Water usage had increased substantially without a corresponding increase in surface water drainage or sewerage, leading to public health hazards.[5] At a time when infectious diseases were common and endemic in Singapore, the public health services must be credited with having contributed most significantly to improvements of the health of the nation by improving environmental health and hygiene, thereby reducing mortality from infectious diseases and improving life expectancy of its citizens.

Curative Services

The period of the early sixties, the years of self-government, and the next couple of decades were characterised by the reorganisation and enhancement of the curative services run by the state, and building the healthcare workforce.

While the preventive services were almost exclusively provided by the state for free as a public good, the private sector played an important role in the curative services.

A number of significant changes took place. These included a new fiscal policy requiring recipients of services to co-pay while the state continued to absorb the major portion of the cost, the development of manpower, and new infrastructure.

Fiscal policy

Among the substantial changes made by the state in the early years was the introduction of fees, initially at the primary care facilities (outpatient dispensaries), and later in the acute hospitals.

While the government was not reluctant to spend for improvement of services, it was felt that there had to be some cost to the individual, without which the value of the healthcare provided would not be recognised or appreciated, and needless demands for healthcare might be made leading to substantial waste. Thus the policy of patients paying for some of the cost of healthcare was introduced from the very early years of internal self-government, even before independence in 1965.

To gradually change the popular concept that medical care was free, a fee system (50 cents per visit) was implemented for the first time in 1960 at the City Council Outpatient Dispensaries (OPDs).[9]

In addition to the City Council OPDs, four (4) new clinics under the Rural Board also charged 50 cents in 1963. From 1964, all OPDs charged 50 cents. In August 1967, a charge of one dollar was imposed for attendance at the clinics that were open on holidays and Sundays.

In 1962 and 1963, the attendances at the OPDs exceeded 3 million, but in 1964 and 1965, the total attendances dipped well below the 3 million mark. The rate of attendance per 1000 population was 1777 in 1962, 1778 in 1963, 1280 in 1964, and 1090 in 1965.

Island and Travelling Clinics which functioned because of need in the rural areas continued to be free.[10]

From December 1964, charges for delivery at KKMH were introduced and set at $10 for Singaporeans and $50 for others.[7]

In 1969, the MOH published a scheme of charges for all services including surgery (Fig. 1.5).[11] Not only were the fees specified for services in government hospitals and OPDs, but the fee limits for some private professional services were also specified. Hospitals had both full paying and "free" wards. For the latter wards, patients had to pay a nominal fee of $1 per day. This marked the end of free inpatient services and the beginning of subsidised wards.

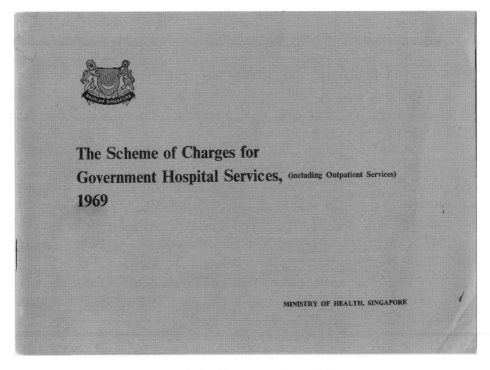

The Scheme of Charges for Government Hospital Services, (including Outpatient Services) **1969**

MINISTRY OF HEALTH, SINGAPORE

Fig. 1.5. The booklet on the scheme of charges.

The Singapore Ministry of Health Report for 1969 states: "From an essentially free medical service, the rapidly rising cost of sickness in recent years and demands of more urgent priorities have necessitated a gradual change in fiscal policy in health resulting in a small part of the total expenditure on health in 1969 being borne by the sick public to whom medical services are provided [...] infectious diseases, TB, leprosy and hardship cases were exempted from payment."[11]

"In that year, 1969, there was a 15% drop in attendance at our OPDs due to the increased charge."[11]

The situation was closely monitored to ensure that individuals in need of health-care were able to access the services.

Development and growth of healthcare professionals

During the colonial era, schools were established to train doctors, dentists, nurses, pharmacists, and radiographers. With an increase in demand for services, the number of healthcare professionals trained was gradually increased and postgraduate training was also instituted.

Hospitals and clinics

In the early years, infrastructure development took the form of expanding existing healthcare institutions and, as infectious diseases were brought under better control, conversion of facilities to acute care needs. One such development was Tan Tock Seng Hospital, which transformed from a hospital largely for patients with tuberculosis (TB) to an acute care general hospital. OPDs were also built to meet the needs of the population.

Public hospital services

In 1965, there were just two general hospitals for acute illness, the General Hospital at Outram Road (Fig. 1.6), (later known as Outram Road General Hospital — ORGH and now Singapore General Hospital) and the Thomson Road General Hospital (TRGH). Together they had 1674 beds (ORGH 1278 and TRGH 396).

Kandang Kerbau Maternity Hospital (KKMH) had 443 beds for obstetrics and gynaecological conditions. Hospitalisations for infectious diseases commanded a large number of beds at that time — 1320 beds at Tan Tock Seng Hospital were allocated for inpatient tuberculosis treatment (about 100 beds were set aside for other adult general medical adult conditions), 61 beds in Middle Road Hospital for venereal diseases, 250 beds for infectious diseases at Middleton Hospital, and

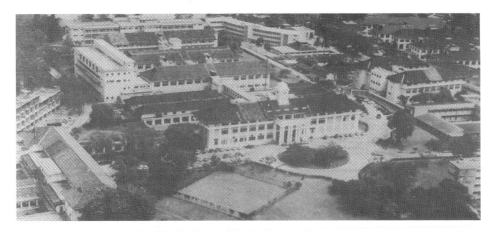

Fig. 1.6. The General Hospital at Outram Road.

Table 1.1. Public Hospitals in 1965 and Their Bed Capacity[6]

Public Hospital Beds Available in 1965		
General Hospital Outram Road	1278	General and acute care beds
Thomson RGH	396	
KKMH (Obstetrics & Gynaecology)	443	
TTSH (Tuberculosis)	1320	
MRH (Sexually Transmitted Diseases)	61	
Middleton Hospital (Infectious Diseases)	250	
Trafalgar Home (Leprosy)	965	
Woodbridge Hospital (Mental Illness)	1869	
Mental Defective Hospital	45	
Chronic Sick Hospital	70	
St Andrew's Orthopaedic Hospital	120	
	6817	

965 beds for leprosy in Trafalgar Home, totalling 2496 beds for infectious diseases. There were also 1869 beds at Woodbridge Hospital and 45 at the Mental Defective Hospital for the treatment of mental illness, 120 beds were available at St Andrew's Orthopaedic Hospital for children's orthopaedic illnesses and 70 beds at the Chronic Sick Hospital (Table 1.1).

Of the some 6800 beds, 2596 were for infectious diseases, 1914 beds for mental illness, and only 1674 beds were allocated for other acute illnesses. TB and leprosy, both chronic infectious diseases, were prevalent and patients required some 2285 beds. New TB cases notified in 1965 numbered 4711 (252 cases per 100,000 population in 1965, current prevalence (circa 2013) being 38/100,000 population), while all TB cases on the register in December 1965 totalled 32,929[6] (giving a prevalence of between 1–2%). Other infectious diseases such as diphtheria (226 cases), typhoid fever (271), amoebic dysentery (328), malaria (201) and poliomyelitis (40) had to be contained as well.

Although in the post war years leading up to independence there was expansion in the number of beds for acute illness, there was a greater increase in beds for infectious diseases, making a ratio of 2 acute beds for every 3 beds for infectious diseases. To see improvements in citizens' health and infectious disease containment, it was necessary to improve living conditions and hygiene, as well as embark on programmes such as vaccination, all of which were pursued with vigour.

It is worth noting that when Thomson Road Hospital was conceived and built, it was meant for managing chronically sick patients who were too feeble to be discharged from the General Hospital at Outram Road. It was only in the years following self-government that Thomson Road Hospital was converted to a general hospital.[6]

A large number of beds was allocated for the treatment of mental illness because the main mode for managing these patients in the past was by institutionalising them.

In the general hospitals, there was already a system of classifying wards into paying and free wards. Those who wished to have extra comfort chose the paying wards and were housed in air-conditioned rooms. Air-conditioning was also made available in a single room in some free wards to enable the most sick to recover under optimal conditions. This practice continues to this day in our public healthcare institutions in the subsidised wards such as the intensive care and burns units.

An Emergency Unit was set up in 1964, and consolidated in 1965, replacing the Casualty Department. It was formed to treat serious medical and surgical cases requiring immediate care before transfer to the wards. It was the beginning of what we now know as "emergency medicine." Prior to this, patients requiring admission were immediately transferred to the wards for treatment.

However half of the cases attending the Emergency Unit were not emergency cases and a third of these non-emergency cases attended after office hours. Reasons given for this phenomenon, which still hold true today, include that OPDs and many GP clinics were closed in the evening and that working parents were unable to take their children to the doctor to seek medical attention during the day. The Emergency Unit was also tasked with developing contingencies to treat cases in the instance of a national emergency.

Usual ER jazz

British military hospitals

There were two military hospitals, the Changi Hospital and the Alexandra Hospital, which continued to be operated by the British for their forces stationed in Singapore, until they left in 1976.

After this, the Changi Hospital was used for the local population. It was closed when the Changi General Hospital was built in 1999.[12]

Alexandra Hospital has continued to function as an acute care general hospital serving the needs of Singaporeans.

Private hospitals

There were already several hospitals listed as private hospitals in 1965 (see Table 1.2 Private hospitals in 1965 and their bed capacity[6]). The Kwong Wei Siu Hospital, the St Andrew's Mission Hospital (for children) and the Singapore Nursing Home were facilities for convalescence rather than for acute care.

Table 1.2. Private Hospitals in 1965 and Their Bed Capacity[6]

Private Hospital Beds Available in 1965	
Gleneagles Hospital (built 1959)	80
Mt Alvernia Hospital	128
Kwong Wei Siu Hospital	454
St Andrew's Mission Hospital (Children)	80
Singapore Nursing Home	54
Youngberg Hospital	67
	863

Outpatient services

The other arm of the curative services involved outpatient clinics, which were the specialty clinics in the hospitals and the primary care services in the community.

The specialist outpatient clinics saw over 1 million attendances annually.

The private sector played a significant role in the primary care sector from the very early years. Most of the doctors in private practice (469 doctors) ran clinics in the community. There were more than 300 private general practice clinics during the flu pandemic in 1957.[13]

The primary care service provided by the state was termed the Outpatient Dispensaries (OPDs), later called the Outpatient Services (OPS). Many of the dispensaries set up before the war were demolished during the war years; these services resumed gradually after the Second World War. In 1955, the services were grouped together as the outpatient services with the headquarters at the General Hospital (at Outram Road) and expanded over the years.[14] In August 1964, the Outpatient Service headquarters which had remained at the General Hospital was closed and moved to Maxwell OPD. By 1965, the government outpatient dispensary services comprised (i) 26 Outpatient Dispensaries (OPDs) across the main island each staffed by one or more doctors; (ii) two island clinics in the larger off-shore islands and three rural clinics staffed part-time by doctors, and five (5) travelling clinics to rural areas staffed by nurses or hospital assistants; and (iii) 5 staff dispensaries staffed by doctors.[6] The attendances at these clinics was in excess of two (2) million. Seven OPDs also offered laboratory tests.

Related services

There were several supporting services that were critical to the functioning of the health services — the pharmaceutical services, the blood transfusion services, and the chemistry department

Pharmaceutical services

Pathology !

This service was responsible for the procurement, manufacture, and supply of medicines, chemicals and surgical instruments and for their sale and use. In the early years, the pharmaceutical laboratory and store had an inventory for about four to six months of supply, costing about 1.5 to 2 million dollars. The laboratory was also responsible for the manufacture of tablets, ampoules and transfusion fluids from imported bulk chemicals and drugs and for the packing of sterile dressings. Checks on sterility and for the active ingredients in the medications were made by the pathology and chemistry department respectively. The Inspector of Poisons also made checks under the Poisons Ordinance and Medicines (Advertisement and Sales) Ordinance. Several convictions took place. A significant gap that was addressed later (1975) was the requirement to register medicines under the Medicines Act.

Blood transfusion services

The blood transfusion services was critical for the hospital services in particular the surgical services at the General Hospital at Outram Road and maternity services at

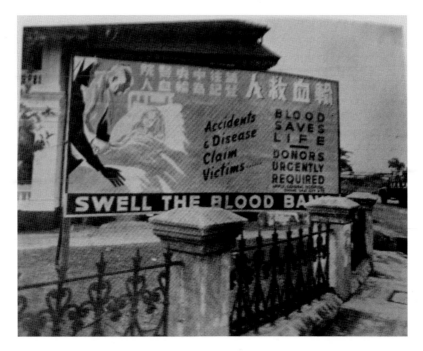

Fig. 1.7.   Blood donation campaign in the sixties.

KKMH. In the early years campaigns had to be held to draw donors and mobile vans were employed to reach out to the donors (Fig. 1.7). The policy of not paying for donors or charging for the blood used, except for processing cost, continues to this day.

Department of Chemistry

In 1961, the Department of Chemistry was brought under the Ministry of Health. It was responsible for chemical analysis of drugs, toxicology, document analysis, and forensic science. Much of their work was used for evidence in court.[6]

Medical Advances in Hospital Services in the Early Years

Many new developments took place in the early years. Investments in specialty care were made regularly and frequently. In most instances the advancements were made essentially by incorporation of expertise developed in Western countries through our specialists who had been trained in overseas centres of excellence (see Health Manpower Development Plan below). This made it possible for Singaporeans to benefit from developments such as cardiac surgery, renal dialysis, coronary care unit, and radiotherapy services in the '60s; organ transplants — starting with kidney transplants, and microsurgery for the reattachment of severed limbs and digits in the '70s; *in vitro* fertilisation — the test tube baby — in 1983, and bone marrow transplant in 1985.

However, one of the most remarkable of these developments in the early years was home grown following research work done in Singapore and contextualised to our population's needs: the preventive strategy for kernicterus.

Kernicterus

Kernicterus is a condition where bilirubin, a yellow pigment from the breakdown of red blood cells, rises to levels that damages the brains of infants, resulting in death or permanent brain damage. In the early years, kernicterus was the commonest cause of death of newborn infants. Following research at the paediatric unit of the General Hospital, it was noted that infants with a deficiency of the enzyme, Glucose-6-Phosphate Dehydrogenase (G6PD), were prone to excessive breakdown of their red blood cells and were particularly at risk. A programme for prevention of kernicterus was unveiled in 1965. The scheme involved the testing for the presence of G6PD in every infant born at KKMH. Infants showing deficiency (absence or low amounts of G6PD) were kept in the hospital after birth for observation and for an exchange blood transfusion if this became necessary. As a result of this scheme, the deaths from kernicterus dropped from 29 in 1964 to 8 in 1965. Most of the deaths persisting after the introduction of the scheme were because parents insisted on taking their child home despite advice, or because they refused exchange transfusion.[6] This work was recognised internationally. As a result of this work, all newborns in Singapore are now screened for Glucose-6 Phosphate Dehydrogenase (G6PD) deficiency.

Health Services — The Latter Years

Many developments contributed to the transformation of the health of the people. Enhancements in the preventive and public health services led to better hygiene and sanitation, enabled clean water supply and delivered vaccination and health education to the people. The well-trained workforce, sound policies, and carefully formulated regulations which ensured high standards of practice, along with the economic success of the nation that enabled modern healthcare facilities to be built, and the restructuring of public healthcare institutions, also contributed to the transformation.

An observer of the development of Singapore's healthcare system would infer that certain principles were in place, many of which may not have been explicitly stated as policies, but which appear to have guided the development of the system. These will be discussed in this section.

1. Expansion and Enhancement of Services

The rapid growth of the economy led to advances in all our healthcare services.

Preventive health services

Health education/health promotion

Health promotion enables people to exert better control of their lifestyle and life choices to achieve optimal health and helps build a healthy population. It is one of the core elements of the health system and is a service that must be revised and expanded regularly.[15]

In response to changing disease patterns over the years, the focus shifted from hygiene and infectious diseases to better nutrition and prevention of chronic diseases. Since the National Healthy Lifestyle Campaign in 1979, through population-wide programmes and programmes tailored for specific groups such as school children, workers or older adults, people have been encouraged to pursue a healthy lifestyle and have been kept informed of the dangers of habits such as smoking and an unhealthy diet. They have also been persuaded to take responsibility for their health — to exercise regularly, build mental resilience and, when appropriate, to go for screening for early detection and management of disease conditions such as hypertension and diabetes. Health services support these initiatives while the social environment is influenced through health promoting initiatives in schools, work places, and community organisations, as well as making healthier alternatives available in the marketplace.

The Health Promotion Board (HPB), a statutory board established in 2001, formed from the merger of various existing departments, has assumed the role of the main driver for national health promotion and disease prevention programmes. HPB implements programmes that reach out to the general population, as well as target groups of children, adults, and the elderly. These programmes include the National Smoking Control Programme, the Workplace Health Promotion Programme, the healthy dining programme, and the integrated screening programme for chronic diseases and some cancers (breast, cervix, and colon). It also administers the school health screening service and school dental service.

In 2013, the Ministry of Health launched an ambitious Healthy Living Master Plan in collaboration with public, private, and community-based agencies. This initiative aims to make healthy living the default choice for Singaporeans by 2020.

School Health Service

The School Health Service has continued to grow and remains largely free of charge. Because of its reach, it is one of the more important preventive services. Today, children in pre-school settings — in kindergartens and child care centres — are under its purview as well.

The School Dental Service has also grown in tandem with the other school health services, expanding its reach to secondary schools. The service, preventive and curative, is provided through in-school dental clinics, mobile dental clinics, and the School Dental Centre at the Health Promotion Board. Dental treatment is provided by dentists or dental therapists. The prevalence of cavities in the permanent dentition of school children has dropped to 23% in 2013.

Public health services

The need for improved integration of many of the Ministry of Health's public health services with other government agencies' programmes led to these services being taken over by related Ministries. The management of environmental health, including Public Health Engineering, Hawkers and Markets, Port Health, and Cemeteries and Crematoria, is now largely under the National Environment Agency (a statutory board of the Ministry of the Environment). Aspects of environmental health which include the management of animals and the sale of food are now under another statutory board, the Agri-Food and Veterinary Authority which is under the Ministry of National Development.

Only the Epidemiology and Disease Control function still rests with the Ministry of Health. While infectious diseases continue to be a significant concern, a large part of the work at the Ministry now includes the monitoring of non-communicable diseases which are the major burden of disease in Singapore. The public health specialists at the Ministry also oversee newer health issues such as performance management of our healthcare institutions and patient care quality assurance and safety.

Curative medical services

Curative medical services are provided by the acute care hospitals, primary care facilities (including outpatient services), and convalescence or rehabilitation facilities.

Acute care hospital services

As it did in the very early years, the state continues to play a dominant role, providing close to 80% of all acute care hospital services. (An account of the role of the private hospitals will be provided later in this chapter).

Public acute hospitals

Eight public hospitals provide acute care. Table 1.3 lists the public acute hospitals and their bed capacity.

Table 1.3.   Public Acute Care Hospitals and Their Bed Capacities

Public Hospital Beds Available in 2013	
Singapore General Hospital	1600
KK Women's and Children's Hospital	830
Changi General Hospital	800
Tan Tock Seng Hospital	1400
Alexandra Hospital	350
Institute of Mental Health	2000
National University Hospital	990
Khoo Teck Puat Hospital	600

• **Singapore General Hospital (SGH) and Singapore Health Services (SingHealth)**
SGH began as the General Hospital, and was the nation's first acute care hospital. In the late 1970s, it began major redevelopment which was completed in 1981. It then took the name Singapore General Hospital (SGH) and has remained the largest general hospital, offering comprehensive tertiary care, except for paediatric services.

Today SGH functions as part of the Singapore Health Services or SingHealth Cluster. Its partner institutions include KK Women's and Children's Hospital, National Heart Centre, Singapore National Eye Centre, National Cancer Centre, National Neuroscience Institute, National Dental Centre, and nine (9) polyclinics.

• **Thomson Road General Hospital/Changi General Hospital**
The Thomson Road General Hospital, built in 1959, was Singapore's second general hospital. It was renamed the Toa Payoh Hospital. In 1999, it was re-sited in Simei as the Changi General Hospital. It continues to provide comprehensive tertiary services and serves the health needs of the population in the eastern part of Singapore.

• **Tan Tock Seng Hospital (TTSH)**
With a reduction in the incidence of tuberculosis in the early post independence years, TTSH reverted to providing general acute care. A new facility with 1211 beds was built on the grounds of the old hospital and opened in 2000. The campus includes the National Neuroscience Institute as a specialty centre and the Travellers, Health and Vaccination centre.[16]

Today TTSH is the main general hospital of the National Health Group cluster. The other healthcare institutions in this cluster include the Institute of Mental Health, National Skin Centre and nine (9) polyclinics.

• The National University Health System

The National University Hospital was the first new hospital to be built following independence. The hospital was completed in 1985 and was built as a University Hospital on the grounds of the National University of Singapore Campus to support the Medical School. It offers a comprehensive range of specialty services and has a number of specialty centres. It has been integrated with the medical and dental schools of the NUS and is now listed as the National University Health System (NUHS).

NUHS and SGH have been designated as Academic Medical Centres and pursue substantial research in addition to the clinical service and educational activities.

• KK Women's and Children's Hospital

The KK Women's and Children's Hospital began as the Kandang Kerbau Maternity Hospital which was built in 1927 for the care of obstetrics and gynaecological cases. In the 1960s, more than 35 thousand deliveries (more than 80% of all deliveries, nationally) took place annually, at the hospital. The hospital was listed in the Guinness Book of Records as the hospital with most births in a year with 39,856 deliveries in 1966.[8] It later underwent major redevelopment, incorporated a paediatric service, and was renamed the KK Women's and Children's Hospital. Today with increased affluence and increased affordability of private care, more than 60% of the approximately 40,000 deliveries annually take place in the private sector with about 10,000 deliveries at KK Women's and Children's Hospital.

• Communicable Disease Centre/Middleton Hospital

Middleton Hospital was built in 1907 as a hospital for the management of infectious diseases. It was renamed Communicable Disease Centre and was incorporated into TTSH in 1985.[16] Plans are now underway to build a National Centre for Infectious Diseases (NCID) on the campus of TTSH.

• Institute of Mental Health (Woodbridge Hospital)

Originally built in 1928 as the Woodbridge Hospital it was redeveloped as the Institute of Mental Health (IMH). IMH was completed in 1993 and is a specialty hospital for mental health.[17]

In 2008 a multi-agency National Mental Health Blueprint was launched. The clinical aspects of the programme including a community-based programme are managed by IMH.

• Khoo Teck Puat Hospital

This is the second hospital (not developed to replace an existing hospital) built following independence, with approximately 600 beds. It opened in the north of Singapore in 2010 as an acute care general hospital.

• Alexandra Hospital

Alexandra Hospital, which was built in 1935 as a military hospital, was taken over from the British in 1971 after the British Military withdrawal; and was converted into a general hospital for acute care.[17] For the past ten years or so it has been manned by staff who have been brought together to run the next hospital to be opened. In this way, the staff of the Khoo Teck Puat Hospital worked as a team even before the hospital was opened. The Alexandra Hospital was occupied by Jurong Health Services prior to the opening of Ng Teng Fong Hospital (run by Jurong Health Services staff) this year. Currently, the hospital is occupied by staff of Sengkang General Hospital while the hospital is being bulit. Another general hospital, Woodlands General Hospital, is at the planning stage.

Specialty centres

Specialty hospitals were already in existence at the time of independence. They included the KKMH (for obstetrics and gynaecological conditions), now KK Women's and Children's Hospital); Woodbridge Hospital (for psychiatric illness); Middleton Hospital for infectious diseases, and Middle Road Hospital (MRH) for skin and venereal disease. New specialty centres were built starting in 1988.

The first of these new specialty centres was the National Skin Centre built in 1988 to replace the Middle Road Hospital that was built in 1945.[17]

The National Blood Centre was also completed in 1988. It housed the Singapore Blood Transfusion Service and the Institute of Science and Forensic Medicine, which was previously known as the Chemistry Department.

The Singapore National Eye Centre was completed in 1990, followed by a series of national centres built on the grounds of the Singapore General Hospital (the National Heart Centre, National Cancer Centre and the National Dental Centre).

In 1999, the National Neuroscience Institute was established at the Tan Tock Seng campus. It now is part of the SingHealth Cluster and operates at both the Tan Tock Seng Campus and Singapore General Hospital Campus.[12]

Today, two specialty centres (University Heart Centre, University Cancer Centre) can be found in the National University Health System.

Private hospitals

Although the private sector had a role from the early days in the provision of tertiary care, it was not until after the opening of the Mount Elizabeth Hospital in 1979 that the private sector's role expanded. The Mount Elizabeth Hospital is Singapore's largest private hospital with a capacity of more than 300 beds. In the early days of the State, the growth of private hospitals was encouraged as an alternative source of medical care for citizens who were able to afford their charges.[11,18]

> "A further easing of the pressure on the resources of the government medical and health services is the growth of medical facilities in recent years in the private sector, both general practice and specialty services."
>
> Singapore Ministry of Health Report 1969

Approximately seventy percent (70%) of in-patients in private hospitals are Singapore residents. However, with the recent growth of the private sector and Singapore Medicine (see below), it has been necessary to moderate some of the growth of the private sector, because of concerns that it has been drawing on the manpower of the public hospitals. Table 1.4 shows the larger private hospitals and their bed capacity.

Table 1.4. The Bed Capacities of the Larger Private Hospitals

Private Hospital Beds Available in 2013	
Gleneagles Hospital	380
Mt Alvernia Hospital	300
Mount Elizabeth Hospital	500
East Shore Hospital	120
Raffles Hospital	380
Mt Elizabeth Novena	250
Thomson Medical Centre (mainly obstetrics)	190

Community hospitals

The Ang Mo Kio Hospital was Singapore's first community hospital and was built in 1993 as part of the State's effort to contain healthcare cost by providing hospital care in non-tertiary facilities. The hospital was part of the Singhealth Cluster from 2000 to 2002 at which point the decision was made to run the hospital as a convalescence-rehabilitation hospital and its administration handed over to a

Voluntary Welfare Organisation (VWO). There are three similar hospitals today run as convalescence-rehabilitation facilities by VWOs — Saint Andrew's Community Hospital, Ren Ci Community Hospital and Saint Luke's Community Hospital.

Primary care services (outpatient services)

The private sector continues to play a dominant role in this sector and continues to grow, taking about eighty percent (80%) of all primary care consultations. There are over 1400 private clinics offering primary care services. Most of these clinics are solo practices which have very few supporting services to enable care for the more complex cases to be undertaken at these clinics. This limitation coupled with payment for care being mainly out-of-pocket, has resulted in a disproportionate number of patients with chronic diseases being seen in the polyclinics (see below).

The state run OPDs and MCH clinics were also increased in number and capacity. Beginning in the 1980s, OPDs and MCH clinics (numbering 41) were consolidated into 16 polyclinics. We now have 18 polyclinics distributed throughout the island. Polyclinics provide a comprehensive range of primary care services including maternal and child healthcare, outpatient medical care, health education, immunisation, laboratory services, and pharmacy services. Some also provide dental, psychiatric, and rehabilitation services. Polyclinics provide twenty percent (20%) of primary care services overall but provide a disproportionately larger percentage of care for patients with chronic diseases. This is in part because care for chronic conditions is more expensive and, until recently, there have been no subsidies at private general practice (GP) clinics. Polyclinics are therefore inundated by large numbers of patients; and managing the more complex cases is a challenge because of the limited time available for consultations. Many such patients are referred to the specialist outpatient clinics, co-located with acute care hospitals for management, where care is generally of a subspecialty nature.

This has now been recognised as an untenable situation, especially considering the increasing longevity of Singapore's aging population, and the increasing burden of chronic disease. To address the situation and to expand both capability and capacity in the primary care sector, the Primary Care Master Plan was launched in 2011. Some of the key strategies in this master plan include: (i) portable state subsidies to off-set out-of-pocket payment, for patients who have been means-tested, so that they may see the neighbourhood GP instead of going to polyclinics that are currently inundated with patients; (ii) Family Medicine Clinics which are state-supported new models of private primary care clinic, with two or more GPs, and supporting services; (iii) Community Health Centres, which are facilities to support solo GP practices with ancillary services. These are recent developments.

With appropriate stewardship, the primary care services can be transformed so that more holistic comprehensive care can be provided at affordable prices for the community.

2. A Well-Trained Workforce

The state has also invested heavily in the training of the workforce so that those in need have the best people caring for them.

Undergraduate and postgraduate training

As a small nation with no natural resources it has been a policy across the whole of government to optimise our human capital. Heavy investments are made to provide excellent facilities and accomplished teachers for our universities, polytechnics, and other training facilities for healthcare professionals. Post-graduate programmes have also been developed.

Collaborations with external universities have been useful to quickly infuse and adapt innovative techniques into our teaching and learning cultures. During the last decade we partnered Duke University, USA, and Imperial College UK, among other universities, to set up our own new medical schools. Similar collaborations with external universities have been set up, where appropriate, for training other healthcare professionals, e.g. for the degree conversion course for nurses who have completed a diploma in nursing.

In addition to formal post-graduate training, healthcare professionals are provided with opportunities to train and hone their skills in specific areas of their specialty at some of the best healthcare facilities overseas under the Health Manpower Development Plan (HMDP). The HMDP which also allows experts to be brought to Singapore for short periods, has contributed immensely to the wealth of expertise in healthcare that now resides in our healthcare system.[19]

Accreditation of overseas schools

We have also welcomed healthcare professionals trained abroad, both citizens and foreigners, to join our healthcare workforce. To ensure maintenance of high professional standards, we review training schools for healthcare professionals in other countries and include good schools in the schedule of the legislation governing a specific healthcare professional group. Graduates of such schools, when offered employment by a healthcare institution accredited as a "learning institution," are able to practice locally, but remain under supervision for two or more years. This period enables us to verify the healthcare professionals' competence and, when necessary, to help them achieve the required practice standards. After having completed the prescribed duration under conditional registration, the healthcare professional is given full registration and may thenceforth practice in any institution.

Service obligation

The service obligation introduced in 1978, now requires all graduates of our local medical and dental schools to serve in the public healthcare institutions for a period of time. The period depends on the course of study and citizenship and varies from 4–6 years. Junior specialists who have benefitted from a HMDP training programme, need to serve 2–3 years. Nurses and other healthcare professionals who receive scholarships or funding for their course, as many do, also have a service obligation to fulfil.

The service obligation ensures that the healthcare professionals who leave to work in the private sector, at the graduate or postgraduate level, are adequately trained. Additionally, it helps retain a significant proportion of healthcare workers in the public healthcare system. In 2013 close to 63% of doctors were in the public healthcare system.[20]

3. Restructuring Public Healthcare Institutions (HCIs)

Public Healthcare Institutions (HCIs) because they are heavily subsidised can become inefficient and wasteful.

The state began restructuring its HCIs, allowing a degree of autonomy, so that HCIs would have greater responsiveness to the needs of the population they served. They were also empowered to pursue strategies to optimise care and yet remain efficient and sustainable — to pursue corporate discipline while retaining the public service mission and ethos. The HCIs providing curative services were the first to be corporatised starting in 1985.

The Health Corporation of Singapore (now called Ministry of Health Holdings) was incorporated in 1987 as a holding company for this purpose. The Ministry commenced the restructuring program for its HCIs in 1988 after the concept was successfully tried out at the National University Hospital for 3 years — since 1985.[21]

National Skin Centre began operations in December 1988 as a restructured institution, followed by Singapore General Hospital in April 1989. Most of the remaining institutions followed and the last HCIs to be restructured were Alexandra Hospital and the Institute of Mental Health in 2000.

Restructuring enabled the hospitals to be more cost conscious and observe stricter financial discipline. The intent was to also minimise cost escalation.

Despite the significant autonomy for operations, the institutions remain wholly owned by the government. The Ministry continues to formulate health policies and guidelines and regulate both public and private healthcare institutions (HCIs). It also technically purchases services from the public HCIs by providing the subsidies for the services the HCIs provide for the public and nurtures a sense of public service ethos among the leadership of the restructured HCIs.

Restructuring enabled a degree of competition between the various public service providers and helped improve the services provided.

While the corporate culture, fiscal discipline, efficiency, and waste reduction improved, the government was conscious of the possibility that these targets were sometimes pursued by the healthcare institutions at the expense of public service. The public service function was sometimes latent or overshadowed. Competition may have contributed to some of these developments.

In 2000, the public HCIs were grouped into two clusters to encourage collaboration and also vertical and horizontal integration of services.[14]

In 2008, Regional Health Systems were started to encourage closer collaboration between regional providers and better opportunities to address existing gaps in regional health services.

HPB and HSA

Following the restructuring of the curative services, most of the remaining services at the Ministry, the public health / preventive services, were also restructured at the turn of the new millennium — in 2001, to encourage corporate discipline. The Training and Health Education Department was merged with School Health Service, the School Dental Service and the Nutrition Unit and formed into a statutory board, the Health Promotion Board.

The blood transfusion services, the scientific services and the pharmaceutical services including health product regulations were merged under a separate statutory board, the Health Sciences Authority.

4. Public Sector Remains Strong and Provides Leadership

Providing a benchmark for healthcare

In today's environment, where medicine is increasingly becoming bottom-line driven (two of our private hospitals are listed in the stock exchange), the public sector provides leadership through its experienced healthcare professionals and plays an important role in preserving the ideals of medicine that include the concept of the healthcare profession being a vocation that is pursued primarily for the benefit of others. A "for-profit" approach may be in danger of creating demand for services which may not be justifiable on the basis of science or cost-effectiveness. As a provider of a significant proportion of healthcare, the public sector must remain vigilant to ensure that healthcare made available through its institutions is anchored in science and remains cost-effective. These institutions have the latest medical technologies and the public trusts them to provide care that is appropriate for their need. The public sector also provides research opportunities for new technology and procedures to be studied for effectiveness.

As the public sector healthcare facilities are almost exclusively, the training ground for healthcare professionals this ethos of service grounded in science and compassion and with attention to cost-effectiveness plays a vital role in inculcating the next generation of healthcare professionals with the right values.

It has been necessary for the public sector to remain dominant and progressive so that quality healthcare is accessible and affordable to the majority of the population. However, it has not been easy to retain staff and talent, and wages have had to be comparable to some extent with those in the private sector.

Manpower retention — Competitive wages

Because of a thriving private sector, especially for specialty services, it has been a constant challenge to retain good clinicians in the public sector to provide the necessary leadership and to also maintain the service standards in the public sector hospitals. Salaries are regularly reviewed to reduce disparities with that of colleagues in the private sector.

In 1984, the Consultation Fee Scheme (CFS) was introduced so that specialists could retain some of the fees earned when seeing private patients. Specialists who opted for this scheme were able to earn up to an additional 60% of their gross annual salary through this scheme.[22]

Many proceduralists, including specialists undertaking radiology, laboratory and other diagnostic examination or procedures, opted for this scheme. For non-proceduralists, the fixed specialist allowance (FSA) was increased.

The CFS has undergone numerous changes. Fees earned were allowed to reach up to 100% of the doctor's salary; and in a subsequent review, the cap to earnings was removed. Earnings by specialists in a department were pooled and weighted towards total work completed, which included care of subsidized patients.

In a subsequent review, specialists were allowed to surcharge up to 200% of the fees as listed in the Scheme of Charges and the surcharge was retained by the specialist. Some restructured hospitals went on to encourage specialists to do after-hours surgery and allowed them to retain most of the fees charged. With the restructuring of the public hospitals the consultation fee scheme was not implemented in the same form in all our public hospitals.

In 2012, it became clear that the direct link to income of doctors led to more after-hours surgery performed and there was concern that the ethos of public service was being eroded by the profit motive. A proposal to replace the CFS with a Service Quality Component that took into consideration other contributions of the doctor has been developed and will hopefully allow for some recalibration of the CFS.

The CFS brought about significant changes to the work attitudes of many specialists. More work was done, bringing benefits like reduced waiting time for elective surgery and procedures, but without careful calibration, the profit motive of some individual doctors will erode the public service ethos of the healthcare services.

However, it must be noted that many excellent clinicians have stayed on in the public sector despite the pay differential, for the meaningful work, collegiality and diversity of pursuits, e.g. as an educator or a clinician scientist, while still being a clinician.

5. High Standards of Service Through Policies and Regulations

High standards of healthcare services have been maintained by legislation and policies governing healthcare facilities and healthcare professionals. The Private Hospitals and Medical Clinics Act requires healthcare facilities to comply with facility standards and stipulates specific categories of healthcare professionals required to run these institutions. The legislation governing healthcare professionals lists the schools whose graduates are recognised for practice in Singapore. It also requires graduates to engage in continuing professional development activities such as attending a required number of lectures at courses or conferences in their specialty periodically, in order to be able to renew their practicing certificates.

Healthcare products in Singapore are carefully regulated, such that products are monitored for adverse events even after they have been registered. Also, when significant events are noted, necessary actions are taken and healthcare professionals are informed. In 2006, this policy led to the discovery of a contaminated eye care solution that triggered its recall, first from the local market and then eventually on a global scale.

6. Retaining Demand-Side Responsibility While Enabling Affordability

Heavy government healthcare subsidises at public healthcare institutions enable access to healthcare for all residents, but avoids creating a welfare state for health. Patients are expected to pay a part of the cost of healthcare services they use. For more expensive healthcare services such as inpatient treatment and, more recently, expensive outpatient treatments such as for drugs for cancers, the government has designed a personal health savings account — the Medisave, to enable patients to pay for their share of these services. The money from this account can also be used to purchase an insurance for catastrophic illness — the Medishield, and also an integrated plan (i.e. Medishield and private plan) for private care if the individual so desires. The funds in the Medisave account can also be used for the immediate family members' needs.

The government has also set up a fund, the Medifund, to help defray the cost for needy Singaporeans who are unable to pay for their share.

These financial schemes have evolved over the years and continue to be recalibrated regularly. For example, while every individual has access to subsidised inpatient care and can choose to use services at the B2 or C Class Wards (the two categories of subsidised wards), the quantum of subsidy has now been recalibrated and calculated based on the individual's financial standing. Previously, anyone could seek treatment in a C Class ward and get an 80% subsidy for the cost of treatment received. With the introduction of the inpatient means test, individuals who are financially well off (the top quintile in terms of income earned) will get a reduced subsidy of 65% instead of 80% when they elect to be treated in a C class ward and 50% instead of 65% when they choose a B2 class ward. Medishield is also being enhanced to Medishield Life, which offers both a higher amount of coverage and a life time coverage for all Singaporeans (including those with pre-existing illness).

The policies will continue to be refined in order to ensure affordability to patients and sustainability of the system. With new challenges new policies will need to be made and implemented.

7. Cost-Effective Healthcare

While allocation of resources for a specific intervention has many considerations such as need and equity, for many years now, whenever possible, a cost-effectiveness analysis is undertaken to assist in the decision.

An area where such analysis has been used with good outcomes has been in subsidy allocation for new drugs. When drugs are approved for subsidy by the state, it has to be clearly shown that the drug addresses a gap in the current therapeutic armamentarium, and that the drug is cost-effective compared to existing drugs.[11] This cost-effectiveness analysis is undertaken by the Pharmacoeconomic Drug Utilisation Unit at the Health Sciences Authority and the analysis defines the cost associated with health gain, the latter usually expressed as quality adjusted life years.

When clinical practice guidelines are written, recommendations, especially for a specific new drug, consider similar cost-effectiveness analyses.

Increasingly, similar analysis is being done to allocate the limited healthcare resources for other areas such as medical devices.

With healthcare being increasingly commodified, suppliers of health services will continue to generate a demand through advertisements and claims of promises and hopes. While cost-effectiveness analysis is increasingly employed to guide decisions, it is not always practical to do this analysis and decisions need to be made taking into account other evidence.

8. Periodic Regular Review and Recalibration of Policies

Recognising that policies are only as good as the stewardship provided for implementation, policies are provided with resources to facilitate implementation and are monitored so that if necessary, adjustments to the policies can be made. Similarly, noting that the healthcare needs of the population or of specific groups of the population undergo change, the Ministry of Health undertakes periodic review of policies, regardless of whether they are thought to be succeeding or not. Feedback from monitoring and evaluation programmes contributes to this review, as does information on changes in the social environment, disease landscape, policies and programmes in other countries, local and international research studies, and advice of international healthcare bodies such as WHO. The Ministry has not been averse to fundamental changes in policies, e.g. the Family Planning and Population Board's policy of family size limitation (two children) was recalibrated to encourage families which could afford more children to have three or more; Singapore Medicine, initially conceived as concerted effort to encourage people from other countries to come to Singapore for medical care was moderated as its momentum may have resulted in more attention being paid to those from overseas seeking medical care than to our own residents. Today, while the private sector continues to pursue this policy of Singapore Medicine, public sector hospitals have put in restrictions to clearly emphasise citizens as their priority.

Conclusion

The transformation of the health of our population did not occur by accident nor was it a result of emulating another country's health system, as no one system will be appropriate for our needs and situation. It was made possible by taking a long-term strategic view. It was made possible by the willingness to learn from the best and local innovation. It was made possible by searching out and painstakingly piecing together the best policies and methods for each individual concern and constantly reviewing and recalibrating policies. Some of the policies were not popular, such as the need to co-pay for care or the service obligation imposed on graduating doctors and dentists, but they have helped us build a sustainable health system and transform the health of our people.

References

1. *The World Health Report 2000 — Health systems: Improving performance.* World Health Organization, Geneva, Switzerland.
2. "Most Efficient Healthcare 2014: Countries." *Bloomberg second annual ranking of countries with the most efficient healthcare.* Available at: http://media.bloomberg. com/bb/avfle/rhpTqieX4Fuc. Accessed 10 Jan 2015.
3. Registrar-General of Births and Deaths, (2014) "Report on Registration of Births and Deaths 2013; Registry of Births and Deaths," *Immigration and Checkpoints Authority.* Singapore.
4. "Government Health Expenditure." *Singapore Health Facts*, Ministry of Health. Available at: https://www.moh.gov.sg/content/mohweb/home/statistics/Health_ Facts_Singapore/Healthcare_Financing.html. Accessed 25 Dec 2014.
5. *Singapore Ministry of Health Report 1961.* Singapore-Malaya Collection, National University of Singapore Medical Library.
6. *Singapore Ministry of Health Report 1965.* Singapore-Malaya Collection, National University of Singapore Medical Library.
7. *Singapore Ministry of Health Report 1964.* Singapore-Malaya Collection, National University of Singapore Medical Library.
8. *Singapore Ministry of Health Report 1966.* Singapore-Malaya Collection, National University of Singapore Medical Library.
9. *Singapore Ministry of Health Report 1960.* Singapore-Malaya Collection, National University of Singapore Medical Library.
10. *Singapore Ministry of Health Report 1967.* Singapore-Malaya Collection, National University of Singapore Medical Library.
11. *Singapore Ministry of Health Report 1969.* Printer: Government Printing Office. Singapore-Malaya Collection, National University of Singapore Medical Library.
12. *Singapore Ministry of Health Report 1999.* Singapore-Malaya Collection, National University of Singapore Medical Library.
13. *Singapore Ministry of Health Report 1957.* Singapore-Malaya Collection, National University of Singapore Medical Library.
14. *Singapore Ministry of Health Report 1955.* Singapore-Malaya Collection, National University of Singapore Medical Library.

15. *Towards better healthcare — Main report of the Review Committee on National Health Policies*. (1992) Singapore-Malaya Collection, National University of Singapore Medical Library.

16. *Singapore Ministry of Health Report 2000*. Singapore-Malaya Collection, National University of Singapore Medical Library.

17. Edmund Wee, ed. (1994) *Pillars of Health*. Epigram Pte Ltd. ISBN number: 9971-913-44-5.

18. *Health — A crucial concern, Excerpts from Ministerial speeches on health 1980–1982*. Published by the Information Division, Ministry of Culture. Singapore-Malaya Collection, National University of Singapore Medical Library.

19. *Singapore Ministry of Health Report 1983*. Singapore-Malaya Collection, National University of Singapore Medical Library.

20. *Singapore Medical Council Annual Report 2013*.

21. *Singapore Ministry of Health Report 1988*. Singapore-Malaya Collection, National University of Singapore Medical Library.

22. *Consultation Fee Scheme; Singapore Ministry of Health Annual Report. 1984*. Singapore-Malaya Collection, National University of Singapore Medical Library.

2 A Brief History of Public Health in Singapore

Joan Sara Thomas,* Ong Suan Ee,†
Chia Kee Seng‡ and Lee Hin Peng§

By nature, public health is a multi-disciplinary and inter-sectoral field that must be seen in the context of the history and development of a country. It is closely tied to socio-economic changes, especially in the case of Singapore, a relatively young nation. The dramatic transformation of this small island nation from a fishing village to a first-world metropolis in less than 200 years is a clear example of this comprehensive development, driven almost entirely by sheer human effort and hard work.

Singapore's population started off as a mixture of indigenous and migrant peoples and remains a multi-ethnic society today. Singapore is unique among the world's developed countries, having achieved significant population health improvements at a relatively low economic cost over a short time span. In the last fifty years, Singapore's rapid socio-economic development brought with it significant improvements in infrastructure and health services. This, in turn, has translated into massive improvements in many health indicators. Average life expectancy increased by 21 years, from 63 to 82.5 years from 1960 to 2013,[1] while infant mortality rate improved from 34.9 per 1000 live births in 1960 to 2.0 per 1000 live births in 2014; now one of the lowest in the world.[2]

*Research Associate, Saw Swee Hock School of Public Health, National University of Singapore.
†Research Associate, Saw Swee Hock School of Public Health, National University of Singapore.
‡Dean and Professor, Saw Swee Hock School of Public Health, National University of Singapore.
§Professor, Saw Swee Hock School of Public Health, National University of Singapore.

[1] Ministry of Health Singapore. (2014) "Population and Vital Statistics." Website: http://www.moh.gov.sg/content/moh_web/home/statistics/Health_Facts_Singapore/Population_And_Vital_Statistics.html
[2] Registrar-General of Births and Deaths, Report on Registration of Births and Deaths 2013; Registry of Births and Deaths, Immigration and Checkpoints Authority, Singapore 2014.

Pre-War Period: 1819–1945

Most documentation of early history and modern medical care in Singapore begins in January 1819, when British explorer Sir Stamford Raffles first landed on the island. At this time, the total population was very small, comprising only a few traders and a handful of fishermen. However, as Singapore established itself as an important trading hub for the region, a steady inflow of immigrants soon begun to flow in from neighbouring countries. By 1850, the population of Singapore had grown to over 52,000.[3] However, arriving with this influx of people were more health needs, compelling the then-British Administration to begin thinking about the need for an island-wide health service.

Dr. Thomas Pendergast, a Straits Settlements' Sub-Assistant Surgeon arrived with Sir Stamford Raffles. Originally based at the General Hospital in Penang, Dr. Pendergast is credited as the person who officially introduced Western medicine to Singapore. He was made Acting Surgeon in-charge of Singapore and became the first Head of the medical department.[4] His main mandate was to take care of the health of his contingent. Over the years, as new regiments rotated in, other regimental medical officers were responsible for the same. Thus, it was the Medical Officers in the Army of the East India Company who arrived when their regiments were posted from India who laid the foundation of early healthcare in Singapore.

Over the years, the Straits Settlements — in particular, Singapore — prospered and its Medical Service began to expand and improve. During this time, army doctors were given the designation of "surgeon"; a title which, at that time, indicated both surgical duties and the status of army medical doctors who would be responsible for both military and civilian health. With a serious lack of trained medical and paramedical personnel on the ground, army medical doctors and their assistant medical subordinates were expected to offer their services in areas most needed. Common medical activities included general hospital work, fighting outbreaks of smallpox and cholera, and treating general wounds and other injuries. Army medical doctors often performed both minor and major operations as well as conducted quarantine activities, port health, and vaccinations. In 1821, Singapore's General Hospital — the first hospital on the island — was built. Staffed by army medical doctors ("surgeons"), its primary goal was to provide medical services to European soldiers, sepoys (local soldiers), and natives.

Soon after the General Hospital was established in 1867, there was a shift in central power and the Straits Settlements were transferred from the India Office to the Colonial Office in London, the United Kingdom. From this point on, all appointments to the Medical Service were made in London.

---

[3] Nah WT, Chew PK. (1972) "A historical review of environmental health work in Singapore." *Singapore Public Health Bulletin.* **10**: 30–34.

[4] Teo, Cuthbert. (2014) "A glimpse into the past: Medicine in Singapore — Part 1." *SMA News.* **46**(5): 24–27.

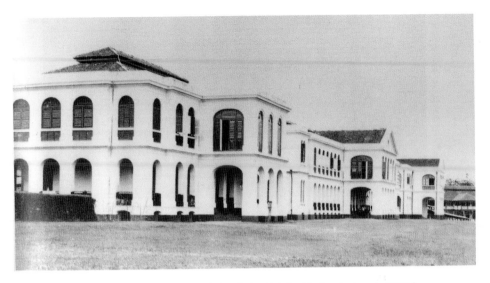

Fig. 2.1. Singapore General Hospital, which had its beginnings in 1821.[5]

During this era of prosperity and rapid economic growth, health needs began to surface in Singapore. As the population began to increase, so did the challenges related to poor sanitation, unclean water, and pollution. Lack of formal regulations in the areas of housing, water, and sanitation quickly resulted in overcrowding of both people and waste. This situation continued up until the 1900s, when concerted efforts were made to improve the Singapore water and sanitation system, resulting in a re-examination of the island's water supply. This review resulted in the first full sewage disposal centre, which was set up in 1906 by the Government.

Singapore's healthcare service began to develop alongside efforts made to deal with the health challenges resulting from new, rapid economic growth. The early beginnings of Western nursing practice began in the early 1900s when English-trained nurses were sent to Singapore to replace nuns, who up till then had been providing basic care services with little formal training.

In 1927, the field of public health nursing developed even further under the guidance of Miss IMM Simmons, the first officially appointed Public Health Nurse in Singapore. Health clinics focused on providing maternal and child health services were opened in response to increasing infant mortality rates and the need for better maternity care for local women. Miss Simmons established the first maternal and child health clinic in rural areas and dispatched a travelling dispensary which allowed treatment to reach sick individuals living far from the General Hospital.

---

[5] *A Legacy in Health: A Photo-Journey Through the History of Primary Healthcare in Singapore.* National Healthcare Group Polyclinics.

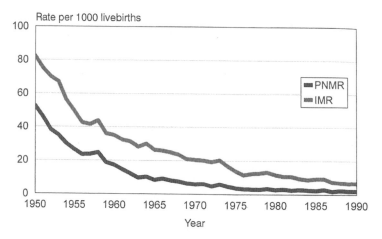

Fig. 2.2. Infant mortality rate (IMR) and post-neonatal mortality rate (PNMR), Singapore 1950–1990.[6]
Source: Registration of births and deaths 1990.

This was a seminal period in the development of maternal and child healthcare, marked by the establishment of the School Health Services (SHS), a government institution acting as the main guardian of the health of schoolchildren. Armed with a staff of two medical officers, approximately 5000 school children were examined in this time of the late 1920s.[7] The SHS continued to operate at a very low key throughout the war years.

Miss Simmons' work improved facilities and services in rural areas, built trust in Western medicine, educated families on maternal and infant health, and sharply reduced the infant mortality rate (IMR) at that time. The IMR is an indicator that is strongly related to structural factors like economic development, general living conditions, social well-being and the quality of the environment; all of which affect the health of entire populations. A declining trend in the IMR is said to reflect an improvement in overall population health.[8] Slowly but surely, Singapore's healthcare system was taking shape.

Post-War Period: 1945–1965

In 1942, medical services came to a standstill as World War II broke out and Singapore fell to the Japanese. The war took a heavy toll on the health of the population,

[6] Seow A, Lee HP. (1994) "From colony to city-state: Changes in health needs in Singapore from 1950 to 1990." *Journal of Public Health Medicine*. **16**(2): 149–158.

[7] Chay SO, Lim C. (1980) "History of the School Health Services in Singapore — Part I and Part II." *The Singapore Community Health Bulletin*. **21**: 36–39, pp. 40–44.

[8] Reidpath DD, Allotey P. (2003) "Infant mortality rate as an indicator of population health." *J Epidemiol Community Health*. **57**: 344–346.

with the impact particularly notable among young children. The SHS post-war reports of 1946–1947 revealed a grim health pattern among schoolchildren, with malnutrition and epidemics of communicable diseases being the most significant problems. Almost 50% of school children examined in 1946 were malnourished and suffered from nutritional deficiencies and infectious diseases, such as measles, poliomyelitis, diphtheria, tuberculosis (TB), and smallpox (with outbreaks occurring in 1946 and 1959).[9]

The twin ravages of TB and malnutrition among children became a further catalyst for development in healthcare services. Free meals and subsidised feeds were introduced in schools to alleviate widespread hunger, and in 1948, nursing personnel were mobilised to slow down the raging spread of TB. Nurses conducted regular home visits to ensure compliance to TB treatment, distribution of supplements like cod liver oil, and offered advice on diet and hygiene.

The political climate of the 1950s and 1960s was quite tumultuous, characterised by the transitioning of power from the colonial government to a national government. The reviewing commission led by Sir George Rendel recommended partial internal self-government for Singapore with Britain retaining control of internal security, law, finance, defence, and foreign affairs in a move later known as the Rendel Constitution. Although the new constitution was far from offering Singapore full independence, election fever gripped the country. In November 1954, the People's Action Party (PAP) came to power led by a young Lee Kuan Yew along with party members, Toh Chin Chye, Goh Keng Swee and S. Rajaratnam. Ending colonialism was the first priority of then-Prime Minister Lee and the PAP.[10] Therefore, *malayanization*, a process by which national workers replaced colonial expatriates, took place throughout much of the 1960s and laid the foundations for an internal self-government. As Singapore's first Prime Minister, Mr. Lee's early policies greatly shaped the nation's modern healthcare system.

Post-Independence: 1965 Onwards

The Government of the day was not a proponent of the welfare state; rather they were convinced that a market-oriented, consumer-driven model of healthcare would serve Singapore far better than the National Health Service-type socialised medicine model. It was therefore decided that within the Singapore healthcare system, the state and individual would share responsibility for healthcare. The individual would be incentivised to take responsibility for their own health, with the government providing a safety net — a move which would also help moderate

[9] Chay SO, Lim C. (1980) "History of the School Health Services in Singapore — Part 1 and Part II." *The Singapore Community Health Bulletin*, **21**: 36–39, pp. 40–44.

[10] Barbara Leitch Lepoer, ed. (1989). *Singapore: A Country Study*. Washington: GPO for the Library of Congress. (http://countrystudies.us/singapore/10.htm).

healthcare costs. Despite the market-oriented model, the Singapore government remained a strong force in actively assessing, controlling and regulating the market, and intervening to address flaws.

The choice between markets or governments is complex and often not pure or binary, but rather a matter of degree and emphasis.[11] In the case of Singapore during these key post-independence years, the government seemed to be doing something right. Two years after independence, the Minister of Health announced that "health would rank, at the most, fifth in order of priority for funds — after national security, job creation, housing and education, in that order."[12] In the 1960s, the Government was largely concerned with aligning itself with its promise and providing basic healthcare. It began mass-inoculation programmes in an effort to battle infectious disease such as tuberculosis, smallpox, diphtheria, and poliomyelitis. It strengthened existing child health programmes by targeting malnutrition with nutritional supplementation schemes. Complementing this, the Government began to push for education, increasing the number of medical professionals and specialists on the island.

By the 1970s, Singapore had become clean, green, and generally free from major communicable diseases albeit with remnants of TB, typhoid and dengue haemorrhagic fever. Rapid industrialisation and social progress gave rise to a demand for better, more specialised medical services. The Government began planning to expand existing medical infrastructure and expertise to meet this increased demand.

Although modernising healthcare systems and infrastructure and increased specialisation of care brought higher costs with them, the Singapore government managed to keep the national health expenditure at approximately three percent (3%) of its ever-expanding GDP throughout most of the 1980s and 1990s. However, the Government was aware that in dollar terms, health care expenditure had been steadily increasing. For instance, between 1967 and 1995, health care expenditure rose seven-fold. This rising trend, coupled with the realisation that increasing life expectancy and rising aspirations would inevitably lead to increasing demands for health care services, catalysed the Government to think about a new approach to more cost-effective provision of healthcare. In the early 1980s, the Government announced its National Health Plan, which detailed expansion of current health care infrastructure planned for the next 20 years. This entailed the expansion and consolidation all primary health care services, outpatient services, infant welfare clinics, and travelling dispensaries into a network of government health clinics, "restructured" public health sector hospitals, tertiary-care specialist centres and private general practitioners. During this period, the number of hospitals grew from

---

[11] Lim J. (2013) *Myth or Magic — The Singapore Healthcare System.* 26.
[12] Yong YL. "Speech by the Minister of Health at the opening of the WHO seminar on health planning in urban development, Singapore." 21 November 1967.

8 in 1957 to 16 in 1965 and 21 in 1990, resulting in a bed-to-population ratio of 3.6 per 1000 persons. By 1994, 20% of primary care and 80% of hospital care was being provided by the government or restructured institutions.[13] The National Health Plan also introduced Medisave — a novel scheme to finance individual healthcare.

Modern Singapore: Emerging Challenges for Public Health and Healthcare

Today, healthcare in Singapore is widely regarded as efficient and widespread. In the year 2000, Singapore was ranked 6th in the World Health Organization (WHO)'s ranking of world health systems (World Health Report 2000). Many of Singapore's health status indicators appear to reflect the robustness of the system and the effectiveness of public health measures undertaken over the past few decades. Infant mortality has declined by 83% between 1980 and 2010,[14] maternal mortality has fallen by 40% between 1990 and 2010,[15] and Singapore's tuberculosis prevalence is the lowest among ASEAN member-states at 40.9 per 100,000 population[16] (for comparison, Cambodia's is 660 per 100,000 population).[17] However, there remain several key population-level trends and challenges that will have significant impacts on not only the Singapore healthcare system, but also public health in Singapore, which warrant closer examination.

Infectious Diseases

Singapore's rapid and systematic economic and infrastructural development was crucial to the elimination of many old-world infectious diseases. For example, malaria was a main vector-borne disease resulting in substantial morbidity and mortality in Singapore in the early 20th century. However, Singapore was declared malaria-free in 1982[18] by the WHO. Today, all of Singapore's reported malaria cases are imported.[19]

Much of the improvements in infectious diseases in infants and children can be attributed to Singapore's comprehensive childhood immunisation programme.

---

[13] (1992) "Towards better health care." *Main report of the Review Committee on National Health Policies.* Singapore.

[14] http://www.oecd.org/els/health-systems/HealthAtAGlanceAsiaPacific2012.pdf

[15] http://www.oecd.org/els/health-systems/HealthAtAGlanceAsiaPacific2012.pdf

[16] https://www.moh.gov.sg/content/dam/moh_web/Publications/Reports/2013/HIV-AIDS%20STIs%20Tuberculosis%20Leprosy.pdf

[17] http://www.oecd.org/els/health-systems/HealthAtAGlanceAsiaPacific2012.pdf

[18] Lee, Vernon J, et al. (2010) "Elimination of malaria risk through integrated combination strategies in a tropical military training island." *Am J Trop Med Hyg.* **82**(6): 1024–1029. Website: http://www.ncbi.nlm.nih.gov/pmc/articles/PMC2877406/

[19] https://www.moh.gov.sg/content/dam/moh_web/Publications/Reports/2013/Vector%20Borne-Zoonotic%20Diseases.pdf

The programme first covered smallpox in 1862, and expanded to cover diphtheria in 1938, tuberculosis in 1957, polio in 1958, pertussis and tetanus in 1959, and measles and rubella in 1976.[20] In 1985, hepatitis B vaccination was introduced into the programme for all babies born to hepatitis B carrier mothers before being rolled out to all newborns from 1987 onwards.[21] The trivalent measles, mumps, and rubella (MMR) vaccine was introduced in 1990 — that same year, mumps, and rubella were made legally notifiable diseases.[22] Many basic vaccinations are provided free for citizens and subsidised for residents at polyclinics, with vaccinations for all school-going children, irrespective of residency status, are provided by the Health Promotion Board's School Health Service. High levels of overall immunisation coverage of above 90% over the years has resulted in polio, neonatal tetanus, diphtheria, childhood TB meningitis, and congenital rubella being virtually eliminated from Singapore.[23]

Despite this, contemporary Singapore is seeing resurgence of infectious diseases of the past, driven by urbanisation and migration trends. In 1960, Singapore's tuberculosis (TB) incidence was 307 cases per 100,000 population. The National TB Control Unit and its active case detection methods helped bring this down to only 56 cases per 100,000 by 1987.[24] Between 1987 and 1998, this incidence remained largely constant, ranging between 49 and 57 per 100,000 resident population.[25] In an attempt to eradicate TB in Singapore, the Singapore Tuberculosis Elimination Programme (STEP) was launched in 1997. The trajectory of STEP is positive. In 2013, the incidence of tuberculosis (TB) among Singapore Citizens and Permanent Residents declined to 36.9 per 100,000 population from 40.9 per 100,000 population in 2012.[26] However, as the number of immigrants who enter Singapore increases, the number of TB cases among non-residents is likewise also increasing. In response to this, the Singapore Ministry of Health (MOH) is taking active measures to strengthen case detection and enhance STEP in meeting future TB challenges.

---

[20] Lieu, Fereen, et al. (2010) "Evaluation on the effectiveness of the national childhood immunity programme in Singapore, 1982–2007." Ann Acad Med Singapore. **39**: 532–541. Website: http://www.annals.edu.sg/pdf/39VolNo7Jul2010/V39N7p532.pdf

[21] ibid. http://www.annals.edu.sg/pdf/39VolNo7Jul2010/V39N7p532.pdf

[22] ibid. http://www.annals.edu.sg/pdf/39VolNo7Jul2010/V39N7p532.pdf

[23] ibid. http://www.annals.edu.sg/pdf/39VolNo7Jul2010/V39N7p532.pdf

[24] Ministry of Health Singapore. https://www.moh.gov.sg/content/moh_web/home/diseases_and_conditions/t/tuberculosis.html

[25] Ministry of Health Singapore. https://www.moh.gov.sg/content/moh_web/home/diseases_and_conditions/t/tuberculosis.html

[26] Ministry of Health Singapore. (2014) "Communicable Diseases Surveillance in Singapore 2013." Annual Report. Website: https://www.moh.gov.sg/content/moh_web/home/Publications/Reports/2014/communicable-diseases-surveillance-in-singapore-2013.html

Dengue

Also, dengue fever remains endemic to Singapore. First recorded in the 1960s as a major cause of childhood death, dengue continues to be a significant public health and vector control issue today. All four dengue serotypes are in circulation in Singapore, with DENV2 being the predominant strain in circulation since 2007.[27] Strict vector controls focused on surveillance and larval source reduction alongside public education programmes and law enforcement to discourage the propagation of *Aedes aegypti* mosquitoes were implemented to combat dengue in Singapore in the 1960s and 1970s. However, after 15 years of low dengue incidence, a resurgence occurred in the 2000s: in 2005, dengue incidence leaped from 9.3 to 312.2 cases per 100,000 resident population.[28] As of 2013, the dengue incidence rate stands at 404.9 per 100,000 resident population.[29]

Singapore's National Environment Agency (NEA) continues to work on controlling dengue transmission via their nationwide adulticide and larvicide control campaign, known as "carpet combing." This approach combines surveillance with community outreach and public education. The number of dengue cases in Singapore remains a pressing challenge, driven by the endemicity of multiple serotypes, low herd immunity, and *Aedes aegypti* adaptation to urban settings. In 2012, 4632 laboratory-confirmed cases of dengue fever/dengue haemorrhagic fever were reported.[30] Although 1059 cases of chikungunya were laboratory-confirmed in 2013[31] — a large increase from the 22 cases in 2012[32] — no deaths were reported from chikungunya fever in either year.

Further, cities such as Singapore are key nodes in infectious disease as they are hubs for national, regional, and global spread; bridge human and animal ecosystems;[33] and are hubs for globalisation processes: changing social, economic, and cultural structures, increasing personal mobility, cross-boundary integration, and extended and

---

[27] https://www.moh.gov.sg/content/dam/moh_web/Publications/Reports/2013/Vector%20Borne-Zoonotic%20Diseases.pdf

[28] "Singapore Dengue Case Study." Website: http://www.oxitec.com/health/dengue-information-centre/singapore-dengue-case-study/

[29] https://www.moh.gov.sg/content/dam/moh_web/Publications/Reports/2014/Communicable%20Diseases%20Surveillance%20in%20Singapore%202013/Vector%20Borne%20-Zoonotic%20Diseases.pdf

[30] https://www.moh.gov.sg/content/dam/moh_web/Publications/Reports/2013/Vector%20Borne-Zoonotic%20Diseases.pdf

[31] https://www.moh.gov.sg/content/dam/moh_web/Publications/Reports/2014/Communicable%20Diseases%20Surveillance%20in%20Singapore%202013/Vector%20Borne%20-Zoonotic%20Diseases.pdf

[32] https://www.moh.gov.sg/content/dam/moh_web/Publications/Reports/2013/Vector%20Borne-Zoonotic%20Diseases.pdf

[33] Horby P, Pfeiffer D, Oshitani H. (2013) "Prospects for emerging infections in East and Southeast Asia 10 years after SARS." *Emerging Infectious Diseases.* **19**(6): 853–860.

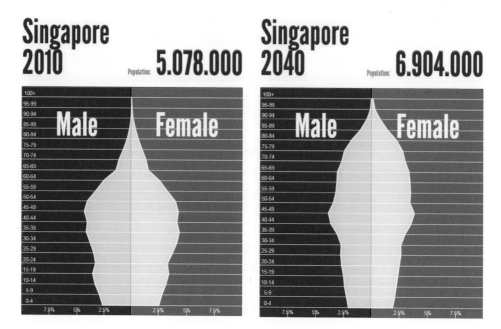

Fig. 2.3. Singapore's demographic profile.[34]

evolving social networks[35,36] — all driving forces of disease dynamics. The "networked disease" lens[37] posits that developed-world cities are key facilitators for the global movement of pathogens; and Singapore's experience with Severe Acute Respiratory Syndrome (SARS) in 2003 demonstrates this. A novel infectious disease outbreak that posed a serious economic, social, and reputational challenge to Singapore, SARS highlighted the abiding importance of isolation, quarantine, and personal hygiene; demonstrated the benefits of a robust and responsive healthcare system; and emphasised the continuing relevance of public health in modern-day Singapore.

Singapore's total fertility rate (TFR), defined as number of children per women aged 15 to 49 years old, stood at 5.1 during the 1960–1965 period. However, over the last several decades, this number has dropped to a fraction of what it was: OECD statistics note that Singapore's 2005–2010 TFR was only 1.3,[38] far below the

---

[34] http://populationpyramid.net/singapore/, created with data from United Nations, Department of Economic and Social Affairs, Population Division. World Population Prospects: The 2012 Revision.

[35] Castells M. (2010) *The Rise of the Network Society: Volume 1 — The Information Age: Economy, Society and Culture,* 2nd Ed. Oxford: Wiley-Blackwell.

[36] Coker RJ, *et al.* (2011) "Emerging infectious diseases in Southeast Asia: Regional challenges to control." *The Lancet.* **377**: 599–609.

[37] Washer P. (2011) "Lay perceptions of emerging infectious diseases: A commentary." *Public Understanding of Science.* **20**(4): 506–512.

[38] OECD and World Health Organization. (2012) *Health at a Glance: Asia/Pacific 2012.* OECD Publishing.

replacement rate of 2.1. There is growing discussion in many low-fertility countries, particularly in Europe, about the negative consequences of having fewer young persons, and the prospects of declining populations. In developed countries in particular, retirement incomes and medical care of the elderly are largely financed by taxes on the younger working population. Low birth rates eventually lead to a smaller working population, and hence a smaller tax base to finance social security payments.

Several attempts have been made by Singaporean policymakers to increase Singapore's low TFR. Some have argued that economic incentives delivered via enhancements of the existing Marriage and Parenthood Package could contribute to an improved TFR. However, existing evidence to support this claim is patchy. Despite two injections of enhancements to the Marriage and Parenthood Package since its introduction in 2001, Singapore's TFR has remained stagnant at 1.2.[39] Also, a 2005 study of Singaporean pro-natalist policies showed that a 1.0% increase in qualifying child relief only resulted in a 1.5% increase in TFR.[40]

Linked to, but distinct from, low TFR is the concurrent Singaporean phenomenon of population ageing. This is occurring at an unprecedented pace in modern Singapore: 8% of the population was aged 65 and over in 2008, this rose to 9.3% in 2011, and is expected to grow to 19% by 2030. Singapore's ageing population is not only growing in size; elderly Singaporeans are also living longer. For the average elderly person in Singapore, life expectancy at age 65 years rose from 16 years in 1990 to 20 years in 2010.[41] As of June 2011, 352,600 of Singapore's 3.79 million residents were aged 65 and over.[42]

Holding current TFR constant and excluding immigration, the government has projected that the number of elderly Singaporean citizens will triple to 900,000 by 2030, and they will be supported by a smaller base of working-age citizens. Currently, old-age support ratio stands at about 6.3 citizens in the working age bracket of 20 to 64 years for each citizen aged 65 and above. By 2030, there will only be 2.1 working-age citizens for each citizen aged 65 and above.[43] Population

---

[39] National Population and Talent Divison. (2013) "Population White Paper: A Sustainable Population for a Dynamic Singapore. White Paper." Singapore: National Population and Talent Divison.

[40] Park C. (2005) "How effective are pronatalist benefits? A literature survey and a study on Singapore's qualified child relief." *Singapore Economic Review.* **50**(1): 9–23.

[41] Department of Statistics Singapore. Website: http://www.singstat.gov.sg/publications/publications_and_papers/population_and_population_structure/ssnsep11-pg1–9.pdf

[42] Department of Statistics Singapore. Website: http://www.singstat.gov.sg/publications/publications_and_papers/population_and_population_structure/ssnsep11-pg1–9.pdf

[43] National Population and Talent Division. (2015) "Our Demographic Challenges and What These Mean to Us." Prime Minister's Office, Government of Singapore. Website: http://population.sg/key-challenges/#.VD9rLmeSzww

ageing comes with myriad health, healthcare, and social challenges. One of the most important of these is arguably a mounting burden of chronic disease in the population.

Chronic Diseases

Singapore's demographic transition, characterised by low fertility and rapid population ageing, is accompanied by a concomitant epidemiological transition: an increase in chronic disease incidence. The 2010 National Health Survey details that Type 2 Diabetes Mellitus (T2DM) among Singapore adults has risen from 8.2% in 2004 to 11.3% in 2010.[44] Cancer has become the number one killer in Singapore, with 58,654 notifications of new cancer cases by year of diagnosis between 2009–2013;[45] and 14 cancer deaths every day.[46] Also, nearly one in three deaths in Singapore is due to heart disease or stroke. Fifteen (15) people die from cardiovascular disease in Singapore every day, and cardiovascular disease accounted for 29.5% of all deaths in 2013.[47]

Cancer, cardiovascular disease, and diabetes are complex, multifactorial diseases that often develop over the course of a long life. As such, many chronic disease sufferers live with disease for a significant proportion of their lives, which contributes to their years of life lost due to disability, lifetime expenditure on healthcare, and productivity losses at work. Singapore's chronic disease burden is exacerbated by a lifestyle transition, characterised by increased sedentary behaviours; decreased physical activity; diets rich in processed, salty, fatty, sugary foods that are often low-cost and convenient, but low in nutrients; smoking; and alcohol consumption. Despite decades of research in the medical sciences that has spurred the development of a cornucopia of chronic disease treatment options, chronic disease prevention remains a major challenge for public health. Much remains to be understood of the interplay of genetic, lifestyle, and environmental factors responsible for the development of these diseases.

The implications of a large chronic disease burden mean that the local health systems paradigm needs to shift towards meeting the care needs and demands more tailored to chronic disease sufferers. Chronic disease patients often experience their diseases over a long duration of time. Many chronic diseases progress slowly

[44] http://www.moh.gov.sg/content/dam/moh_web/Publications/Reports/2011/NHS2010%20-%20low%20res.pdf

[45] Singapore Cancer Registry. (2013) "Trends in Cancer Incidence in Singapore, 2009–2013." *Interim Annual Registry Report.*

[46] Ministry of Health, "Singapore Health Facts, Principal Causes of Death," updated 30 Jan 2012.

[47] Ministry of Health Singapore. (2014) "Principal Causes of Death." Website: http://www.moh.gov.sg/content/moh_web/home/statistics/Health_Facts_Singapore/Principal_Causes_of_Death.html

and continuously over extended periods of time, decreasing patients' quality of life, increasing risk of comorbidities and risk of premature mortality (from comorbidities or acute events linked to chronic disease status), and causing significant economic repercussions for the individual, their families, and society as a whole. The health-care that they will require, as such, will be long-term and not acute-centric. Primary healthcare will play an integral role in the follow-up of chronic disease patients, ensuring adherence to regular treatment regimens, and acting as key nodes to link patients to the appropriate specialist care according to their individual needs. Additionally, greater attention needs to be placed on chronic disease prevention as research has shown that many chronic conditions can be prevented, delayed, or slowed down through proactive prevention measures.[48]

This chronic disease burden has serious implications for healthcare expenditure at the national level and for the population: Will the burgeoning number of chronic disease sufferers be able to afford the healthcare that they require over the course of many years of their lives, bearing in mind increased healthcare costs over time — and can Singapore's healthcare financing system rise to meet this swelling demand?

Healthcare Financing

The Singapore healthcare system is fundamentally grounded in the provision of social safety net protection: all Singaporeans are entitled to basic medical services at government polyclinics and hospitals, where rates are regulated and subsidised. However, to reduce over-utilisation of healthcare services, the policies that govern Singapore's healthcare system are underpinned by a strong principle of personal responsibility for one's health — that is, irrespective of subsidy levels, no healthcare service is provided free of charge, even within the public healthcare system.

3M: Medisave, Medishield, Medifund

Singapore's healthcare system is financed primarily via a combination of government subsidies, out-of-pocket payments, and compulsory savings from payroll deductions, known as "Medisave." Introduced in April 1984, it mandates a contribution of between 6.5 to 9.0% of income into a personal Medisave account. An individual's Medisave funds can be used to meet personal or immediate family member's hospitalization, day surgery, and certain outpatient expenses. However, limits have been set on the amount of Medisave that can be expended.

---

[48] Kathleen Strong, Colin Mathers, Stephen Leeder, Robert Beaglehole. (2005) "Preventing chronic diseases: How many lives can we save?" The Lancet. **366**(9496): 1578–1582.

Medishield is the second layer of social security offered by the Singapore healthcare system. It is an insurance scheme designed to meet large Class B2 and C hospitalisation bills. Introduced in 1990, MediShield operates with deductible and co-payment features, reinforcing the notion that patients should assume a degree of personal responsibility for their health and concomitant medical expenses.

A third layer of social safety net is Medifund, a government-established endowment fund aimed at helping needy Singaporeans who are unable to afford subsidised medical bill charges, despite Medisave and MediShield coverage. Recognising that healthcare costs increase with an ageing population, the government carved out a portion of Medifund to create Medifund Silver in 2007. Medifund Silver was launched with a start-up capital sum of $500 million to deliver targeted assistance to needy, aged Singaporean patients.

Medishield Life: One step closer to universal health coverage?

In response to ever-louder public concern about the affordability of healthcare over time, the Singapore government will be implementing Medishield Life at the end of 2015. Medishield Life, an augmented version of the existing Medishield, seeks to offer better protection and higher payouts to patients, so they will have less Medisave and/or out-of-pocket payments for large medical bills. Medishield Life is an opt-out system that will be automatically extended to all Singapore citizens and permanent residents, including the very elderly (i.e. those above the age of 90) and those with pre-existing conditions.

Although yet unannounced, the government has reassured the public that MediShield Life premiums will be affordable and can be fully paid by Medisave. The government has also endeavoured to keep premiums affordable by offering premium subsidies to low- and middle-income households, special premium subsidies to the Pioneer Generation, added premium support for the needy who are unable to afford their premiums after premium subsidies, and transitional subsidies to facilitate population-level shifts from Medishield to Medishield Life.

Overall, Singapore's healthcare financing system in the public sector relies primarily on government subsidies, supplemented by individuals' Medisave, insurance and out of pocket payment. This has kept Singapore's healthcare spending low (3–4% of GDP) compared to that of many other developed countries like the US and UK. The implementation of Medishield Life will have a significant impact on the total percentage of GDP spent on healthcare.

Health Systems Reform and the Regional Health System (RHS)

As Singapore has progressed from Third World to First, it has also reaped the benefits of development and growth. Singaporeans today have long lives — life expectancy at birth in 2013 was 82.5 years,[49] among the highest in the world. However, Singapore may not be exempt from global trends that point to the fact that although we are living longer, we also accumulate more years of life lost due to illness and disability. Analyses of the Global Burden of Disease Study of 2010[50] found that around the globe, the average man spends 10.7 years suffering from poor health while the average woman spends 13.3 years. The main contributor to these figures is increasing chronic disease burden in our populations. As such, the clear and present danger confronting us is the ability of healthcare systems to cope with this demand. Understandably, the focus of many economies is on treating, managing complications and rehabilitating patients with chronic illnesses. However, Singapore has recognised that the challenges that lie ahead may not be resolved through mere expansion of the healthcare system and its facilities.

Singapore today has a mixed healthcare delivery model. The public sector dominates the acute hospital care sector, delivering 80% of the care. The primary care sector is dominated by private sector providers, which account for about 80% of the market. In the step-down care sector (e.g. nursing homes, community hospitals, and hospices), service provision is mainly provided by voluntary welfare organisations, most of which are funded by the government for their services rendered to patients.

Although the MOH regularly evaluates and adjusts healthcare policies to regulate the supply and cost of healthcare services in the public sector, private healthcare costs remain largely unregulated and subject to market forces. The private healthcare sector is a growing force in Singapore, providing care to the privately insured, foreign patients, or public patients with the means to afford substantial out-of-pocket payments for healthcare services.

The traditional healthcare model in Singapore is reactive and structured to respond best to episodic care — this has nurtured an episodic relationship between the patient and the health system. That is to say, hospitals, clinics, and other healthcare

---

[49] Ministry of Health Singapore. (2014) "Population and Vital Statistics." Website: http://www.moh.gov. sg/content/moh_web/home/statistics/Health_Facts_Singapore/Population_And_Vital_Statistics.html
[50] Murray C, Vos T, Lozano R, et al. (2012) "Disability-adjusted life years (DALYs) for 291 diseases and injuries in 21 regions, 1990–2010: A systematic analysis for the Global Burden of Disease Study 2010." The Lancet. pp. 2197–2223.

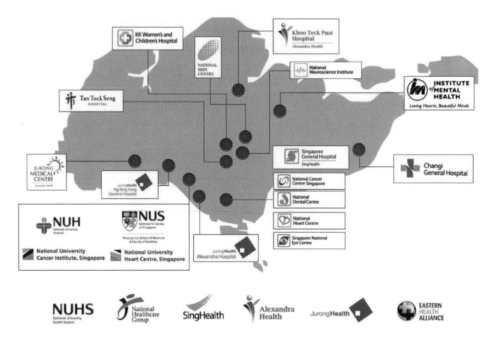

Fig. 2.4.　Healthcare institutions of Singapore.

facilities are primarily utilised by patients when they experience acute, short-term illnesses (e.g. coughs and colds) or sustain trauma (e.g. falls and injuries). In 2012, there were a total of 10,756 hospital beds in the 25 hospitals and specialty centres in Singapore. The eight (8) public hospitals comprise six (6) acute general hospitals, one women and children's hospital, and a psychiatric hospital. All public hospitals are "restructured," meaning that they operate as government-owned corporations instead of typical public hospitals, which are owned by government and receive government funding.

This traditional acute-centric healthcare model has facilitated nationwide excellence in episodic and reactive clinical care. However, it does not — and arguably, cannot — serve the needs of chronic disease patients as competently. The acute-centric system, as it stands in Singapore, today is not sufficiently integrated with social resources within the community that are beneficial, and to an extent essential, to improving the health, welfare, and well-being of chronic disease sufferers who live and work within society.

Recognising these in the current healthcare model, the growing need to cater to chronic disease sufferers, and the need to develop a healthcare system that can deliver care that is appropriate to patient need, delivered in the appropriate setting which is accessible to the patient, at an appropriate and affordable cost, the Singapore government has begun rolling out the Regional Health System (RHS).

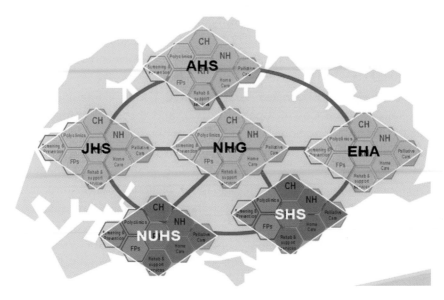

Fig. 2.5.   Singapore's Regional Health Systems as of 2014.

Source: Singapore Caregiver Online, http://sg-caregiver.com/transformations-in-public-hospital-landscape/regional-health-system/#!prettyPhoto

The RHS is an evolving concept that can be broadly described as acute hospitals and other healthcare providers within a geographical region working together to deliver patient centric care that is accessible, appropriate to patient need, affordable, and sustainable. The RHS aims to coordinate services seamlessly in order to care holistically for the population within a community setting and across the entire health spectrum. One of the main provisions of the RHS is to deliver high-quality, accessible, and affordable primary care that provides early detection and early management of chronic diseases, so as to prevent complications and unnecessary admissions into acute care hospitals.

The RHS spans the entire healthcare continuum, from health promotion through to episodic care, integrated care, and chronic care that is continuous and extends beyond acute hospitals and into the community. This will include primary care, nursing homes, rehabilitation centres, home care, community hospitals, and hospices. Under the RHS, public healthcare institutions are divided into six broad clusters, each serving the island's north, east, west, and central zones. Each cluster is anchored by a Regional Hospital (RH) as follows:

- National Healthcare Group: Tan Tock Seng Hospital, Institute of Mental health, 9 NHG Polyclinics, National Skin Centre

- National University Health System: National University Hospital NUS Yong Loo Lin School of Medicine, NUS Faculty of Dentistry, and the Saw Swee Hock School of Public Health (SSHSPH), National University Cancer Institute, National University Heart Centre
- Alexandra Health: Khoo Teck Puat Hospital, Yishun Community Hospital, Admiralty Medical Centre (opening 2017), and the Woodlands Integrated Health Campus (operational from end December 2015 to 2022)
- SingHealth: Singapore General Hospital, KK Woman and Children's Hospital, Sengkang Health, National Cancer Centre Singapore, National Dental Centre Singapore, National Heart Centre Singapore, National Neuroscience Institute, Singapore National Eye Centre, 9 Singhealth Polyclinics, and Bright Vision Community Hospital
- Eastern Health Alliance: Changi General Hospital, St. Andrew's Community Hospital, and partnerships with SingHealth Polyclinics and the Salvation Army Peacehaven Nursing Home
- Jurong Health System: Ng Teng Fong General Hospital, Jurong Community Hospital, and management of Jurong Medical Centre and Lakeside Family Medicine Clinic

Once fully operational, the government aspires that the RHS will be able to reduce fragmentation of care and instead deliver healthcare that is appropriate to patient needs, as well as encourage collaboration between different healthcare sectors to help patients move smoothly across different care settings as needed and ensure that patients receive appropriate care by way of shared clinical pathways, so they can stay healthy and better manage their conditions over the long term.

Healthcare Manpower Challenges

As part of enhancing the healthcare system and developing the RHS, new acute and community hospitals, as well as medical centres, will be built. These developments will allow the health system to support a larger, older population — one that is estimated to rise from 5.8 to 6 million by 2020 — while alleviating the strains that the system currently faces.[51]

While this is a welcome and necessary development, there remain long-standing concerns regarding the healthcare workers needed to man these new facilities. There are only three medical schools in Singapore that take in a select number of students. Also, while many local students go abroad to study medicine, not all of them return

---

[51] National Population and Talent Division. (2013) "Population White Paper: A Sustainable Population for a Dynamic Singapore. White Paper." Singapore: National Population and Talent Division.

to serve the local healthcare system. We must also consider the temporal factors that influence the rate at which doctors enter the healthcare system: as medical school takes four to five years, there will be a significant time lag associated with the entry of qualified doctors entering the public healthcare framework.

Additionally, few local institutions offer degrees in nursing and other allied health fields such as physiotherapy and radiology — fields that will increase in prominence and need as the Singaporean population ages and the burden of chronic disease increases. The need for geriatric, rehabilitative, and palliative care professionals, as well as social work and elder care workers will also rise. Thus far, immigration has helped alleviate some of these woes; Singapore has actively courted and brought over skilled healthcare professionals from neighbouring countries such as Malaysia and the Philippines. However, this policy may contradict the government's recent assertion that Singapore "cannot allow in unlimited numbers of foreign workers" so as to not "be overwhelmed by more foreign workers than we can absorb."[52]

In the context of Singapore desiring to "reduce reliance on foreign workers in the long run,"[53] the healthcare sector may be limited, in spite of its vast infrastructural improvements and enduring need for healthcare manpower. Overcoming these conjoint challenges is essential to ponder, as the robustness of the Singaporean healthcare system — from hospitals and facilities to manpower — has great implications for the well-being, economic productivity, and prosperity of the Singaporean population as a whole. Perhaps most importantly in the case of healthcare, emphasis should be placed not only upon the quantity of healthcare professionals who staff these premises, but also the quality of care that they provide to Singaporeans.

The Enduring Challenge of Public Health and Disease Prevention

Although the case for prevention has strengthened over the years, marked by impressive accomplishments in preventing disease and reducing mortality, challenges in justifying cost of prevention over cost of treatment continue to slow down the widespread covering of effective prevention programs. A treatment service must only be shown to be reasonably effective in addressing a given disease. For a preventive service, however, an ironclad argument must be marshalled regarding its effectiveness in delivering the desired health outcome and it must also demonstrate that the cost of delivering the service is less than the cost of treating the preventative

---

[52] National Population and Talent Division. (2013) "Population White Paper: A Sustainable Population for a Dynamic Singapore. White Paper." Singapore: National Population and Talent Division.

[53] National Population and Talent Division. (2013) "Population White Paper: A Sustainable Population for a Dynamic Singapore." White Paper. Singapore: National Population and Talent Division.

condition. The important aspect of this equation is that no value is given to the state of better health achieved by the person served by preventing a disease.[54]

The world today is more complex, interconnected, and interdependent than ever before and our approach to public health challenges has to evolve. Broadly stated, the first phase of public health (Public Health 1.0) can be characterised by improvements in health that occurred largely as by-products of industrial and economic development. Examples of this include better housing, clean water, and improved hygiene and sanitation practices. Many years later, the landscape changed again and became largely defined by a biomedical approach to Public Health. This second phase, Public Health 2.0, was thus characterised by identifying single major risk factor of a particular disease. For example, small pox is caused by the variola virus and vaccination has successfully eliminated the virus globally; mesothelioma is due to asbestos exposure and can be controlled by the control of occupational and environmental exposure. Today, we are entering the third phase of public health development, Public Health 3.0. This phase is characterised by common diseases that are due to multiple factors ranging from biomedical to socio-economic-environmental and other system level factors interacting in adaptive manner. The prevention of these common diseases like diabetes, hypertension, cancer, and heart diseases cannot be targeted at single factors. Moreover, there are multiple stakeholders, levers, and barriers that have to be managed simultaneously. PH 3.0 requires us to embrace and understand complexity science and implementation science. It requires many disciplines outside the traditional medical and healthcare domains: urban planning, behavioural science, economics, sociology, engineering, marketing, business administration, and so forth.

The case of prevention is critical for the future of public health in Singapore. Building upon its rich past from the days of Sir Stamford Raffles, Singapore has entered Public Health 3.0 and older paradigms are beginning to shift to new ones, focused on the need for effective, innovative prevention efforts across all sectors of the nation.

An Integrated, Comprehensive Approach to Public Health and Healthy Living

The case of type 2 diabetes mellitus (T2DM)

In 1975, the prevalence of T2DM was a mere 1.9%. By 2010, the prevalence had increased to 11.3%. In 2020, burden of disease forecasts show that Singapore will have 500,000 diabetics a number set to rise to 1 million by 2050.

---

[54] McGinnis JM. (1985) "The limits of prevention," *Public Health Reports.* pp. 255–260.

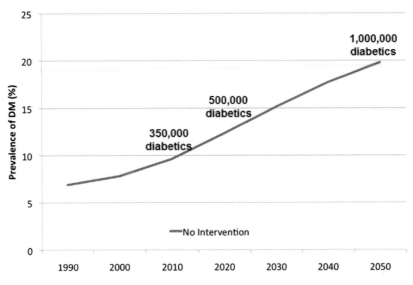

Fig. 2.6. Projected Diabetes Burden in Singapore.[55]

*This projection uses agent-based simulations incorporating demographic, obesity trends, ethnicity, and genetic factors

With its high level of co-morbidity, this forecasted increase in burden of disease of Diabetes will place an overwhelming demand on Singapore's healthcare system. It is clear that the time has come to not simply only increase capacity of the healthcare system or to turn our current basin into a bath tub. Rather, we must learn to slow down the rate of increase or the flow in the number of diabetics in Singapore. The key was to shift this patient care to the primary healthcare system and to increase our efforts in prevention. By improving the efficiency and quality of care, as well as focusing on prevention, the onset of complications and disabilities can be delayed. The compression of morbidity, a hypothesis put forward by James Fries of Stanford University, refers to the shortening of the number of years lived with disability before death by delaying the first onset of chronic diseases. However, we need effective preventive measures to do this, which must be intentional, implemented with clear leadership and vision, and involve multiple stakeholders and sectors to have greatest impact.

One example of this is the Healthy Living Master Plan (HLMP). The HLMP is the Singaporean government's vision to ensure that all Singaporeans have access to a healthy lifestyle. The Master Plan acts as a roadmap aimed at keeping Singaporeans healthy and disability-free for as long as possible. It consolidates healthy living

[55] PHMA team — Saw Swee Hock School of Public Health, National University of Singapore, 2015.

initiatives from public agencies and the communities ensuring that opportunities (infrastructure and programmes) for healthy living are pervasive and convenient, and that nudges are available to drive intrinsic motivations of individuals and influence behaviour change. The government is aware that dictating healthy living is not productive and instead has taken a whole-of-society approach. This involves plans to seek synergistic efforts to bring about healthy living options, through connections across government agencies, across the community, and between the community and the government. The first step was a public consultation exercise, earlier this year, which welcomed the views and feedback on how the nation can achieve and promote healthy lifestyles.

Total Workplace Safety and Health (TWSH)

Nationally, chronic diseases such as diabetes are forecasted to rise significantly. With the extension of the retirement age and a rapidly ageing population, the prevalence of chronic diseases in the Singaporean workforce has become an area of great concern. These demographic and health changes, have catalysed a shift in Singapore's perspective on workplace health management. The Ministry of Manpower (MOM) has been actively encouraging industry ownership and empowerment of workplace safety and health (WSH) management through greater risk management and prevention, which has resulted not only in a shift in industry mindset, but also significant improvements in WSH standards across the board.

As Singapore's workplace conditions improve, WSH risks are shifting away from traditional occupational hazards such as physical injuries towards other causes which impact employees' health, well-being, and ability to work. Therefore it is imperative that the Singapore workplace health management mindset continues to move towards viewing workplace health and safety as two integrated, interrelated issues, and towards not just making the physical work environment safe and healthy for workers, but also towards fitting the work environment to workers' capabilities and limitations. This has become increasingly important in the light of a rapidly ageing population and workforce. The "greying" of the labour force is an inevitable result of sustained low fertility as well as accelerated population ageing. There are concerns about the consequences for worker productivity and mobility of an older work force, as it appears likely that reduced worker mobility will result from a higher average age of workers. While the medium- to long-term economic consequence of this trend is potentially an inhibited ability of labour markets to adjust to changing economic conditions, we must also consider the public health consequences of an aged workforce. With unhealthy lifestyle behaviours, extended life expectancy, and the extension of retirement age, as is happening here in Singapore, employers are weighed down by the increasing number of workers suffering from chronic diseases. The employee's health has implications on the cost of business such as direct costs of healthcare expenditures, and lost productivity through absenteeism and presenteeism.

In response to these needs, the National University of Singapore's Saw Swee Hock School of Public Health (SSHSPH) has pioneered and spearheaded efforts towards the implementation of total and integrated Workplace Safety and Health services in Singapore. Total and integrated WSH is a more holistic approach managing three components of workplace safety and health, namely occupational safety; occupational health; and wellness (chronic disease management and health promotion) in workplaces. Using modelling and simulation anchored in current literature, SSHSPH estimated that out of the 350,000 diabetics living in Singapore today, 150,000 are in the working population. These 150,000 working diabetics are costing Singapore more than S$1 billion per year in health costs related to diabetes alone. The strain on already limited healthcare resources is evident.

With a growing recognition of the need for a new approach to prevention in the workplace, TWSH is grounded in rigorous evidence-based research of its relevance, feasibility, and cost-effectiveness, and brings together the Ministries of Health and Manpower, Health Promotion Board, and Workplace Safety and Health Council.

Conclusion

Public health development in Singapore has been characterised by steady and systematic developments that began by targeting disease related to development, sanitation, and hygiene, and have since evolved into efforts to develop a national healthcare system commensurate with the country's socioeconomic development and responsive to community needs. As a young nation, Singapore recognises the need to be innovative and develop new solutions, anticipating upcoming population health issues and needs in order to meet the myriad health and healthcare needs of the present century.

3 Evolving the Governance of Public Healthcare Institutions — A Continuous Improvement Journey

Elizabeth Quah* and Neo Boon Siong[†]

Introduction

Traditional economic theory posits that the "invisible hand" of the market is best able to allocate goods and services, via a pricing system. Government planning, on the other hand, suffers from the problems of inefficient allocation, and an inability to change in response to fast-changing conditions. In the provision of healthcare services, both government and markets are imperfect. Market imperfections such as patient-provider-payor split, could result in sharp increases in healthcare costs, without significant improvements in healthcare outcomes. At the same time, lower income groups may not have access to needed services. These factors result in the public sector directly providing healthcare services in a number of countries. In others, hybrid models have developed, whereby state-run insurance schemes or state financing enable low cost subsidised healthcare services to be provided via the public and private sector.

Singapore has a hybrid healthcare system. In primary care, about 80% is provided by approximately 1500 fee-for-service general practitioner (GP) clinics, with the remaining 20% provided by public sector polyclinics which deliver subsidised healthcare services. Of recent years, the government has allowed access to subsidised healthcare services from the private GP sector. The reverse applies for acute hospital care, where the seven public sector hospitals[1] account for 80% of the national supply

*Group Director in the Ministry of Health, Singapore.

[†]Professor at the Nanyang Business School, Nanyang Technological University.

[1]Singapore General Hospital, National University Hospital, Tan Tock Seng Hospital, Changi General Hospital, Khoo Teck Puat Hospital, Alexandra Hospital and Kandang Kerbau Women's and Children's Hospital. The public sector also operates a psychiatric hospital, the Institute of Mental Health.

of acute beds, with the private sector taking up the remaining 20%. Finally, the intermediate and long-term care (ILTC) sector is run predominantly by community groups and voluntary welfare organisations (VWOs), several of which receive Government subsidies for needy patients.

This chapter explores how the governance structure of the Singapore healthcare system has evolved over time, and how the current structure of Regional Health Systems aims to address the challenges posed by an ageing population and the increasing fragmentation of healthcare provision, driven by advances in medical science and technology. It describes how MOH leverages upon market levers as far as possible to address government imperfections whilst at the same time reinforcing its strategic role in the governance of healthcare entities to better align them to their public mission in the provision of healthcare services to all Singaporeans.[2]

Corporatisation

Prior to self-government and Independence, healthcare in Singapore was delivered by a mix of providers — community-run healthcare facilities, hospitals run by the colonial government for the British servicemen and local community, and traditional medicine healers. Over time, the system shifted towards the British national health system whereby hospitals and primary care clinics were government-owned and government-run, funded via general taxation. Whilst user-charges were introduced in 1960, these were relatively low. Subsequently, during the 1970s, healthcare expenditure increased by four times, driven by increasing hospital admissions. Concerned that citizens may have taken subsidised healthcare for granted, the National Health Plan (1983), amongst other things, laid out the principles of a revised healthcare financing system, based on not only government subsidies, but also co-payments by patients, and the introduction of a new Medisave scheme, pegged at "C" class rates, to help Singaporeans pay for their own hospitalisation expenses. The new healthcare financing system aimed to put the financing of the healthcare system on a more sustainable basis whilst at the same time promoting affordability for all Singaporeans.

At the same time, in keeping with the direction of the NHP, MOH explored how the healthcare system could be organised and governed for greater efficiency and responsiveness to public needs. It took inspiration from reforms in other countries,

---

[2] A more detailed case study of the transformation of Singapore public healthcare institutions can be found in the paper, "Transformation of Singapore Healthcare from 2004 to 2013," by Neo Boon Siong and Leong Ching with the assistance of Wong Hui Zhen, Melinda Elias and Bernard Toh, published by the Healthcare Leadership College of the Ministry of Health Holdings Pte. Ltd. This paper draws on the case study and frames the governance of Singapore public healthcare in how it attempted to calibrate the market with government intervention and to play to the strengths of each.

such as the UK under Prime Minister Margaret Thatcher, and the US under President Ronald Reagan. These countries were similarly embarking on corporatisation or privatisation of core government services. Through this process, governments would be able to "steer" rather than "row," to concentrate on policy formulation and regulation, with the corporatisated or private entities focusing on the more efficient delivery of services. In this manner, governments could also distance themselves from the political heat of service provision, particularly for social and health services.

In the 1980s, the Singapore Government started corporatising public services. Eventually, the corporatisation efforts would cover public hospitals, telecommunications, energy supply, port services and public works. In healthcare, the intent was that market competition among corporatised hospitals would result in greater efficiency, nimbleness and responsiveness to meeting the needs of the public.

An initial pilot, namely the establishment of the National University Hospital (NUH) as a corporatised entity in 1984, was assessed to have successfully achieved more responsive service, innovative management and public acceptance of price adjustments. MOH then proceeded to corporatise the rest of the government-run hospitals — SGH in 1989 and the most of the other hospitals in the 1990s.[3] MOH addressed public concerns that corporatisation would result in increasing the cost of healthcare, by reassuring the public that the corporatised, or "restructured" entities would still retain their public service mission:

> "Our programme is, in fact, not to privatise the hospitals in the sense of selling the hospitals to private companies and let them try to survive as viable independent units. **The whole objective of our programme is, in actual fact, to restructure the hospitals, allow it to operate as autonomous units free from the constraints of Civil Service regulations. In this way they will be able to plan their management system, recruit the necessary staff, remunerate them, come out with systems that are efficient, since they do not have to comply with the very detailed regulations under the Civil Service.** [...] Although hospitals have been restructured, [...] there will always be subsidised rates to cater for the low income group in Singapore who cannot afford to pay the full cost of hospital care."
>
> — Acting Minister for Health Yeo Cheow Tong,
> Parliamentary Speech, 25 March 1987

The restructured hospitals (RHs) were given broad autonomy under a holding company, Health Corporation of Singapore (HCS), to manage areas such as finance,

---

[3] Tan Tock Seng Hospital (TTSH), Toa Payoh Hospital, and Changi Hospital (now merged to form Changi General Hospital (CGH) and Kandang Kebau Hospital (KKH).

human resource, medical care and research, for greater operational flexibility. Each RH had its own Board of Directors with MOH representation for governance and oversight purposes.

At the same time, given Singapore's small population, low-volume and complex treatments were consolidated in six national specialty centres.[4] This allowed for economies of scale to be realised and for scarce specialist talent to be brought together in one centre of excellence, thus allowing for development of the specialty, research, and the training of the next generation of specialists.

The strategic intent — that corporatisation would drive greater competition, and efficiency amongst hospitals was reiterated in the White Paper on Affordable Health Care (1993).

> *"We must rely on competition and market forces to impel hospitals and clinics to run efficiently, improve services and offer patients better value for money. When hospitals are insulated from price signals and market forces, the potential for inefficiency and waste is enormous."*
>
> *— White Paper on Affordable Health Care, 1993*

Overall, the restructuring exercise was beneficial. Hospitals innovated, pushed for greater efficiency in resource allocation and utilisation, were able to respond quickly to the needs of patients and were better able to review their personnel policies to attract and retain staff. Each developed their own sense of identity and corporate ethos.

However, as hospitals focused on achieving their own individual goals and objectives, they began to see each other as competitors for patients and for talent, rather than collaborators in delivering public healthcare services. Under the White Paper, hospitals were allowed to attract unsubsidised A and B1 ward patients, and to keep the revenues. To do so, hospitals began to offer new services, or introducing new medical technologies. In some institutions, doctors' compensation mechanisms also allowed doctors to retain a share of their earnings from private patients, thus giving them an incentive to treat private patients. Subsidised patients could also benefit from these new services offered.

However, such competition had its downsides. Hospitals pushed to introduce new services, even though this could encroach on the role of the national centres, and even though it was unlikely that they could attract sufficient cases to sustain a service. Competition for scarce specialist talent to run such services also resulted in pushing up salaries, so smaller, less well reputed hospitals which were less

---

[4] National Skin Centre; Singapore National Eye Centre; National Cancer Centre; National Heart Centre; National Dental Centre; and National Neuroscience Institute.

attractive to unsubsidised patients also had difficulties attracting good doctors. A new balance had to be struck, between the centralised system of the past and the highly autonomous model of individually corporatised hospitals.

Two Clusters

In 2000, the Government sought to achieve this new balance with the restructuring of Alexandra Hospital (the last remaining government-run hospital), Woodbridge Hospital (now renamed the Institute of Mental Health) and the government polyclinics and to reorganise all the restructured institutions under two clusters — the National Healthcare Group (NHG) and the Singapore Health Services (SingHealth). The strategic intent was to allow the various institutions under each group to provide vertically integrated care for patients — from primary care, to acute care, and to tertiary care — and reap some economics of scale as part of a larger cluster. Through the clusters, MOH aimed to achieve a better balance between competitive and co-operative behaviour, leading to better service and lower cost.

A Group Chief Executive Officer (CEO) was appointed for each cluster. The CEOs of the individual hospitals reported to the Group CEO, but still enjoyed a fair degree of operational autonomy. HCS remained the holding company for the two new clusters, but was renamed as MOH Holdings Pte Ltd (MOHH). In a separate exercise, MOH also created two new statutory boards — the Health Promotion Board, to take care of health promotion and to run student health services; and the Health Sciences Authority, responsible for blood collection and banking, pharmaceutical and product regulation, and forensic services.

To address abiding concerns on the "profit-maximising" role of a corporatised entity, MOH also re-positioned SingHealth and NHG as "not-for-profit" entities, to clearly signal that the restructured hospitals still had to follow their public mission.

> "I want to make our position on this explicit. SingHealth and NHG would therefore be repositioned as not-for-profit entities. As not-for-profit entities, their main objective is not to maximise profits, neither are they under pressure to pay dividends to their shareholders. To underscore this "not-for-profit status", the Minister for Finance has agreed to exempt the two clusters from paying corporate tax. Instead, the tax savings and any surpluses generated as a result of their efficiency gains will be ploughed back for medical research, training and patient care... By modelling themselves as not-for-profit organisations, our restructured hospitals will have a different organisational culture from the private hospitals. Our restructured hospitals will continue to preserve their sense of public

service. Let me clarify that not-for-profit does not mean that our restruc-
tured hospitals do not have to worry about costs. The not-for-profit
organisation must still exercise financial prudence, cost their services
accurately, control their costs and improve productivity... "

— *Minister for Health, Lim Hng Kiang, Parliamentary Speech,*
10 March 2001

The clusters were able to achieve some economies of scale and scope. Since 2003, the SingHealth Group Procurement Office has achieved a combined savings of more than $150 million.[5] Common electronic medical records (EMR) systems were also introduced, enabling patient records to be shared across institutions within each cluster. There was also greater scope to share clinical best practices, e.g. protocols to reduce hospital-acquired infections.

But, other challenges emerged. In its 2003 report, the Economic Review Committee (ERC), set up by the government to review Singapore's economic strategies, recommended, among other things, the inclusion of the healthcare sector as part of overall efforts to expand an export-oriented services. This led to a drive to actively promote Singapore's healthcare services overseas — covering both private and public sector hospitals. Clusters began accepting more private foreign patients, which also helped generate additional financial revenue for the clusters. This accentuated the competition over specialist talent. Signals from the Ministry reflecting the concern over long-term sustainability of national healthcare spending and the establishment of block budgets also led the clusters to watch their finances, and bottom-lines.

At the same time, with such a wide span of functions, it was difficult for the large clusters to provide the necessary governance oversight and direction, as well as management attention to implement well the different strategic initiatives. The large geographical footprint of the two-cluster system meant that they would have to deal with too many stakeholders, and were thus unable to build relationships and develop the trust required to succeed in chronic disease management.

Reforming Governance

MOH thus embarked on a two-fold effort to reform and strengthen the governance of the healthcare clusters. First, the public hospital's mission had to be clarified and realigned to MOH's broader directions and goals. Second, to strategically reorganise the public healthcare sector to tackle the challenges of an ageing population. These strategies have resulted in the evolution of the delivery system

---

[5] As reported in Parliament, 22 February 2010.

from two clusters to six regional healthcare systems — a structure that is paradoxically, both more and less centralised — with six rather than two entities, but all six more aligned to a national healthcare vision.

> "The Ministry went back to first principles, took a fundamental review and concluded that the intent was for government hospitals, regardless of how they were structured, to serve Singaporeans... [the clusters] are owned by the Ministry of Health to perform a political and social function, not an economic function. The purpose of corporatisation was really to allow the institution to run more flexibly and more efficiently. It wasn't for [them] to become a business. So along the way I think we decided that we needed to reform the governance of the public hospitals."
>
> — Then Permanent Secretary Ms. Yong Ying-I, in a 2012 interview

When the two clusters were first established, MOH had set out a Service Level Agreement (SLA) which aimed to set out performance targets and objectives in return for government subvention. Implicit in the work on the first SLA was that MOH's relationship with the operating entities was primarily structured via a contractual agreement reviewed at regular intervals.

However, beyond the SLA, and other regular meetings between the Ministry and the cluster/hospital leadership, there was no formal institutional structure for the ministry to set out the operating mandate and priorities for the clusters as these evolved annually. The challenge for MOH was how to strengthen the governance and accountability structure for the public sector hospitals, whilst maintaining the autonomy of the individual clusters, and their Boards of Directors. Three key measures were undertaken:

- *Engagement of Cluster Boards* — Whilst the Minister for Health appointed the Chairman and the Members of the Cluster Boards, there was limited engagement between the Boards and the senior management of MOH. Today, the MOH representative is a member of MOH's senior management, at the Permanent Secretary or Deputy Secretary level. Board members are invited to the Ministry's annual Workplan Seminar and other key events. Through such interactions, Board members are updated on MOH's key priorities and directions.
- *Development of the Accountability Documents* — A suite of accountability documents have been drawn up to define the relationship between MOH and the clusters: the Policy Agreement (signed over 2009/2010), a standing document which sets out the public mission of the clusters and demarcates the roles and responsibilities of MOH and the clusters vis-à-vis each other;

the three-year Service Level Agreement, which formalises the performance outcomes required of clusters for funding received; and the Statement of Priorities, which lays out the immediate year's priorities and key performance indicators.

- *Involvement in Key Appointments* — MOH's approval is required in the appointment of the Chief Executives and Chairmen of the Medical Boards (CMBs) of the clusters and public sector healthcare institutions. MOH also gives annual inputs on the contributions of the CEOs and CMBs to national healthcare initiatives, e.g. participation in key committees, leadership of major national initiatives.

In parallel, MOH also embarked upon a major initiative to improve upon the performance measurement and management of public sector institutions.

In 2008, the Ministry developed the National Standards for Healthcare (NSHC) with the primary objective to ensure public institutions provide care that was appropriate to patients' needs, based on current evidence and clinical knowledge across the continuum of healthcare. Prior to the NSHC, hospitals were monitoring a handful of clinical indicators, but these were not standardised across hospitals, hence it was not possible to facilitate "like-for-like" comparisons across hospitals. Also, while institutions may have had existing committees/departments which monitor quality and performance, an overarching framework was needed to coordinate NSHC-related quality improvement efforts. This led to MOH establishing the Healthcare Performance Offices (HPOs) at every institution in 2009, to support local implementation of NSHC.

Concurrently, the Ministry implemented a performance measurement framework which comprised a series of cascading scorecards starting from the National Health System Scorecard, to provider/specialty-level scorecards. The scorecards took reference from internationally accepted indicators and definitions, in particular those developed under OECD's Healthcare Quality Indicator project. The National Health System Scorecard enables Singapore's performance to be compared internationally with other countries while the Public Hospital Scorecard complements the National Health System Scorecard by facilitating comparison of how institutions performed vis-à-vis with one another.

The Public Hospital Scorecard indicators covered both the clinical quality (i.e. output and outcomes of care) and the patient (i.e. patient satisfaction) perspectives. They were further tied to either strategic targets that articulated long-term outcome or performance targets, which were established in accordance to institutions' prevailing level of capacity and capability. The annual Public Hospital Performance Report reviewed performance across public acute hospitals by

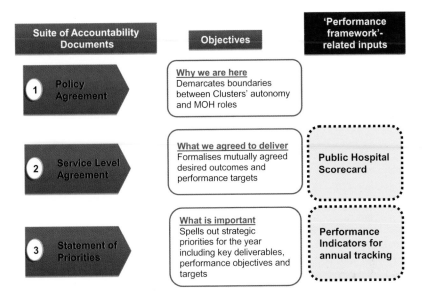

Fig. 3.1. MOH's accountability documents and the Public Hospital Scorecard.

highlighting areas in which hospitals were doing well and areas to be improved. The exercise of cross-comparison across healthcare institutions drove goal setting for institutions to push for continuous improvement and innovation to close gaps. Lastly, the Public Hospital Scorecard was embedded within the SLA and SOP (Fig. 3.1 depicts how the SLA and SOP and the Public Hospital Scorecard complement each other), providing MOH with the institutional basis to set meaningful performance goals for the institutions, based on both clinical quality indicators, and patient satisfaction indicators, in alignment with the public mission of the public sector institutions. More recently, MOH has been working with the HPOs to identify 3–5 *"Indicators of concern"* for their own institution based on their performance *vis-a-vis* other institutions and their own performance over time, and to develop Action Plans for improvement in these areas. The HPO's Action Plans, and Progress Updates on these Plans are discussed at various platforms including annual MOH-Cluster Meetings.

In addition, the Government has taken the lead to publish more healthcare information to reduce the information asymmetry, empower patients and enable the market to function better. Since 2003, total hospital bill sizes for top medical conditions has been published on MOH's website. Starting with public hospitals, the data now includes private sector hospital information. To provide additional transparency, MOH began to publish the cost of performing 65 common surgical procedures (previously included within the total bill size) for public hospitals on its website in September 2014.[6] This will provide more information to empower patients to make informed decisions, and allow market forces to work more efficiently.

Six Regional Health Systems

The new governance framework provided MOH with the institutional mechanisms and levers to foster greater alignment between the ministry and the healthcare clusters, whilst the public hospital scorecard created a platform for a meaningful discussion on hospital performance and avenues for improvement to take place. But, to what end? How did MOH see the healthcare sector developing in order to meet future healthcare needs?

The transformation of the healthcare system since 2004 may be understood as a response to the past experience of the hospital corporatisation and two-cluster system. It may also be understood in the light of three recent, significant developments affecting healthcare.

First, Singapore experienced rapid population growth in recent years, with the population exceeding five million for the first time in 2010. This led to the need to build new healthcare infrastructure and training new healthcare professionals. As new towns grew up around Singapore, e.g. in Sengkang and Punggol, there was also a need for hospitals to be better distributed across the island, when previously, hospitals were all situated in the eastern, southern and central parts of the country.

Second, the rapidly ageing population gave rise to a growing chronic disease burden. This pointed to a need for better and more integrated primary, intermediate and long-term care services.

Third, advancements in medicine were leading to increased specialisation and sub-specialisation. Whilst beneficial in opening up new care and treatment options for patients, this resulted also in increased fragmentation of healthcare delivery with patients seeing numerous specialists, with no one doctor coordinating care for the patient. The GP landscape in Singapore was fragmented and lacked the right incentives to shift their attention towards providing adequate chronic care management and coordination in the primary care setting. The nursing homes and day centres — predominantly run by VWOs — struggled with shortages of skilled professional and administrative manpower, and the perennial need to raise funds. As relatively small organisations, they were unable to reap the benefits of

---

[6] Subsequently, on 3 October 2013, the Parkway Pantai group announced that its four private hospitals in Singapore (Gleneagles Hospital, Mount Elizabeth Hospital, Mount Elizabeth Novena Hospital and Parkway East Hospital) would publish historical prices of 30 of its more common procedures on their hospital websites.

economies of scale. As such, they faced challenges in maintaining and raising the standards of care.

In short, while the healthcare system was generally producing good health outcomes, it was optimised for the delivery of tertiary care and not the long-tail chronic care required for an ageing population, nor the long-term primary care relationships needed to manage chronic diseases. These three developments in population growth, ageing, and geographic distribution, required extensive outreach to the primary care and long-term care providers working within the community.

Six regional health systems, each covering on average slightly less than one million people, were therefore initiated to enable the bulk of healthcare needs of residents to be met by the healthcare providers within each region. By reducing the size of each catchment, and organising the healthcare delivery systems at the regional level, it would be easier to integrate care services around between the public sector hospitals and polyclinics on one hand, and the private sector primary care providers, VWO-, and privately-run long-term care providers, on the other.

> *"We have established regional clusters to build partnerships and seek synergies beyond the public healthcare sector. With an ageing popula-tion and increased prevalence of chronic diseases, we are strengthening community-based prevention, management and rehabilitation services, most of which are delivered by the private and charity sectors. **There is a need for more proactive and coordinated joint management of patients by healthcare players from all three sectors.***
>
> — *Minister Khaw Boon Wan, Response in Parliament,*
> *22 February 2010*

The six healthcare clusters were put in charge of organising and integrating the health providers within their region. Mr. Khaw believed that the clinicians within the hospitals had to "provide intellectual leadership and own the solution" for integrated care. The public sector acute hospital acted as the anchor of the RHS, and a bridge to and between key healthcare partners in the region. This included primary care partners such as the general practitioners, and ILTC partners such as community hospitals, nursing homes, and hospices. While the mission of the hospitals had been to ensure that the patient was treated well in the hospital, Mr. Khaw put forth a challenge to the clinicians to "run a hospital without walls," and to "share a common mission with GPs, nurses and other healthcare professionals to ensure that our patients remained healthy".[7] Together, the institutions were to

---

[7] Minister Khaw Boon Wan, in a 2012 interview.

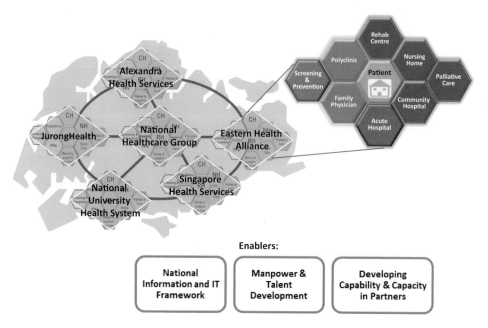

Enablers:

| National Information and IT Framework | Manpower & Talent Development | Developing Capability & Capacity in Partners |

Fig. 3.2.   Organising the Regional Health Systems.

take a patient-centric approach, as opposed to the traditional institution-centric approach (see Fig. 3.2).

Of the six healthcare clusters, two were tasked to develop as Academic Medical Centres (AMCs), responsible for cultivating research excellence and nurturing clinician-scientists, in addition to their service and teaching missions. In 2008, the National University Health System or NUHS was incorporated as a joint venture between the National University of Singapore and MOHH. NUHS grouped the National University Hospital (NUH) with the National University of Singapore's (NUS) Yong Loo Lin School of Medicine, Faculty of Dentistry and the Saw Swee Hock School of Public Health under a common governance structure. The other AMC is located in SingHealth, which combined clinical expertise in SGH and KKH with the education and research capabilities of the Duke-NUS Graduate Medical School (established in 2005). The AMCs initially started off with the development of their research and academic mission, in support of their clinical mission. However, over time, it became clear that the two tertiary hospitals anchoring the AMCs — namely SGH and NUH — were both significant providers of healthcare services within their individual regions, and as such had to also develop their own regional health strategies. Thus the AMCs' research mission must also be applied within the broader context of the RHS.

The Regional Health Systems are still in their early stages of development. The initial stage was one of generating new ideas and piloting new initiatives. From the experience garnered during this stage, MOH has established a set of priorities for the RHS to work on. These priorities include the development of programmes to address the needs of frequent admitters to the hospitals, to facilitate "right-siting" of care from the acute hospitals back to the community, and to develop capabilities in the primary care or ILTC partners.

Other governance, funding, and operating principles also need to be worked out. Unlike a hospital-based system, whereby patients are treated for each of their conditions on a discrete basis, a regional health system operates on the premise that patients move from one provider to another, to receive care appropriate to their condition and state of health. Variations in treatment protocols and in financing systems become more apparent to the patient, and can cause confusion to patients and providers alike. The public does not see six individual RHSes, but one public healthcare system.

For the MOH, one key challenge in RHS development continues to be striking the appropriate balance with providing regional health systems the autonomy to continue to innovate and be creative in trying out new services, while ensuring fundamental systems and operating principles are aligned across all RHSes.

Strengthening the Horizontals

With the creation of the six healthcare clusters, it was also apparent that in order to prevent fragmentation and diseconomies of scale from creeping in, certain areas and functions would need to be undertaken or coordinated centrally, rather than by individual clusters. There were two main areas identified: corporate management functions; and national-level promotional and developmental activities for the ILTC and primary care sectors. For the former, MOH decided to expand MOH Holdings (the holding company for all six clusters) to undertake such systems-level strategising and operations. A separate IT services company, Integrated Health Information Services (IHiS), was also established to provide specific IT services to clusters, consolidating the IT capabilities of the clusters in the process. To take on the role of championing the ILTC and primary care sectors, MOH set up the Agency for Integrated Care (AIC).

MOHH and IHiS — Supporting the clusters and MOH

Following the establishment of the two clusters in 2000, MOHH was a shell company with the majority of corporate HQ functions being undertaken within the SingHealth and NHG corporate headquarters. MOHH was briefly rejuvenated to support the public healthcare sector in promoting its medical tourism activities, but this role diminished as the "reclustering" initiatives began to take precedence. Today, MOHH focuses on systems-level coordination in manpower and talent development, IT, and infrastructure development.

For manpower and talent development, MOHH coordinated overseas recruitment efforts, centralised employment of junior doctors and dental officers and the administration of scholarships for the healthcare family and leadership development. It has embarked on talent and leadership development programmes to instil public healthcare ethos and values among medical staff and leaders.

To support the growth in healthcare facility development, MOHH set up a team to take charge of the entire process of infrastructure development from planning and design, to project management and delivery, management of the tender process, and engagement with authorities and certification of works done. The MOHH team also serves as a central repository of best practices learned from the team's experience as well as from overseas.

In IT infrastructure development, MOHH decided to take an incremental approach. Integrated Health Information Systems Pte Ltd (IHiS) was created in 2008 as a MOHH subsidiary to bring together in one organisation around 600 staff from the IT departments of all restructured hospitals to help integrate, deliver and manage IT systems across all public healthcare institutions and optimise workflow and processes. As MOH's agent, MOHH also took the lead in developing a National Electronic Health Record (NEHR) that provides NEHR users access to key medical information of patients across all public healthcare institutions and, increasingly, across private sector providers as well.

Lastly, MOHH undertakes central treasury management on behalf of the clusters. It currently manages S$1 billion of the public healthcare family's accumulated surpluses. It also centralised the internal audit function across the public healthcare sector, leading to the development of a 30-person team that included specialised areas such as IT audit and forensic audits.

Agency for Integrated Care (AIC) — Developing and championing primary and community-based care

In 2009, MOH set up the Agency for Integrated Care (AIC) to work with the community in developing capacity and capability in primary care, integrated long-term care, and community mental health. Dr. Jason Cheah, CEO of AIC characterised its scope as "generally dealing with patients and providers outside the acute hospitals" and its function as "ensuring better coordinated care and enabling things to happen for patients who are living in the community."

AIC's origins actually date from the early 1990s, when there was a small depart-ment in MOH for "care liaison services" which provided information and referral services for patients. This continued with the two-cluster system in 2000, with the organisation based in NHG, but operating across the two clusters. The needs of an ageing population, rising public expectations as well as the increased complexity of care, have all pointed to a need for a larger coordinating and organising function, leading to the establishment of AIC.

AIC has been working hard to engage different groups of stakeholders to win their trust and to promote its common vision of integrated, patient-centric care. AIC has been helping bridge some of the gaps among acute hospitals, GPs and other VWO-operated services to enhance integrated patient care in the community. AIC also must help develop new viable care models to support care integration and find partners who are prepared to try out these new care models, refining both the business and care model along the way.

Conclusion

Healthcare is complex by nature and is often fragmented due to care being delivered by many specialised professionals and institutions. The delivery of healthcare services is deeply emotive for the patient, and complicated by the asymmetry of information between doctor and patient. There is a potential for over-consumption when the costs are borne by a third party (government subsidies or insurance coverage). Thus, it is an issue with high public concern, visibility, and political salience.

The organisation of Singapore's public healthcare system has evolved over the years as MOH seeks on one hand, to find an optimal organisation and governance structure to drive productivity, innovation, and cost-effective, value-based care provision; and on the other, ensuring that public sector healthcare institutions stay true to their public mission of providing quality care to all Singaporeans.

Early reform efforts aimed to address *government imperfections* and *harnessing market forces*, by corporatising the hospitals, and setting them to "compete" with the private sector. The fundamental principle — that corporate discipline will help providers seek cost efficiencies, and that the demands of the patients will drive the development of new services, remain relevant. Public healthcare hospitals and polyclinics will always have a critical role to play in ensuring that benchmarks are set for the private sector — in terms of sustainable pricing, and standards of service delivery. But competition between the hospitals was for the limited pool of higher income patients, in procedures and services where margins were higher. In a supply-constrained environment where the number of doctors and hospital beds were controlled by MOH, the competition was focused on attracting medical talent, especially specialists, bidding up salaries and benefits.

The next stage of reform thus focused on *reducing market imperfections* — on adjusting the balance between competition and collaboration amongst public sector entities, through forming the two clusters; there were efforts to embark upon care integration by including polyclinic groups within each cluster. To make markets work better, MOH also sought to increase transparency of information on pricing and healthcare outcomes.

But markets on their own focus more on the provision of high-end, high-yield acute care and specialist services. They are inadequate in raising standards, and under-invest in developing healthcare services, for example, in critical services such as nursing homes, or community-based day care. It is the task of MOH to ensure that there is sufficient attention and sustainable investment in areas which will allow the healthcare system to meet the longer term healthcare needs of the population. The vision to build up preventive healthcare and community based care will mean less income, and fewer patients, for acute care hospitals than would otherwise be the case. Thus it is not feasible for the private sector hospitals in Singapore to be the main drivers of changes which would adversely affect their bottom line.

Thus in this new stage of development, MOH sought to build upon the *strengths of government* to embark on our care transformation journey — government's traditional role in longer term planning and institutional redesign, and the public sector healthcare institutions' deep expertise and resources to drive care transformation and change. There is a new policy focus on long-term care, primary care and the treatment of chronic diseases. New models of care and care integration are being piloted within the context of the regional health systems. Singapore's compact size and highly networked systems also provide the operational nimbleness to bring about the transformation of the system.

The *strengths of the market* — to improve efficiency, and productivity to rein in rising healthcare costs, and to make the best use of limited resources — remain important. But, at the core of each public institution, must still be the ethos and values which undergird a vital, publicly funded service.

> *"This goal of instilling discipline remains relevant and it will play an important role in moderating the growth of healthcare cost. **Our public healthcare institutions must have a public mission with corporate discipline, and not act as if you have a corporate mission with public sector discipline!**"*
>
> — *Minister for Health, Mr. Gan Kim Yong, MOH's Annual Workplan Seminar 2013*

Lastly, the relationships between MOH and MOHH, and the public sector healthcare clusters, have also evolved together over time, with a growing appreciation of the relative weaknesses and strengths of both markets and government in delivering public services. From initial efforts to structure a transaction-based, arms-length relationship, based on contractual service agreements, the new governance framework emphasises alignment of vision and strategies between MOH and the clusters, at the Board and management level. A broader definition of successful performance and greater rigour in outcome measurement have also provided the basis for "competition" in the context of a publicly funded, not-for-profit healthcare system. The search for efficiency gains and resource optimisation will also continue. Where the earlier corporatisation exercises had led to considerable improvements in operational efficiency, the current focus on more holistic, integrated care for patients requires an operating environment that emphasises greater standardisation and inter-operability. This could require closer cooperation and collaboration *between* providers, including re-centralisation of functions such as IT architecture, remuneration policies and leadership development, to improve care delivery and achieve systems-level economies of scale.

Going forward, the challenges become more complex over time as the governance arrangements must extend to include non-public sector players within the regional health systems, each with their own corporate structures and incentives. Some are profit-driven, private sector entities; and others are VWOs, structured and operated as charities or societies. Given the multiplicity of roles and functions in each RHS, and the different level of capabilities for each provider, we will learn more lessons on what should be the optimal number, size and mode of operation for the RHSes. In short, MOH may need to continue to innovate, to develop new policy and governance levers to achieve its objective of improving care outcomes via the regional health systems, whilst keeping healthcare services affordable for the individual and sustainable for the country in the long term.

4 Paying for Healthcare

Lai Wei Lin*

One of the foremost public policy challenges around the world is ensuring population access to affordable and good quality healthcare that is sustainable for the country. The unique nature of healthcare makes financing it challenging. Healthcare needs vary greatly over one's lifetime and across individuals; it is unpredictable when illness will strike. Hence, costs need to be socialised or risk-pooled across the population to ensure affordability for the patient. Instead of the patient paying, the payer may be the government, in instances where taxes collected are used to subsidise healthcare services; or an insurer, who collects premiums to pay for the insured's healthcare. The objective is the same — for others who are not ill to pay for the bulk of the patient's treatment cost and ensure affordability, with the government or insurer playing the role of intermediary.

Once a third party payer insulates patients from the real cost however, moral hazard arises. Providers can more easily offer more tests and treatment or charge more, and the patient would have little incentive to question. There is also great information asymmetry between the patient and his doctor. Patients depend on their doctors to advise them on the appropriate treatment, and in their anxiety may seek, or be encouraged to pursue, more expensive options at all costs, without evidence that outcomes will be better. The third-party payer ends up bearing higher costs, with limited benefit in patient outcomes. Costs inevitably spiral up as patients come to expect more treatment or faster access. The third party payer, who is an intermediary after all, then needs to raise the necessary revenue to pay for it.

This is why the design of healthcare funding is central to every healthcare system. Good design ensures affordability of care, while incentivising the provision of appropriate care to avoid runaway costs, which is ultimately borne by the entire society.

*Deputy Secretary, Ministry of Health, Singapore.
The author would like to thank Ms. Joanne Chiew for her excellent support in undertaking research and editorial work for this chapter, as well as Ms. Lavinia Low for her forthcoming assistance with various data points.

Evolution and Innovation — Adding the 3Ms to Subsidies

Although the end-objective is always the same, countries design their healthcare financing systems differently depending on their socio-political context, their populations' attitudes and expectations concerning healthcare and how healthcare practice is changing, all of which evolve over time. What is ideal in one context or at one time may not be ideal in another, and what is "right" is often a moving target. This is no different in Singapore.

Singapore's early healthcare system was based on taxed-financed subsidies, similar to the United Kingdom's National Health Service (NHS). The first major financing reform was the introduction of Medisave in 1984. This was followed by the introduction of MediShield in 1990 and Medifund in 1993, but subsidies have remained the foundation of how healthcare is financed. Copayment has also remained an important principle, as it engenders personal responsibility for one's health, and manages against potential over-consumption of healthcare services.

The Subsidy and 3Ms Framework

Singapore has a multi-payer healthcare financing framework, where a single treatment episode can be covered by multiple schemes/payers.

Heavy government subsidies are available for all basic healthcare services. At the public hospitals, all Singaporeans can choose subsidised inpatient care, and also subsidised specialist outpatient care if they have an appropriate referral from primary care. Patients can also choose private (i.e. non-subsidised) services. Polyclinic and emergency services are subsidised for all patients. Portable subsidies for the lower- to middle-income are available at private General Practitioner (GP) and dental clinics under the Community Health Assistance Scheme (CHAS) and for long-term care.

Individual responsibility remains important, hence, patients copay part of the treatment cost. Subsidies account for a large part of how healthcare is financed, with the remaining bill payable by MediShield or other insurance, the patient's Medisave/cash, and Medifund if necessary.

Medisave is part of the Central Provident Fund (CPF) framework and a compulsory individual healthcare savings scheme for all working Singapore Citizens (SC) and Permanent Residents (PR). All workers and employers contribute part of the monthly salary into the worker's CPF account. The employee and employer CPF contribution currently totals up to 37% of the gross monthly wage, with 8 to 10.5% (more than one-fifth) going to Medisave, to support CPF members' and their families' healthcare needs.[1] The CPF Board pays interest on the Medisave balance, similar to other accounts.

Enforcing regular savings via Medisave ensures that the patient and his family have savings to tap on should they need healthcare, reducing their cash outlay. Uses of Medisave are specified — for hospitalisation, selected outpatient treatment (e.g. cancer, kidney dialysis, specific chronic diseases, scans), selected preventive care (e.g. vaccinations), and premiums of approved insurance plans. Medisave contributions and savings are sized for subsidised care, and therefore the dollar limits for Medisave use are likewise based on subsidised care.

MediShield, which is run by CPF Board, complements Medisave by focussing on larger subsidised hospital bills and outpatient treatment (e.g. cancer, kidney dialysis). MediShield payouts are subject to deductibles (for inpatient stays), co-insurance and claim limits.

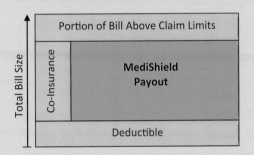

Coverage is automatically extended to all SC and PRs at certain milestones — for example, at birth or when they make their first CPF contribution from work — but one can opt out of the scheme at any time. MediShield premiums can be paid for by Medisave and are age-based (i.e. they reflect health risks of the age cohort). To moderate the increase in premiums as one ages, those in the working ages pay ahead for part of their old-age premiums, so as to more evenly distribute their premiums over their life time. Those who wish to stay in private ward classes can buy additional private insurance coverage.

Patients' bills reflect the total cost of their treatment, as well as their share of the bill after government subsidies and insurance payout. Because of Medisave, most patients pay little to no cash for their hospital stay. In 2013,

---

[1] Other CPF accounts are the Ordinary Account, which can be used for the housing purchases, education, and investments; and the Special Account, which is dedicated for saving for retirement.

8 in 10 subsidised inpatient bills incurred less than S$100 cash, with many paying $0 cash. On average, 4% of the total cost of subsidised inpatient care was paid for using cash.

Medifund is a safety net for patients who cannot afford their bills, after subsidies and insurance/Medisave. Medical social workers assess the patient's need, based on the bill size versus the family's income and savings. Many needy patients receive full Medifund assistance for their bills.

A similar framework of subsidies, savings and insurance applies for long-term care, though Medisave use is more limited. It can be used for premiums for the national long-term care insurance scheme, ElderShield, day rehabilitation services and palliative care. ElderShield is currently offered by 3 different private insurers, with benefits specified by the government. Cash payouts are currently $400 per month for 72 months for those who cannot perform at least 3 out of the 6 Activities of Daily Living.[2] Coverage is automatically extended to SC and PRs when they reach age 40, and they can opt out. Unlike MediShield, ElderShield premiums do not rise with age and are payable until age 65 only. ElderShield can be described as a form of "prepaid premium" for protection against disability that typically occurs well into old age.

Advent of Medisave

In the early 1980s, the trend of rising healthcare costs internationally prompted a review of how healthcare in Singapore should be financed. In its review, the Singapore government continued to reject the idea of a "cradle-to-grave welfare health system," which it thought disregarded the fact that resources are finite.[3] It however sought to re-calibrate the cost-sharing arrangements for healthcare, across individuals, employers and the government.

Medisave has remained one of the greatest innovations in Singapore's healthcare financing framework. Built on the idea that "a small but regular saving set aside every month should ensure that most Singaporeans will be able to pay for their own hospitalisation expenses,"[4] Medisave supports the principle of copayment and reinforces the role of personal responsibility in saving for healthcare needs.

---

[2] Washing, dressing, feeding, toileting, mobility and transferring.

[3] Goh, Chok Tong (1981), Speech by Mr. Goh Chok Tong, Minister for Health and Minister for Trade and Industry, at the Singapore Medical Association Annual Dinner, 10 May 1981.

[4] Blue Paper on the National Health Plan 1983, Ministry of Health. *NHP: National Health Plan: A Blue Paper*, February 1983. Singapore: The Ministry of Health, February. 1983.

That Singaporeans get to keep the remaining balance in their Medisave Account for their own or their family's future use[5] also provides an incentive to stay healthy as much as possible, and not over-consume on treatment.[6]

Over the years, Medisave use has been expanded beyond inpatient care, to include selected outpatient treatments like chemotherapy, dialysis, chronic disease treatment, as well as preventive care.[7] The rationale for extending Medisave use to the outpatient setting, was to support early treatment of chronic disease so as to reduce costly complications and hospitalisation later. From time to time, withdrawal limits have been raised to keep pace with inflation, and contribution rates increased in tandem with expansions of Medisave coverage. This ensures sufficient Medisave savings for one's retirement healthcare needs. The current Medisave contribution rates are 8 to 10.5%, up from 6% at the start.

The government also supplements Singaporeans' Medisave savings, with special attention to the poor and elderly. The lower-income receive top-ups into their Medisave accounts under the Workfare Income Supplement scheme — a wage credit scheme for older low-wage workers — to help them accumulate savings for their retirement healthcare needs. In 2012, the Government introduced annual Medisave top-ups for eligible elderly (85% of all elderly) under the GST Voucher Scheme. Newborns now also receive a $3000 grant in their Medisave accounts to help pay for their healthcare costs, such as insurance premiums and vaccination costs. Besides regular top-ups, there are also ad-hoc Medisave top-ups for Singaporeans from time to time.

While the idea of individual Health Savings Accounts has gained prominence internationally, Singapore remains the only country in the world to have implemented it on a nationwide, mandatory basis. Introducing Medisave was a major and far-sighted move in the 1980s, made easier by the existing CPF framework of monthly contributions for retirement savings. Medisave has been important in retaining the individual's ownership of his health and healthcare consumption. During old age, which is when one consumes the bulk of healthcare services, Medisave savings make it possible for patients to continue to pay for a small part of their healthcare needs, and reduces the excesses that often result from a comprehensive third-party payer system.

Risk-pooling Through MediShield and Other Insurance

However, Medisave alone proved insufficient to adequately cover patients against the high variance of healthcare expenses. A rare but large healthcare bill of say,

---

[5] Currently, about 35% of Medisave dollars spent by elderly patients are from their immediate family member's account, which shows the effective reach of Medisave savings beyond the individual.
[6] Opening Speech for Parliamentary Debate on National Health Plan, 1983.
[7] For example, antenatal care, outpatient scans, palliative care, day rehabilitation services.

S$10,000 after subsidy, which is above the 99th percentile of subsidised hospital bills in 2014, could deplete a significant part of one's Medisave savings.

This was why a basic insurance scheme — MediShield — was introduced in 1990. MediShield helps to stretch the Medisave dollar to cover large bills. Like any insurance scheme, annual premiums are paid into a common pool and then used to pay for the unfortunate small group of patients who incur large bills during the year. This also reduces the need for Singaporeans to over-save for the large but rare bill. MediShield coverage was initially conservative, but its benefits have been regularly enhanced over the years. It currently focuses on inpatient treatment and expensive outpatient treatment like dialysis and chemotherapy.

From the outset, the Ministry was conscious about getting the insurance design right, to "avoid unrestricted and open ended medical insurance practised in the US, which leads to the provision of unnecessary medical services and escalating premiums."[8] Therefore, the key tenets of the MediShield design included annual deductibles (for inpatient stays/day surgery) and co-insurance of 10% to 20% to be paid by the patient using Medisave or cash. The deductibles (currently S$1500/S$2000 for Class C/B2 respectively) have attracted criticism from those who prefer complete peace of mind and first dollar coverage. However, this is an essential part of MediShield's design, to focus on "catastrophic" larger bills, leaving Medisave to cover smaller dollar amounts, and reduce the risk of moral hazard. First-dollar coverage also results in higher premiums, which need to be paid for from one's Medisave in any case. The Ministry has therefore chosen to retain the copayment elements and spend increased premium dollars on improving the payouts for the small number of sicker patients, even though this is undoubtedly less popular. The importance of patient copayment, including via high-deductible insurance plans complemented by savings accounts, in managing costs is borne out by research.[9]

MediShield currently covers more than 90% of the population, achieved through systemic "auto-coverage" of SCs and PRs at key life milestones at birth and when entering the workforce. This aims to catch the population as early as possible, before they develop medical conditions which may attract exclusions. MediShield will be replaced by universal, mandatory MediShield Life coverage in end-2015 and close the remaining coverage gap.

---

[8] Ministry of Health, Singapore. "Affordable Health Care" (1993). (https://www.moh.gov.sg/content/dam/moh_web/Publications/Reports/1993/Affordable_Health_Care.pdf)

[9] Brook et al., "The Health Insurance Experiment: A Classic RAND study speaks to the current health care reform debate," published 2006 (http://www.rand.org/pubs/research_briefs/RB9174.html). Buntin et al., "Consumer-Directed Health Care: Early evidence about effects on cost and quality," Health Affairs 25, no. 6 (2006). (http://content.healthaffairs.org/content/25/6/w516.full.html)

Private Insurance Plans

Each year, about 40% of patients choose opt for private ward classes (Class B1, Class A) in the public hospitals or private hospitals. Such bills can be more than 3 times those in the subsidised wards (Class C/B2), and MediShield coverage will not be sufficient. They can purchase additional private insurance, the most common being the Integrated Shied Plans (IPs) which ride on top of MediShield. IPs were introduced following a major reform of MediShield and the private health insurance market in 2005, to integrate the private plans with MediShield. To avoid the insurance companies cherry-picking the better risks into their risk pools, leaving MediShield with a poor risk-pool, MediShield was structured as the base of all such private plans i.e. the private plans had to be integrated with MediShield. 60% of Singaporeans are currently enrolled in an IP.

IPs also have deductibles and co-insurance, and like MediShield have guaranteed renewability. This means that policyholders who fall seriously ill cannot, at the annual renewal, be dropped from coverage or risk-loaded due to their newly diagnosed condition. These requirements are imposed by the Health Ministry, as part of the conditions for allowing IP premiums to be paid for with Medisave. Medisave use for premiums are subject to withdrawal limits, given that IPs are mostly targeted at non-subsidised treatment.

Competition among the insurers has led to product innovations over time, with two notable shifts. First, almost all active plans are now on an as-charged basis with no reimbursement limits. Second, cash "rider" plans to cover the entire deductible and co-insurance are widely available, though these are distinct from the IPs and do not come under the Health Ministry's regulation. Many buy riders for first-dollar, full insurance coverage, for complete peace of mind. However, IPs are expensive (see Table 4.1), and with the lack of safeguards there has inevitably been a surge of claims, leading to escalating premiums. Those entering their 50s and 60s in particular may have to start paying cash for part of their IP premium, when it exceeds the Medisave withdrawal limit for premiums. Riders are also expensive, and can cost more than $1500 in cash for those in their 60s and more than $4000 at the oldest ages.

There are private insurance options that are not integrated with MediShield, such as group insurance coverage purchased by companies for their employees. However, many such workers still enrol in MediShield and IPs, so that they remain insured even when their current employment ceases or they retire. There are tax incentives to encourage employers to offer their workers portable medical benefits, for example, by supplementing their employees' Medisave savings or paying for their MediShield and IP premiums.

Table 4.1.   Comparison of 2014 MediShield and IP Premiums for Selected Plan Types and Age Groups

Age Group (Age Next Birthday)	MediShield Premiums (S$)	As-charged IP Premiums (S$)	
		Public Hospital Class A	Private Hospital
31–40	105	208–267	277–383
51–60	345	666–825	955–1205
71–73	560	1859–2339	2572–3000
86–88	1190	4039–5563	5758–7597

The Medifund Safety Net

With Medisave and MediShield, the majority of Singaporeans are adequately protected. In 1993, the Government established Medifund as a safety net, to help needy patients pay for their healthcare bills. Medifund can fully cover a needy patient's bill, such that he pays nothing. Given that Medifund can be used to cover patient bills in full, it was important to retain discipline and sustainability in how the assistance funds are used. Hence, it was designed as an endowment fund, with only the interest income from the fund available for use each year. In this way, the principal is protected and can continuously generate interest for future use. During years of budget surpluses, the government has topped up the principal sum, as a way of redistributing the benefits of economic growth to needy Singaporeans. This has enabled the sum of annual Medifund assistance to grow from S$5 million at inception to S$130 million in FY13. In addition, Medifund applications are reviewed by Medifund Committees comprising representatives from the community, professionals, and other individuals with relevant expertise. This committee reviews the patient's and his family's circumstances, as well as the social workers' recommendations, before making the final decision on whether to assist the patient, and by how much.

Medical social workers assess each patient and make a recommendation to the Medifund Committees, which are made up of community leaders, professionals, etc., for their consideration. Patients known to be needy, for example, those on social assistance schemes, are automatically approved for Medifund help. While Medifund is targeted at the lower-income, case by case assessment allows flexibility for the middle-income to also receive assistance, depending on the size of their bills and their other financial commitments.

A Progressive and Equitable System of Subsidies and Copayment

Equity is one key measure of a good healthcare system. This means the rich and poor alike can access the care that they need. Unlike most healthcare systems which set uniform charges, the Singapore system has evolved to differentiate charges, based on the patient's and his family's ability to pay.

In 1 January 2009, means-testing for subsidised wards was introduced — where a patient's subsidy would vary according to his income, or if he had no income, the Annual Value (AV) of his residential property. This was a landmark move as it introduced progressivity in direct subsidies and charges for a widely used healthcare service. Prior to this change, only subsidies for selected services (e.g. in long-term care) were differentiated. Although higher-income patients can continue to choose the subsidised wards, receiving 65% subsidy in Class C, they pay more than lower-income patients, who receive 80% subsidy. It was a gentle step to differentiate subsidies, as more than 90% of subsidised inpatients continue to receive the maximum subsidy. More changes in 2014/2015 followed, to differentiate charges in the subsidised specialist outpatient clinics (SOC), and for outpatient medications. Again, access to subsidised care was retained for all Singaporeans with appropriate referrals, but higher subsidies were given to the lower- and middle-income. This approach is a contrast to other healthcare systems where there is progressivity only at the point of paying taxes or premiums.

Almost all healthcare services now have differentiated charges, except for polyclinic services and Accident and Emergency (A&E) services. Other than differentiation by means, subsidies are also differentiated by citizenship and residency status, with permanent residents enjoying lower subsidies than citizens and foreigners enjoying no subsidies at all. Differentiated subsidies and charges require strong administrative support to ensure that patients receive the subsidies that they are eligible for, without hassle at the point of care.

Portable subsidies for Non-government Providers in Long-term Care and Primary Care

While the subsidy framework was well-established in the government polyclinics and hospitals from the early days, long-term care services have mainly been provided by Voluntary Welfare Organisations (VWOs), with funding from government subsidies and charity dollars. Subsidy support has been steadily enhanced in recent years, to cover more types of services, including those run by private operators, a wider segment of the population and a higher proportion of the costs. Currently, two-thirds of elderly are able to enjoy subsidies for a spectrum of long-term care services. Since 2012, there has also been substantial expansion of portable subsidies in primary care for lower- to middle-income Singaporeans via CHAS. With 1500 private GP and dental clinics in the scheme, CHAS has enabled the Ministry to tap on the capacity in the private sector, to supplement subsidised services at the government polyclinics.

Strengthening Coverage and Collective Responsibility

In 2013, the Ministry of Health began a major review to future-proof the financing framework for the ageing population. With chronic diseases more prevalent, and more elderly living into their late 80s and 90s, some in frailty, the Ministry determined that outpatient and long-term care were areas worthy of review. Over time, the cash out-of-pocket payments could become large on a cumulative basis and pose a burden to the elderly and their families. Changes had already been made in 2012, with the introduction of CHAS and enhanced subsidies for long-term care.

With the review, further changes were made to expand the reach of CHAS, enhance subsidies for specialist outpatient care and for medications for the lower- and middle-income, and broaden Medisave use. An $8 billion Pioneer Generation (PG) Package to honour Pioneer Singaporeans[10] who contributed to Singapore's nation-building, was also introduced. Pioneers receive additional subsidies for outpatient care, cash assistance if they are disabled, Medisave top-ups and special premium subsidies when MediShield Life is introduced. As Medisave was introduced only later in the working lives of Pioneers, they are unlikely to have accumulated sufficient Medisave for their retirement healthcare needs. The Package thus sought to relieve their healthcare expenses. Finally, another significant outcome of the review was to move to universal insurance coverage under MediShield Life. This closes a gap in MediShield coverage for the remaining population, and the existing insured who have exclusions. There are also significant enhancements to benefits.

Taken together, these changes mark a shift in the healthcare financing philosophy towards greater government responsibility, with a higher government share of healthcare spending through more subsidies, and greater collective responsibility through insurance risk-pooling under MediShield Life. With these changes, as well as greater Medisave savings and usage, patient copayment, especially in cash, is lowered.

The World Health Organisation (WHO) has a framework that describes healthcare financing coverage in terms of — (i) population coverage; (ii) services coverage;

---

[10] The Pioneer Generation refers to those born on or before 31 December 1949 (65 years old or older in 2014) and became a Singaporean citizen on or before 31 December 1986.

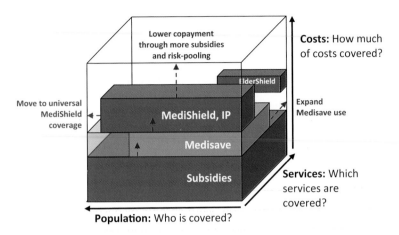

Fig. 4.1. Dimensions of healthcare financing coverage. *Adapted from The World Health Report: Health systems financing: the path to universal coverage (WHO, 2010).*

and (iii) dollar coverage (see Fig. 4.1). Viewed through this lens, the 2013/4 review improved the dollar coverage in outpatient and long-term care, through subsidies, and for inpatient and expensive outpatient treatment, through MediShield Life. Greater Medisave use and Medifund support also improved the dollar coverage more generally. While the option of subsidies in the public institutions has always been universally available to all patients, and most Singaporeans can access their own or a family member's Medisave, the move to MediShield Life will achieve universal *insurance* coverage.

Future strides in improving affordability will be to expand service coverage as healthcare practice evolves, and ensure that dollar coverage keeps pace with increasing costs and utilisation. With healthcare increasingly being delivered in the outpatient setting, and more elderly requiring long-term care, funding for long-term care and outpatient care will continue to warrant close review. The Government has committed to a review of ElderShield, which will address the needs of the future elderly. In the meantime, support for long-term care has been enhanced for the current elderly through a myriad of schemes, such as the Seniors Mobility and Enabling Fund which provides support for mobility aids, and a grant for employing Foreign Domestic Workers (FDWs). In the reviews ahead, there will be continued tension around how much healthcare risk ought to be socialised via subsidies and insurance, and how much individual responsibility and copayment to retain. The choice is not just one of how total costs are shared out, but may itself cause the total bill to be higher than it would otherwise be. For example, there is a risk that an insurance-based system could lead to a blunting of price signals at point of use, and cause both providers and users to increase utilisation.

Medisave will continue to be a key plank in the financing system, so that society can retain the discipline of copayment but in an affordable way. To keep it simple and easy to administer, it is sized based on the use of subsidised healthcare services, and a "typical" patient in terms of intensity and frequency of usage. If the savings are spent on items beyond what they were intended for, they will be insufficient for healthcare expenses in old age. However, there will be constant tension between this approach and the fact that patients' means and healthcare needs vary across the population and across ages. Singaporeans have different perspectives of their expected healthcare use and life expectancy. Some argue that they have more than enough and wish to use more of their Medisave now, to pay for more types of treatment, non-subsidised treatment or even non-treatment needs, while others have fear that their Medisave savings will not be enough, given that most of their expenses will be at end of life, and healthcare costs are constantly rising. No matter how much customisation we can build into the Medisave, it will always be "too much" for some and "too little" for others. Policy-making is the fine art of trying to optimise across such tensions.

Another area to address is the private IPs, and Government's role in providing assurance for those who opt for non-subsidised or private services. IP policyholders have voiced concerns about their rising premiums, which insurers have explained are a result of rising claims and treatment costs.[11] This is exacerbated at the older ages, when premiums are higher and policyholders have to pay an increasing cash amount for the premium. At the same time, policyholders complain about insurers' strict underwriting standards, resulting in exclusions for what they consider are minor conditions. While many Singaporeans buy IPs and view them as important for their peace of mind, it was found that for more than half of the hospitalisations in 2013 where the patient had an IP plan for non-subsidised wards, the patient opted for a subsidised ward instead. More education is needed so that consumers understand that MediShield is part of an IP, appreciate what additional insurance coverage the private plan provides on top of MediShield and at what additional cost, and make more informed and considered purchases. On the supply side, more intervention from insurers may be needed to better manage payouts and premiums.

As coverage is expanded to enhance healthcare affordability (i.e. expanding the blue box of pooled funds in Fig. 4.1), national spending (the whole box) will inevitably rise as patients will be able to afford more care. Singapore's healthcare system has been efficient and the country is fortunate to have the fiscal resources to afford the recent expansions in healthcare coverage. As overall healthcare spending grows, it is even more critical to expand coverage prudently and with appropriate safeguards, as there is no turning back thereafter.

---

[11] Ng, Magdalen. "Health insurance cost to rise from March." *The Straits Times*. 3 February 2013.

National Health Expenditure (NHE)

Singapore has been both lauded and criticised for spending a small percentage of its GDP on health (currently 4.2%). In comparison, most OECD countries spend about 9% of their GDP on health, while Asian economies like Korea, Hong Kong and Taiwan spend between 5% and 8%. However, Singapore has performed respectably in overall health outcomes, making it an effective and efficient system.

Singapore's absolute NHE rose at a rate of 9% per annum in the last decade,[12] and this is expected to continue. Singapore's population is relatively young, with only 9% of the total population being elderly, compared to 12% to 15% in Korea, Hong Kong and Taiwan. Once Singapore's NHE is expressed on a per capita PPP$ basis, its level of spending is more similar to other Asian systems. As Singapore's population ages, the share of GDP spent on NHE will likely go up, as the elderly incur much higher healthcare costs than the young.

As a result of the copayment philosophy and patients being able to choose private or non-subsidised services, government's share of national healthcare expenditure is about 40%. However, a significant portion of the remaining expenditure is borne by government-instituted schemes such as Medisave, MediShield, ElderShield and IPs, as well as employer medical benefits, leaving the out-of-pocket share, which includes both cash and some unknown third-party payers, at slightly under 40%.

Managing Costs, Navigating Choices

It is never easy to find the right balance across the key priorities of access, quality and affordability in healthcare. Too affordable, and demand grows, lengthening wait times. To reduce wait times, we need to invest more resources in the healthcare system, to maintain quality of care and outcomes. Therefore, there is a fourth, important consideration that underpins these three priorities — sustainability.

Every country needs to ensure that healthcare is not only affordable to patients, but also affordable to the society that pays for it. It is also important to ensure that what can be paid for today can continue to be paid for tomorrow. Often, it is the younger generation that shoulders the disproportionate costs incurred by the eld-

---

[12] Singapore Parliamentary Report (Sitting date: 13 May 2013), Vol. 90. Title: Healthcare Spending and Funding Sources. Link: http://sprs.parl.gov.sg/search/topic.jsp?currentTopicID=00000068-WA&current PubID=00000021-WA&topicKey=00000021-WA.00000068-WA_3%2BhansardContent43a675dd-5000-42da-9fd5-40978d79310f%2B

erly, and with an increasing old-age dependency ratio, this burden will continue to increase even if expenditure does not. Sustainability should also not be measured in dollar terms only, but in overall resources consumed. For Singapore, human resource is particularly limited and precious.

Everyone has to agree what the optimal balance among the four priorities is as a society, regardless of who the patient is — a stranger whom he is paying for via taxes or insurance premiums, or his loved one, whose treatment will be paid for by others.

> *Design a whole system so the different parts complement one another and make wise trade-offs between outcome and costs, in order to make individual and collective choices which we cannot avoid making. Nothing is for free, there is always a limit to resources, choices have to be made, trade-offs have to accepted.*
>
> *— Prime Minister Lee Hsien Loong, Universal Health Coverage Meeting, 10 February 2015*

Ultimately, as it is society who bears the cost, the government's role is to design a system that maximises the value and health outcomes from the available resources. Given the market imperfections in healthcare, the government needs to incentivise the right behaviour on the part of providers and patients, provide central planning and coordination to ensure efficiency, build capability for the future, and educate patients.

Common Healthcare Tradeoffs

to ensure affordability for both the patient and society

— Cap the growth of services, and ration by queues. Providers have to be adept at identifying and prioritising the urgent cases to the top of the queue to be seen more quickly, so as not to compromise their care. However, for many other patients, they may be faced with queues and longer waiting times.

— Newer and more expensive treatments are not brought in or so readily available.

— Have the future generation pay, but this may become untenable as the population ages and the dependency ratio worsens. In some cases, affordability and sustainability may be achieved at the present time, but there is under-investment in building capacity and capability for the future.

*The key question of health care financing is who pays for it — individuals, the Government, insurance companies, or employers. This belief is mistaken, because no matter who pays for health care in the first instance, ultimately the burden is borne by the people themselves. If the Government pays, it must collect taxes from the people to do so. If insurance companies pay, they must collect premiums from those who are insured. If employers pay, they must add this to their wage costs, and trade it off against other components of the wage package. **The real issue is therefore not who pays, but which system best encourages people to use health care economically, and encourages health care providers to minimise costs, inefficiency and over-servicing.***

— *White Paper on Affordable Healthcare, 1993*

Patient Copayment

The Singapore system is known for its emphasis on the principle of copayment as a way to retain discipline on healthcare costs. This is evident in many aspects of policy design — that the patient continues to copay a certain part of his bill after the subsidy, and insurance features like deductibles and co-insurance. In addition, dollar limits on the use of Medisave and MediShield help to curb over-charging and over-servicing, as charges beyond the limits will have to be paid for by the patient himself.

When healthcare is free, patients tend to consume more healthcare resources than necessary, because a third party pays. For example, the provider may prescribe more tests, even if these have little real additional value in managing the patient's condition. For providers that have autonomy and flexibility in pricing their services, comprehensive coverage by subsidies or insurance can present an opportunity for them to charge more, or sell additional services that are not necessary. All this will be less likely if patients have to copay part of their healthcare bill.

"The ideal of free medical services collided against the reality of human behaviour, certainly in Singapore. My first lesson came from government clinics and hospitals. When doctors prescribed free antibiotics, patients took their tablet or capsules for two days, did not feel better, and threw away the balance. They then consulted private doctors, paid for their antibiotics, completed the course, and recovered. I decided to impose a charge of 50 cents for each attendance at outpatient dispensaries."

— *Mr. Lee Kuan Yew, Singapore's first Prime Minister*
Excerpt from "From the Third World to First: The Singapore Story, 1965–2000," 2000

Critics have noted that as patients have little control over their healthcare consumption, which is largely determined by their health condition and what doctors order, the copayment can become a financial burden. However, patients' decisions, preferences and behaviours can have an impact on costs in simple ways. For example, they may ask for more medication to "stock up" only to have it go to waste, or visit the Emergency Department — where there are dedicated, specialised resources to treat the urgently ill — for non-urgent conditions like the common flu. In short, those who want higher than necessary levels of service or more creature comforts have to be prepared to pay more. At the same time, Medisave savings and the Medifund safety net are in place to help patients afford the treatment that they need.

Influencing Practice

Copayment cannot be the panacea to managing healthcare costs. Guidelines are also needed on what are clinically and cost effective treatment options, drugs, and so on, which balance quality, outcomes and overall cost to the system.

One way in which Singapore has instituted this is via the Chronic Disease Management Programme (CDMP), where Medisave use is subject to disease management protocols. Using Medisave use as a lever to hold providers to this standard of practice ensures that patients' precious Medisave dollars are spent wisely. It not only discourages non-essential components of treatment, but also specifies important components of treatment or secondary screening that ought to be provided, without which the overall effectiveness of the patient's care would be compromised.

In the area of drugs, only those assessed to be clinically and cost effective are included in the Standard Drug List, and subsidised. The list of subsidised drugs on the SDL is reviewed on an on-going basis to take into account changes in clinical practice, advances in medical science, and evolving needs of patients. The assessment is done objectively and professionally by the Drug Advisory Committee (DAC) which comprises senior clinicians, and is chaired by the Director of Medical Services in the Ministry of Health. The DAC considers three main factors when determining whether a drug can be subsidised, with inputs from other clinicians. First, whether the drug is essential for the treatment of medical conditions that are important causes of morbidity and mortality in Singapore. Second, whether the drug offers a major improvement in efficacy and effectiveness compared to existing subsidised drugs. Third, whether there is sufficient evidence of long term safety and cost-benefits of the drug. With the difference in subsidy coverage, the price differential between an SDL drug and its non-SDL alternative will widen and induce doctors and patients to choose SDL drugs.

Health Technology Assessment (HTA) is an important capability to have, grow and apply, so that new treatments, technologies and drugs can be evaluated and judicious decisions made about which to be covered under their national schemes. Given how rapid medical advances are, this helps to avoid a situation where precious health dollars are spent on new and unproven or less effective treatment. However, the extent of its impact is limited to how much actual practice in the public and private sectors is influenced by the guidelines. Patients also need to accept such assessments and understand that newer or more expensive is not always better.

A question that has arisen is whether these assessments should be limited to subsidised practice only. Currently, doctors retain autonomy over prescribing practice and patients can still access non-standard drugs if they are willing to pay the full price. Often, this results in private patients having greater choice of drugs. However, it can be argued that an emphasis on clinically and cost-effective care is beneficial for all patients, regardless of subsidised or private.

Reimbursement Design

Another important aspect of cost management is the design of hospital funding. Reimbursement to the public hospitals comprises diagnosis related group (DRG) based funding for inpatient and day surgery services and piece rates for outpatient attendances, with the costs and funding rates determined through regular, detailed costing exercises. The DRG approach for inpatient and day surgery care bundles related types of services necessary for the management of a particular condition and pays a standard averaged rate regardless of the intensity of the treatment or the acuity of the individual patient. This disincentivises providers from over-servicing, for example, by arbitrarily keeping the patients in the hospital for longer than necessary. Clinical outcomes are also monitored to keep a careful watch on potential under-servicing. Funding hospitals at the average cost also drives cost discipline and efficiency, and a focus on providing value-for-money services.

At the same time, cost-recovery ratios for the different types of services are closely monitored to ensure that patients pay only the target copayment (which is based on the patient subsidy rate), with government funding to the hospital to cover the rest. Between costing exercises, funding amounts are incremented annually, often matching or lagging volume and cost growth. Hospitals have to mind their costs, because the dollar funding from the government is fixed, and they also cannot exceed the target copayment levels to recover any shortfall from the patient. There is then incentive for the hospitals to constantly review and streamline processes, which in many cases also improves the patient experience.

The current hospital subvention framework will need to continue to evolve as the care model evolves, with the Regional Health Systems playing a stronger role in integrating care across different providers. For example, if different patient types, needs and the desired outcomes can be articulated, there is opportunity for payments across providers (e.g. inpatient, specialist outpatient care, home care) to be bundled into a single rate, instead of funding each type of service that is rendered. This enables providers to come together to re-organise the way care is provided for better outcomes or for more cost-effective care, or both.

Governance and Systems Design

The fact that the bulk of tertiary care is delivered in publicly-owned entities helps to keep a lid on costs. There is oversight of the public hospitals' leadership and management practices, distribution of resources across subsidised and non-subsidised patients and greater opportunity to influence practice to ensure a focus on cost-effective care. Centralisation of aspects of hospital management — for example, drug procurement — also allows savings to be reaped. Highly specialised services are restricted to designated centres, and purchase of expensive equipment centrally scrutinised, taking into account national capacity already available.

The public sector also has a useful influence at the systems level. William Haseltine, in his book Affordable Excellence,[13] quotes former Minister Khaw Boon Wan as saying that a dominant public sector is necessary to set the boundaries and ethos for the entire system, which should not only be about maximization of profits. If subsidised and quality care in the public sector is a reasonable and available alternative, private providers will need to ensure that they do not price themselves out of the market. The Ministry also publishes hospital bills on its website for common medical conditions and surgeries, by ward classes and hospital. This enables patients to compare costs across both public and private providers and inject greater price-consciousness among consumers and price-competitiveness among providers.

However, as the Ministry seeks to tap on private sector capacity in more ways, it will need to grow subsidy provision or insurance coverage for privately provided services and strengthen its levers over private practice. In sectors where the public sector accounts for a small share or none at all, for example, primary care and long-term care, prices need to be monitored, otherwise private providers may opportunistically raise their prices at each revision of subsidy rates. In the hospital sector, there is scope to relook IP coverage and encourage the adoption of features that help to contain costs, to address public concern about rising premiums.

---

[13] Haseltine, William A. *Affordable Excellence: The Singapore Healthcare Story*. Washington, D.C.: Brookings Institution, 2013. Print.

At the national level, the Ministry monitors and manages the bed and doctor supply carefully, as supply-induced demand can easily fill excess capacity in the system. There is detailed workforce planning to determine the number of healthcare professionals required in the system, and coordinate the training capacity in universities, polytechnics and teaching hospitals. Once new capacity is injected into the system, there has to be close monitoring of utilisation as there is a risk that the new capacity will be quickly taken up due to over-servicing and over-consumption.

> "…even expanding the healthcare system's capacity to meet future needs may find ourselves chasing our tails, stimulating supply-induced demand and increasing the need and demand for healthcare. Once equipment and facilities are available, they will be fully used. It is very hard to run a hospital with beds kept empty. It is very hard to have a MRI and to say this patient does not need a scan. Patients get used to higher standards of healthcare and faster responses even when these are not medically essential and later on if you come back to more normal standards, there is a reaction. So slack capacity is quickly taken up, and we end up having to build more hospitals, more clinics, provide more services, need more doctors, spend more money."
>
> — PM Lee, Universal Health Coverage Meeting, 10 February 2015

The public institutions have also invested in many initiatives to evolve their model of care — for example, to reduce a stable patient's visits to the specialist, and build up primary and community-based care. This ensures more efficient use of specialist resources and lowers cost of care, and is also more convenient for patients. Many enablers — the National Electronic Health Records, targeted funding for workforce capability building, etc. — are instrumental in making this possible.

… But Continuous Building for the Future

In many cost-constrained systems, capacity and capability building for the future may inadvertently become compromised. In healthcare, a mis-step in this direction can have serious consequences, due to the lead time required to build capacity. For example, it takes 10 years of education and training before one can become a specialist, and continued years of practice thereafter to excel and lead in the field.

Singapore has been careful to continue to invest in building capabilities, like workforce development and research. For example, the hospitals receive additional support for the cost of training and even absentee payroll in some cases, to send their staff overseas for fellowships and attachments, and to strengthen skills upgrading and clinical training. Many more local and overseas, undergraduate and postgraduate scholarships are now available, to attract talent to the healthcare sector.

In the costing and funding of hospitals, depreciation of equipment and other fixed assets are factored into their annual budgets, and in turn patient charges and government funding. Over time, these accumulate as reserves and are tapped on to pay for asset replacement. This financial discipline in determining all the costs incurred in running the hospital ensures timely replacement of equipment and long-term sustainability. The hospitals are also able to use their surpluses for other strategic activities such as teaching and research, which is a form of investment in the future.

Conclusion

Singapore's multi-payer approach to financing and strong element of progressivity in the copayment for healthcare services, with the needy able to access healthcare services free, are its unique features. The system has also undergone constant innovation and improvisation to improve coverage for the people.

Singapore's healthcare spending will certainly rise rapidly as its population ages. As the Government considers further expansions of subsidy and 3Ms coverage, it will also need to consider how coverage can be expanded in the private sector with adequate controls to manage costs and affordability for patients, and the difficult tradeoffs of managing cost and influencing patient choice.

As Singapore celebrates its 50th birthday, the next chapter will see a need for the Government to continue to play an important role to ensure affordability, as well as to design the system and incentives to focus on providing appropriate, cost effective care, in order to ensure a sustainable healthcare system for the current and future generation that does not consume a disproportionate share of the nation's and families' resources.

5 Healthcare Regulation

Harold Tan,[*] John C.W. Lim,[†] Se Thoe Su Yun,[‡]
Suwarin Chaturapit,[§] Melissa Tan,[¶] Eric Chan,[‖]
Ng Mui Kim,[**] Cynthia Kwok,[††]
Sia Chong Hock,[‡‡] Foo Yang Tong,[§§]
Wang Woei Jiuang[¶¶] and Dorothy Toh[‖‖]

Introduction

The state of health regulation in Singapore has evolved in tandem with the changing healthcare landscape over the last several decades. Healthcare services have modernised and are more sophistically structured today to serve the complex health needs of the population. The profile of risks in healthcare have also morphed, moving from

[*] Director, Regulatory Compliance and Enforcement Division, Ministry of Health, Singapore.

[†] Deputy Director of Medical Services (Industry and Research Matters), Office of the Director of Medical Services, Ministry of Health, Singapore.

[‡] Deputy Director (Biosafety), Biosafety Branch, Ministry of Health, Singapore.

[§] Senior Consultant (Administration and PEDU), Health Products Regulation Group, Health Sciences Authority, Singapore.

[¶] Senior Manager (Hospital Services), Hospital Services Division, Ministry of Health, Singapore.

[‖] Senior Manager (Hospital Services), Hospital Services Division, Ministry of Health, Singapore.

[**] Senior Assistant Director (Investigation), Regulatory Compliance and Enforcement Division, Ministry of Health, Singapore.

[††] Deputy Director (Regulatory Policy), Regulatory Policy & Legislation Division Ministry of Health, Singapore.

[‡‡] Senior Consultant (Audit and Licensing), Health Products Regulation Group, Health Sciences Authority, Singapore.

[§§] Director, Clinical Trials Branch, Premarketing Division, Health Sciences Authority, Singapore.

[¶¶] Director, Medical Devices Branch, Premarketing Division, Health Sciences Authority, Singapore.

[‖‖] Acting Assistant Group Director, Vigilance, Compliance & Enforcement Division, Health Sciences Authority, Singapore.

basic sanitation and hygiene issues to issues concerning advanced treatment methods and medication errors. There are also emerging issues pertaining to the dignity of care of elderly residents in nursing homes and psychosocial as well as ethical implications of assisted reproduction and organ donation. The threat of emerging infectious diseases and biosafety concerns demand that the scale and scope of public health preparedness and protection as well as health regulations be accelerated and broadened significantly. This chapter focuses on the developments in a few key areas of health regulation and documents some of the emerging and ongoing issues that continue to demand significant regulatory attention, relating to the development of regulatory and enforcement capabilities in the Health Ministry to cope with the ongoing regulatory challenges.

Licensing and Regulation of Healthcare Services

Apart from health services run by the Ministry of Health, all other healthcare services were basically unregulated prior to 1993. There was no licensing system to ensure that such services were provided in hygienic premises with proper equipment. Furthermore, the quality of staff providing the services could not be assured as there was no legal structure to formally recognise qualified staff or require a minimum level of staff competency to provide the healthcare services.

In 1980, the Private Hospitals and Medical Clinics (PHMC) Act[1] was passed in Parliament, thus establishing a regulatory framework that required all "private hospitals" (including "nursing homes" and "maternity homes"), "medical clinics" and "clinical laboratories" to be licensed. Further deliberation and planning was undertaken to determine the scope of regulation needed. In 1993, the PHMC Act was implemented to license and regulate only "western" mainstream medical services, while exempting services that use traditional healing methods.[2] Following the reorganisation ("restructuring") of the government healthcare services in the 1980s and 1990s, the public sector hospitals and polyclinics became corporatised entities which were then brought under the ambit of the PHMCA.

Since the implementation of the PHMC Act, MOH has been licensing all medical and dental clinics, hospitals, nursing homes and clinical laboratories (Fig. 5.1). Most of the healthcare facilities are issued 2-year licences which are renewable. Prior to the renewal of licence, each healthcare facility and its services would be subject to re-inspection and evaluation. The PHMC Act and its subsidiary legislation promulgated the minimum standards for maintaining a healthcare service. These standards relate mainly to the general maintenance of the facilities, medical record keeping, drug storage, infection control, medical and nursing manpower, and fire safety. Healthcare institutions that do not meet the minimum standards would be required to rectify their deficiencies or face the prospect of having their licences shortened. In cases where deficiencies are repeated or serious, the healthcare institution could even be fined and/or have its licence suspended or revoked.

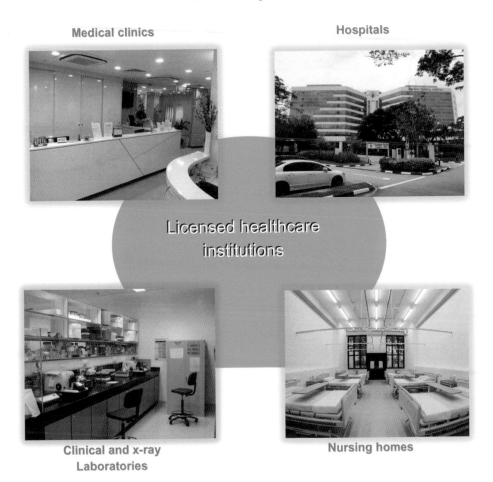

Fig. 5.1. Licensed healthcare institutions in Singapore.

Our system of licensing, inspection, and audit of healthcare institutions have served us well for the last two decades since the inception of the PHMC Act and has contributed to the overall improvement of clinical service and patient safety. The system is regularly reviewed to ensure that it remains effective and relevant to the developments in the healthcare sector, such as in health technology and organisation of services. The Ministry recently reviewed the licensing system with the aim to encourage greater compliance among healthcare institutions and enhance the quality and safety of healthcare services. It has introduced an incentive in the form of a 5-year licence for clinics with a good compliance record. This provides significant savings for licensees who perform well. Random inspections would still be done to ensure continuing compliance. This new "risk-based" licensing system has been implemented for medical/dental clinics, and is currently being monitored. If the outcomes are good, the system will be extended to other types of healthcare institutions such as clinical laboratories and nursing homes.

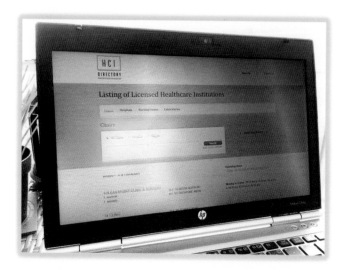

Fig. 5.2.   Online directory of local licensed healthcare institutions.

The Ministry also recently enhanced its electronic licensing portal and database system for healthcare institutions, as well as the online directory of these institutions. The enhanced licensing system, known as eLIS, helps to improve the efficiency of licence processing and overall experience of licence applicants.[3] The system also helps staff better manage the collection and evaluation of licensing data. Meanwhile, the enhanced online directory[4] of HCIs provides the public with more information about the healthcare institutions' services, including their opening hours, doctors in charge, and range of services (Fig. 5.2).

Regulation of Aesthetic Practices

Over the last decade, we have observed the emergence of minimally invasive aesthetic procedures and their rising popularity with healthcare consumers. Many of these aesthetic procedures are widely practised in other developed countries, such as Botox injections, chemical peels, intense pulse light (IPL) therapy, and laser skin resurfacing (Fig. 5.3). Given that this area is relatively new and the need to ensure that these aesthetic procedures are carried out safely for patients, safe practice standards had to be set. In 2008, the Academy of Medicine and College of Family Physicians developed the Guidelines on Aesthetic Practices for Doctors,[5] which was endorsed by the Singapore Medical Council. These guidelines were complemented by new licensing terms and conditions[6] imposed by the Ministry to regulate low-evidence aesthetic practices as well as liposuction, which is an invasive and high-risk procedure. An Aesthetic Practice Oversight Committee (APOC) was also set up to provide professional regulatory oversight to ensure that doctors comply with the minimum standards. Licensing inspectors from the Ministry would conduct periodic checks on clinics and hospitals to ensure

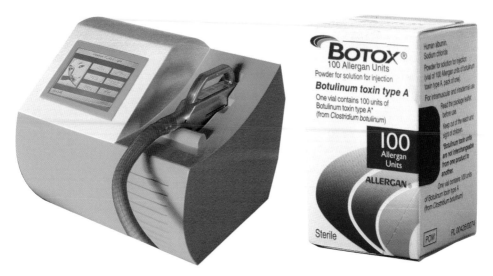

Fig. 5.3. (*Left*) Use of Intense Pulse Light for facial rejuvenation; (*Right*) Botulinum Toxin Type A injectable.

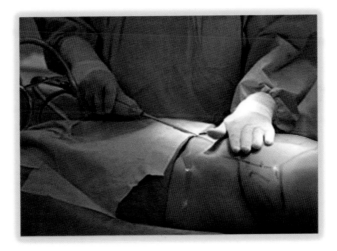

Fig. 5.4.   A liposuction procedure in progress.

that aesthetic services are provided by licensees in accordance with the guidelines and requirements. Doctors who did not comply with these standards were referred to the Singapore Medical Council for review, while non-compliant licensees faced enforcement actions. Overall, the regulatory framework has kept aesthetic services in check and has ensured that appropriate measures were taken when necessary.

Liposuction is an invasive aesthetic procedure that became increasingly popular over the last 7–8 years (Fig. 5.4). There were concerns that some doctors performing liposuction were not properly trained, since liposuction was not part of the medical training curriculum for doctors. These doctors would normally attend a few days of liposuction workshop offered by medical device companies before they start providing the service. This was clearly inadequate. Furthermore, there were concerns that patients might be pressured by liposuction providers to undergo the procedure without having adequate opportunity to consider the risks thoroughly.

In view of the above concerns, the Ministry imposed new licensing terms and conditions on clinics providing liposuction to protect patients[7]. Under these licensing conditions, doctors have to observe and perform a minimum number of liposuction procedures under preceptorship before they can be accredited to perform the procedure independently. An Accreditation Committee for Liposuction (ACL) was established to oversee the accreditation of liposuction practitioners. Liposuction that involves removing more than 1 litre of fat may only be performed in ambulatory surgical centres or hospitals. Liposuction providers are required to grant patients a 7-day cooling off period for them to consider carefully before consenting to the procedure. All healthcare institutions are to report to the Ministry any major complication associated with liposuction. These are some of the key measures taken to ensure the safety of liposuction practices in Singapore. The liposuction regulatory framework is still regularly reviewed to keep pace with technological advancement in liposuction techniques and changing nature of risks.[8]

Regulation of Human Organ Transplantation

The need for organs especially kidneys was identified as early as in the 1960s. For kidney failure patients, transplantation offered an opportunity for an improved quality of life. It was then estimated that approximately 800,000 kidney donor pledgers were required to support an effective kidney transplantation programme.[9] Regarding the need for organs, the Medical (Therapy, Education, and Research) Act (MTERA)[10] was passed in 1972 to allow for persons to pledge to donate their organs and tissues for the purposes of therapy and transplantation, education or research after they passed away. This is an opt-in scheme which allows any person who is 18-years-old and above and who is not mentally disordered to give all or any part of his body for treatment, education, or research upon his death. In cases where a person had not pledged his organs under MTERA before passing away, family members of the deceased can donate his organs under MTERA upon his death if they wish to do so.

Following the introduction of the MTERA, campaigns were conducted to enlist persons to pledge their organs (Fig. 5.5). However, after 15 years, only 27,000 pledges were received.[11] The Law was deemed ineffective in supporting the needs of the people. After further review and examining how other countries were dealing with similar organ shortage issues, the Human Organ Transplant Act (HOTA) was enacted in 1987 with the aim of making provisions for the removal of kidneys for transplantation and concomitant prohibition of organ trading. This Act, unlike the

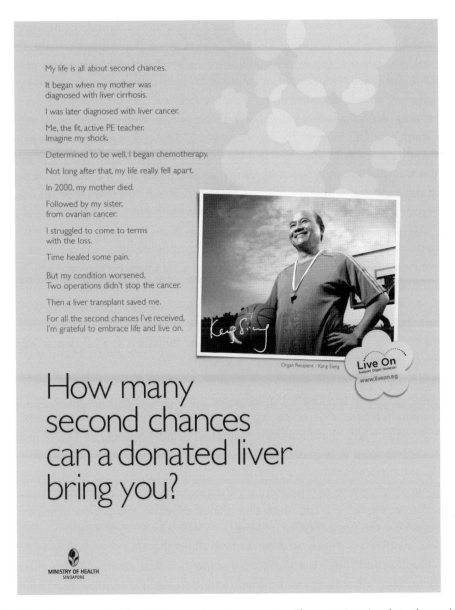

My life is all about second chances.

It began when my mother was
diagnosed with liver cirrhosis.

I was later diagnosed with liver cancer.

Me, the fit, active PE teacher.
Imagine my shock.

Determined to be well, I began chemotherapy.

Not long after that, my life really fell apart.

In 2000, my mother died.

Followed by my sister,
from ovarian cancer.

I struggled to come to terms
with the loss.

Time healed some pain.

But my condition worsened.
Two operations didn't stop the cancer.

Then a liver transplant saved me.

For all the second chances I've received,
I'm grateful to embrace life and live on.

Organ Recipient - Keng Siang

Live On
Support Organ Donation
www.liveon.sg

How many second chances can a donated liver bring you?

MINISTRY OF HEALTH
SINGAPORE

Fig. 5.5. A poster on the "Live On" organ donation campaign. The campaign aimed to educate the public on the Human Organ Transplant Act and rally all Singaporeans to support and embrace organ donation.

MTERA, was based on the concept of "presumed consent," i.e. the HOTA is an opt-out legislation. This meant that kidneys from victims of fatal accidents could be removed for transplantation if the victims had not registered their objection to organ donation in their lifetime. A grace period was introduced for Singaporeans to decide if they wanted to opt-out of the legislation before the Act was implemented.

The HOTA was subsequently amended a few times. Notably, the Act was amended in 2004 to include additional organs beyond kidneys, i.e. liver, heart, corneas, and those of regulatory significance — which included regulation of living donor organ transplantation. Prior to the 2004 amendments, living donor kidney transplantation was regulated under a professional circular which restricted donors to first and second degree relatives of the recipient. Potential donors were referred to a Transplant Coordinator for social, psychological, and emotional assessment, and would also have to undergo detailed medical assessment to confirm suitability for the transplantation procedure. When amendments to the HOTA to regulate living donor transplants were being considered, it was felt that aside from living related organ donation, living unrelated organ donation could be allowed with strict safeguards and regulations under the law in place. This would ensure effective and enforceable control of the donation and transplantation processes. It was also determined that requests for organ transplants would best be evaluated by Transplant Ethics Committees (TECs) to ensure that specific ethical issues pertaining to each request could be adequately assessed and discussed. The amended HOTA included safeguards for the Ministry to regulate and replace the TECs should any of the TECs be deemed as not discharging their functions in accordance with the HOTA or in a satisfactory manner.

In 2009, further efforts were made to strengthen the TEC framework, including instituting national panels from which TEC members should be appointed; and comprising independent medical practitioners and laypersons to conduct unbiased evaluations and safeguard the donors' interest. Guidelines for the TEC and transplant centres were also issued to help TEC members make careful decisions on transplant applications.

Other amendments of regulatory significance were the inclusion of enforcement provisions in the Act in 2008, which determined the roles and powers of inspectors, provisions on the protection of informers, as well as raising the penalty on organ trading syndicates. These amendments marked the Ministry's commitment to take tough actions against organ trading practices. The 2008 organ trading case involving Tang Wee Sung[12] was a grim reminder that our country is not immune to the risk of organ trading practices becoming rife on our shores (Fig. 5.6). It highlights the need for continuing vigilance on the part of our regulatory agencies and regular review of the HOTA to ensure that regulatory controls remain robust and effective.

Since the HOTA amendments in 2004, we have seen an increase in the number of living donor organ transplants carried out in Singapore. It is crucial that TEC members continue to maintain a high level of competency and vigilance when evaluating transplant requests. In this regard, TEC members undergo a training programme to help equip themselves with the skills necessary for such evaluation.

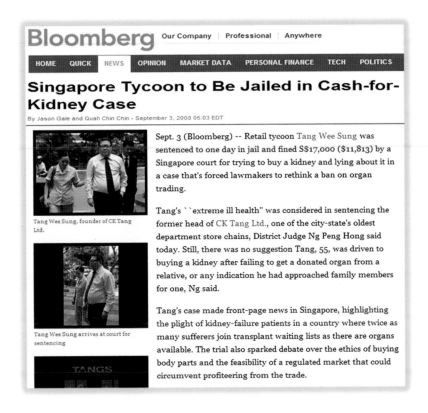

Fig. 5.6. Extract of an internet news report on the organ trading case involving Tang Wee Sung in 2008.

Regulation of Biological Agents and Toxins

The Biological Agents and Toxins Act (BATA)[13] was enacted in 2005 with the aim to prohibit or otherwise regulate the possession, use, import, transhipment, transfer, and transportation of biological agents and toxins, as well as to provide for safe practices in their handling. This legislation was necessary, given Singapore's development as a biomedical science hub and the emergence of more laboratories handling biological agents that pose significant public health risk (Fig. 5.7). The laboratory-acquired SARS infections in Singapore, Taiwan, and China are a testimony to such hazards. Some biological agents such as *Bacillus anthracis* (bacteria that causes anthrax) have been used historically as biological weapons and could potentially be abused;[14,15] this risk is real especially in the wake of global terrorism. These global security threats, including the 2001 anthrax scare in the USA,[16] made it even more imperative for Singapore to develop stringent and robust controls on the possession and use of biological agents and toxins.

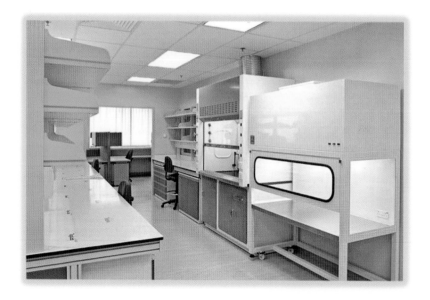

Fig. 5.7. A biosafety research laboratory at Science Park, Singapore.

Under the BATA, biological agents and toxins are classified into different schedules according to their respective biosafety risks (individual versus community) and biosecurity risks. This is to allow the Ministry to calibrate regulatory controls of the biological agents according to their differential risks. Biological agents under the Second Schedule such as the Ebola virus, Nipah virus, and smallpox virus pose the highest individual and community biosafety risk as well as biosecurity risk. This is followed by biological agents under the First Schedule which generally have a lower community biosafety risk. Under this Schedule, some agents have higher biosecurity risks (e.g. *B. anthracis*, SARS-CoV) than others (e.g. *M. tuberculosis*, HIV). Biological agents under the Third and Fourth Schedules are generally of moderate individual risk and low community risk, with minimal biosecurity risk (e.g. *Salmonella sp.*, Hepatitis B virus, *Legionella sp.*). Eight microbial toxins are included under Fifth Schedule for regulatory control as these pose significant biosecurity risks.

Generally, all the Scheduled agents are not allowed to be imported unless permission is granted by the Director of Medical Services, MOH. They are also prohibited from being transported through mail or public transport. The possession of biological agents under the First and Second Schedule, and toxins under the Fifth Schedule are strictly controlled while special approval is needed to use biological agents under the Second Schedule (e.g. for research). All biological agents under the First and Second Schedules may only be handled or stored in facilities that are certified as Biosafety level 3 (BSL-3) or above. For First Schedule-Part II and

Second Schedule biological agents, the additional criterion is that the facility must also be protected and security-cleared. Protected place and security-clearance are also requirements for facility storing and handling of Fifth Schedule toxins. The certification of BSL-3 facilities is done by MOH-approved third-party certifying bodies and takes into consideration engineering controls, facility design, laboratory practices and equipping, and administrative processes.

The BATA also prohibits non-peaceful use or manipulation of any biological agent/toxin, not limited to those under the Schedules. Stiff penalties such as fines amounting to $1 million and/or life imprisonment could be imposed on offenders convicted of offences under the BATA.

Development of Enforcement Capabilities in MOH

MOH administers more than 20 primary legislations that regulate healthcare premises, healthcare professionals, and professional practices. Prior to the setup of the MOH enforcement unit, the responsibility of enforcement rested with the various policy divisions driving the regulations as they possess the relevant subject matter expertise. This led to policy officers in the policy divisions doubling up as investigators, which was not ideal as the policy officers lacked the investigation experience to conduct proper investigations that could withstand scrutiny in the event of a prosecution or court trial. The lack of proper investigation protocols and procedures was further compounded by the absence of operational intelligence that could tap on the established databases of other law enforcement agencies, such as the Police, the Central Narcotics Bureau, and the Ministry of Manpower, to support the enforcement and investigation of breaches of MOH's legislations.

MOH subsequently undertook a major review which led to the development of a dedicated enforcement unit. Two senior Police officers were seconded from the Singapore Police Force to set up the unit in June 2008. To benefit from the investigation experience of the Police and bridge the expertise gap, retired Police officers were recruited as Investigation Officers and Field/Operations Officers in the newly set up unit. The Enforcement unit has since undergone two re-organisations together with other regulatory functions of MOH. Currently, it is part of the Surveillance and Enforcement Branch under the MOH Regulatory Compliance and Enforcement Division. The unit comprises 20 personnel and is headed by Senior Officers seconded from the Singapore Police Force. The functions of the unit include surveillance, operations, and investigation. The unit works closely with other law enforcement agencies such as the Police, Singapore Customs, Health Sciences Authority and Ministry of Manpower to conduct various enforcement operations. For example in 2010, the Enforcement unit worked with HSA's enforcers to bust a syndicate that was peddling codeine-containing cough mixtures in Geylang and Peninsula Plaza.[17] Other operations include tracing of tuberculosis patients who default on treatment orders, HIV-infected persons who risk the lives of others through irresponsible sexual behaviours, and persons involved in illegal online selling of contact lenses. The Enforcement unit is also responsible for investigating offences pertaining to healthcare laws under MOH's purview, such as those relating to illegal clinics, doctors or other healthcare practitioners, suspected organ trading, and errant advertising of healthcare services.

To help enforcement officers manage and track various investigations, a web-based intranet system known as the Health Regulation Investigation and Management System (HERIMS) was set up.[18] HERIMS is benchmarked against the Police's Criminal Investigation Management System. The system ensures that investigation procedures are properly carried out and also serves as a repository for all investigations and operations to enable more efficient referencing of past cases. It is anticipated that MOH's enforcement capabilities will continue to grow and strengthen in the face of emerging areas in healthcare that warrant regulation and enforcement for patient safety and public interests.

Regulation of Health Products

Medicinal Products

The regulation of health products in Singapore has evolved significantly over the last 50 years, in tandem with the development of Singapore's healthcare system and regulatory infrastructure. In the earlier years, before the implementation of medicinal product registration under the Medicines Act in 1987, the Inspectorate Section of the then-Pharmaceutical Department of the Ministry was the regulatory unit responsible for the enforcement of the following pieces of legislation:

- **Sale of Drugs Act (Cap. 282)** — This Act was originally part of the Sale of Food and Drugs Ordinance of 1914 that was separated into two pieces of legislation, namely the Sale of Food Act and the Sale of Drugs Act in 1971. The objective of the Act was mainly to safeguard consumers from harmful adulterated drug products, products containing prohibited substances, and products with false or misleading statements on the packages.
- **The Poisons Act (Cap. 234)** — This Act originated from the Poisons Ordinance 1938. The Poisons Act requires a person to hold a "Poisons Licence" before he can import, possess for sale, or sell substances listed as poisons in the Poisons List. The Poisons Act is still relevant and useful today in dealing with illegal products containing scheduled poisons.

- **The Medicines (Advertisement and Sale) Act (Cap. 177)** — This Act came into operation in 1956 to prohibit advertisements relating to certain diseases listed in the Schedule and those relating to medical services, as well as prohibition of advertisements relating to abortion. The Act also required disclosure of compositions of items recommended as medicines.

The key areas of regulatory focus were on preventing illegal supplies of poisons, especially Schedule 3 poisons that were prescription drugs, and curtailing misleading advertisements which were rampant in the early '60s and '70s.

The enactment of the Medicines Act in 1975 was one of the key milestones in the history of health products regulation in Singapore. It provided for a comprehensive regulatory framework for the control of medicinal products, including licensing of medicinal product importers, manufacturers, assemblers, and wholesale dealers; registration of premises operating as retail pharmacies; and regulation of medical advertisements and promotion of sales of medicines. The Act also provided for licensing of each medicinal product before being legally supplied in Singapore. The provisions under the Medicines Act were implemented in phases to allow time for the various stakeholders to meet the new requirements. The requirement for all medicinal products to be registered, unless they were legally exempted, posed to be the main challenge, and it was implemented over three years from 1987 to 1990. The Drug Administration Division of the Ministry's Pharmaceutical Department was the regulatory unit responsible for implementation.

With the expanded regulatory functions and responsibilities, the Pharmaceutical Department was renamed the "National Pharmaceutical Administration (NPA)" in 1999. On 1 April 2001, a new statutory board was established under the Ministry. This was the Health Sciences Authority (HSA) which consolidated NPA together with four other specialised Ministry departments, namely the Centre for Drug Evaluation, the Product Regulation Department, the Institute of Science and Forensic Medicine, and the Singapore Blood Transfusion Service (Fig. 5.8). Under HSA, the national health product regulatory functions were carried out by the Centre of Drug Administration and the Centre for Medical Device Regulation. In 2006, these two centres became HSA's Health Products Regulation Group (HPRG). The establishment of HSA was a very significant milestone at the turn of the century. In addition to medicines regulation, HSA also housed the national blood service and the country's forensic science, forensic medicine, and analytical chemistry testing capabilities. With HSA's formation, the development of human resources and scientific capabilities needed for health product regulations in an era of rapidly advancing bio-medical science was able to grow at a much faster pace. Nonetheless, given Singapore's size and human resource constraints, innovative approaches to regulation also had to be adopted because it was never tenable to just keep increasing headcount.

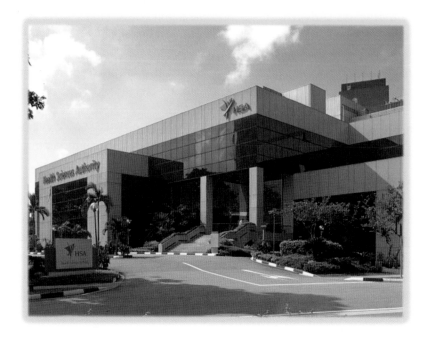

Fig. 5.8.   Health Sciences Authority at Outram Road.

HSA has promoted greater transparency of submission processes and evaluation routes. This included clarity about which products underwent full evaluation if they had never been licensed elsewhere, in contrast to the majority of products going through abridged assessments if there was valid reference data from approvals in other jurisdictions. This has been an aspect of Singapore's regulatory system lauded by international counterparts and agencies like the World Health Organisation (WHO). Through collaborations, memoranda of understanding, information exchange, and training with major international drug regulatory agencies such as the US Food and Drug Administration (FDA), the UK Medicines and Health products Regulatory Authority (MHRA), Australia's Therapeutic Goods Administration (TGA) and Health Canada, HSA has been able to leverage on global cooperation to effectively strengthen Singapore's health products regulatory processes to protect public health in spite of its relative small regulatory group.

Developments in Good Manufacturing Practice (GMP)

A key aspect of medicines safety relates to the quality of products and how they are manufactured. Good Manufacturing Practice (GMP) is critical for setting and regulating the standards of production.

From 1 January 2000, Singapore became the first Asian member of the Pharmaceutical Inspection Cooperation Scheme or System (PIC/S). This was a major step in boosting the robustness of health products regulation and recognition for Singapore's internationally benchmarked framework. One of the biggest spin offs from being a PIC/S member was the signing of the bilateral Singapore-Australia Mutual Recognition Agreement (MRA) on GMP Inspection in February 2001. The signing of this MRA was facilitated by the PIC/S membership of both Australia and Singapore. With this MRA, Australia's TGA does not need to send its GMP Auditors to inspect manufacturers in Singapore and vice versa. More than 15 pharmaceutical companies in Singapore and many more in Australia have benefited from the MRA. The companies include manufacturers of Active Pharmaceutical Ingredients, innovator drugs, generic drugs, and herbal medicines.

Within the Association of South-East Asian Nations (ASEAN), an ASEAN MRA Taskforce on GMP Inspection was formed in 2005, with Singapore and Malaysia as Chair and Co-Chair. By 2009, this Taskforce had delivered an ASEAN Sectoral MRA on GMP Inspection for Manufacturers of Medicinal Products which was signed by the Economic Ministers of all 10 ASEAN Member States on 10 April 2009. This ASEAN Sectoral MRA is benchmarked to the PIC/S framework, and came into force from 2012. Singapore, Malaysia, and Indonesia, by virtue of their PIC/S membership, have commenced implementation of this MRA by accepting one another's GMP inspection reports without the need to duplicate inspections. The benefits of the ASEAN Sectoral MRA include avoiding duplication of GMP inspections; saving time, resources, and costs for regulators and the pharmaceutical industry; facilitating trade in medicinal products; quicker access to medicinal products by patients; and increased business competitiveness of ASEAN vis-à-vis other industrialised countries.

Regulation of Clinical Trials

Before a new drug substance can be approved for use as a medicinal product, its safety, quality, and efficacy have to be demonstrated through a series of rigorous clinical trials. Clinical trials are an essential part of the health products' regulatory process. As such, regulation of clinical trials was one of the first areas to be introduced in 1978, shortly after the Medicines Act came into force. The Ministry established the Medical Clinical Research Committee to oversee the conduct of clinical drug trials in Singapore. In 1998, the clinical trials regulations were revised to establish a legal framework for Good Clinical Practice (GCP) to align with international best practice. The conduct of a clinical trial in accordance with the principles of GCP helps to ensure that the safety and interests of trial participants are protected, and that scientific data generated from the trial are valid and accurate. With HSA's establishment, the conduct of clinical drug trials in terms of assessing the safety of the investigational product and related study protocols, as well as conducting GCP inspections, are now regulated by HSA's Health Products Regulation Group (HPRG).

Over the past 15 years, there has been remarkable progress in Singapore's Biomedical Sciences Initiative since it launched. The research ecosystem system, fuelled by biotechnological advances that have led to the discovery of ever increasing disease-relevant molecular information heralding a thrust toward precision medicine or personalised medicine, has created an environment conducive for early drug development to take place in Singapore. Coupled with a sound healthcare infrastructure and science-based regulation, these key elements together with the inclusion of GCP in the legislation, have facilitated the conduct of drug development by global pharmaceutical companies in Singapore. Early phase clinical trials on new innovative drugs initiated locally have constituted a sizeable proportion of trials conducted in recent years. The soundness of the regulatory framework not only continues to ensure safeguarding of patients' interests and safety, but will also enable progress in early phase clinical trials of precision medicine and downstream drug registration, including novel products to treat diseases which are relatively more prevalent in Singapore.

The Health Products Act and Medical Devices

As only medicinal products can be regulated under the Medicines Act, a new piece of legislation was needed to provide for the categorisation of health products according to their different characteristics and uses. The new Health Products Act was passed in Parliament in 2007, with medical devices and cosmetic products listed in the First Schedule. This piece of legislation has an innovative structure in minimising mandatory requirements in the main Act, and allowing more details to be fleshed out in the Regulations for the different product categories. This allows for a more responsive risk-based regulatory approach in that subsidiary legislation can be amended more promptly to appropriately address risk profiles of products as biomedical science and technology change over time. Higher risk products are regulated more tightly while a lighter touch is applied for lower risk products; and this approach also applies within each product category.

The regulatory control of medical devices (Fig. 5.9) in Singapore was implemented in three phases from November 2007 to January 2012, starting with the implementation of post-market obligations for dealers to report adverse events within certain timeframes, to notify HSA before initiating product recalls, and to keep records of complaints and product distribution. From January 2012, all medical devices imported and supplied in Singapore had to be listed on the Singapore Medical Device Register, unless they were exempted from registration or had been authorised through one of the authorisation routes implemented to facilitate certain

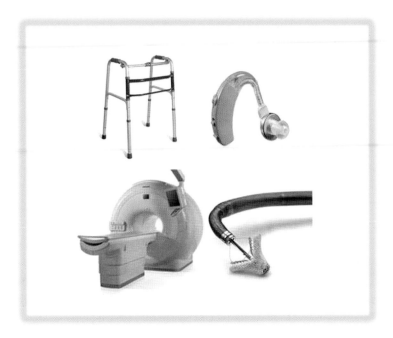

Fig. 5.9. Medical devices cover a broad range of products from low risk devices like the walking frame and hearing aids to higher risk devices such as computer tomography (CT) scanners and percutaneous cardiac valve repair instruments.

types of imports such as medical devices imported for non-clinical use. A series of initiatives were implemented from 2012 to reduce administrative burden, shorten evaluation turnaround times, and lower regulatory fees. For example, Class A medical devices, except for sterile devices, are now exempted from registration.

HSA continues to make improvements and refinements to the medical device pre-market framework to ensure its effectiveness and relevance in this era of fast paced technological innovation, while ensuring HSA's primary mandate of upholding public health and patient safety. In striving to achieve a "Smart Regulation" philosophy — to effectively protect public health, enable efficient healthcare delivery, and enhance public confidence — the roles of pre- and post-market regulation must be well-balanced, coordinated, and complementary in adding value to the framework.

Strengthening of Pharmacovigilance Activities

Singapore joined the WHO International Drug Monitoring Programme in 1993 as its fortieth member after the successful implementation of adverse drug reaction monitoring programme in Singapore by the Ministry's Pharmaceutical Department. The adverse drug reaction programme has been expanded by HSA's Vigilance and

Compliance Branch to cover a full range of pharmacovigilance activities, including in-depth risk assessment, risk communication, and risk minimisation. The scope of safety monitoring has been expanded to include the whole spectrum of health products, including medical devices, vaccines, and novel health products such as cell and tissue therapies.

Over the past 11 years, the number of adverse event reports for marketed pharmaceuticals, complementary health products, and medical devices has risen 30-fold, from slightly over 600 in 2001 to more than 20,000 from 2011 onwards. The majority of cases were reported directly by healthcare professionals in public hospitals and primary care clinics. In addition, Singapore has taken the world lead in terms of the number of valid individual case safety reports (ICSRs) per million inhabitants submitted to the WHO's global database; there are now more than 3000 ICSRs per million inhabitants, an indicator of the comprehensiveness of the country's vigilance system. An effective communication system has been developed by the Ministry, clinicians, and HSA's vigilance team to facilitate timely dissemination of important safety information to healthcare professionals and stakeholders (Fig. 5.10). All registered healthcare professionals can be notified within a few hours.

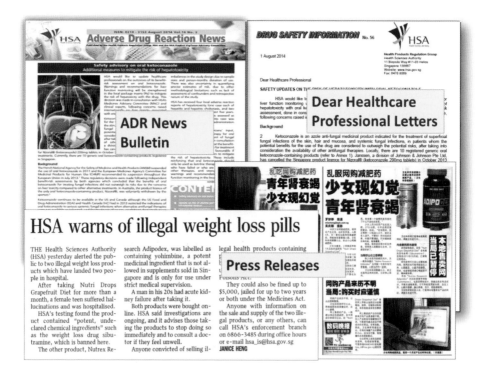

Fig. 5.10. HSA routinely communicates safety risks to healthcare professionals and consumers through Adverse Drug Reaction Bulletins, Healthcare Professional Letters and Press Releases.

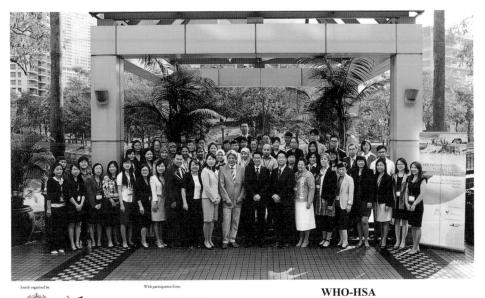

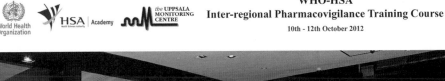

WHO-HSA
Inter-regional Pharmacovigilance Training Course
10th - 12th October 2012

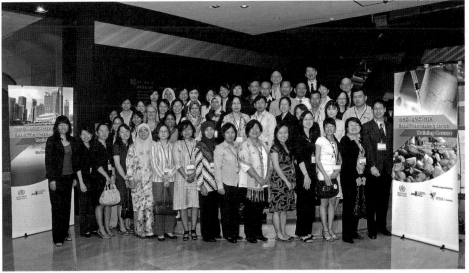

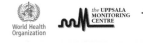

WHO-UMC-HSA
Basic Pharmacovigilance Training Course
31 May - 4 June 2010

Fig. 5.11. The Health Products Regulation Group, HSA, collaborated with the World Health Organization (WHO) to organise inter-regional pharmacovigilance training in Singapore in 2010 and 2012.

A pharmacogenomics team was formed in 2007 to collaborate with several public sector hospitals to investigate possible genetic associations behind serious skin reactions. This project led to the recommendation for genotyping of the HLA-B*1502 allele before initiation of carbamazepine therapy[19] in new patients of Asian ancestry as the standard of care in Singapore. There has been no carbamazepine-induced serious skin reactions in patients screened for HLA-B*1502 since the genotyping recommendations were rolled out on 30 April 2013.

Moving forward, to further strengthen the protection of public health, a provision will be included in the new Health Products (Therapeutic Product) Regulations under the Health Products Act to provide HSA with the mandate to direct the company which has registered a therapeutic product to implement risk management plans to minimise risks relating to the unsafe and inefficacious use of therapeutic products.

Moving Ahead

All in all, Singapore's health products regulatory system has seen remarkable development over the years. It is recognised internationally for using strong scientific basis regarding decisions, the soundness of its systems, and the innovativeness of approaches that continue to serve as an example and benchmark for developed and developing countries' regulatory agencies (Fig. 5.11). This is testimony to the hard work and strong commitment to scientific professionalism and innovation of all the regulatory staff who have worked in the Ministry's Pharmaceutical Department and its successive organisations to the present day Health Products Regulation Group in HSA.

Acknowledgements

Public Health Group, MOH
Regulatory Policy and Legislation Division, MOH
Regulatory Compliance and Enforcement Division, MOH
Hospital Services Division, MOH
Health Products Regulation Group, HSA

References

1. Attorney General Chambers. (2014) *Private Hospitals and Medical Clinics Act*, Singapore Statutes Online. Website: http://statutes.agc.gov.sg/aol/search/display/view.w3p;page=0;query=CompId%3A9a09e1b8-082f-4dfa-8dc0-738b7e4aacd5;rec=0;resUrl=http%3A%2F%2Fstatutes.agc.gov.sg%2Faol%2Fbrowse%2FtitleResults.w3p%3Bletter%3DP%3Btype%3DactsAll

2. Source: Ministry of Health Singapore, 2014.

3. Ministry of Health Singapore. (2014) *E-Licensing for Healthcare (eLIS)*. Website: https://elis.moh.gov.sg/elis/

4. Ministry of Health Singapore. (2014) *HCI Directory.* Website: http://hcidirectory.sg/hci-directory/

5. Singapore Medical Council. (2014) "Guidelines on Aesthetic Practices (Oct 2008)," Website: http://www.healthprofessionals.gov.sg/content/hprof/smc/en/topnav/guidelines/guidelines_on_aesthetic_practices.html

6. Ministry of Health Singapore. (2014) "Circular on Amendment of Clinic and Hospital Licence under PHMC Act: Regulation of List B Aesthetic Procedures, Annex B: Additional Terms and Conditions for Medical Clinics or Hospitals performing List B Aesthetic or Equivalent Procedures imposed under Section 6(5) of the Private Hospitals and Medical Clinics Act (2008)," *eLIS*. Website: https://elis.moh.gov.sg/elis/publishInfo.do?task=download&pkId=120

7. Ministry of Health Singapore. "Licensing Terms and Conditions on Ambulatory Surgery — Liposuction (2010)." *eLIS*. Website: https://elis.moh.gov.sg/elis/publishInfo.do?task=download&pkId=113 .

8. The licensing terms and conditions for liposuction have been further revised. The revised conditions, *inter alia*, require all liposuction procedures to be performed only in ambulatory surgical centres and hospitals, and that *all* liposuction practitioners except hospital-based personnel must be accredited by the Accreditation Committee on Liposuction. The revised licensing conditions took effect on 1 March 2015.

9. Source: Ministry of Health Singapore, 2014.

10. *Medical (Therapy, Education and Research) Act*, Singapore Statutes Online, 2014. Website: http://statutes.agc.gov.sg/aol/search/display/view.w3p;page=0;query=CompId%3A57f7ffd6-6599-4c21-a2a7-80a4de6b129d;rec=0;resUrl=http%3A%2F%2Fstatutes.agc.gov.sg%2Faol%2Fbrowse%2FtitleResults.w3p%3Bletter%3DM%3Btype%3DactsAll

11. Source: Ministry of Health Singapore, 2014.

12. Tang Wee Sung, a prominent social figure who was suffering from a kidney ailment, was imprisoned and fined for his role in a high profile organ trading case which involved his nephew-in-law Whang Sung Lin and the latter's friend Wang Chin Sung, both of whom were also convicted and imprisoned for their offences under HOTA. The foreign prospective donor Sulaiman and his friend Toni were also convicted for organ trading and sentenced accordingly.

13. Singapore Attorney Generals Chamber. (2014) *Biological Agents and Toxins Act*, Singapore Statutes Online. Website: http://statutes.agc.gov.sg/aol/search/display/view.w3p;page=0;query=CompId%3Ab2d7ac29-fe83-4843-ae69-4dddb52ca194;rec=0;resUrl=http%3A%2F%2Fstatutes.agc.gov.sg%2Faol%2Fbrowse%2FtitleResults.w3p%3Bletter%3DB%3BpNum%3D1%3Btype%3DactsAll

14. Spencer RC, Wilcox MH. (1993) "Agents of biological warfare." *Rev Med Microbiol.* **4**: 138–43.

15. Spencer RC. (2003) "Bacillus anthracis." *J Clin Pathol.* **56**(3): 182–187.

16. Warrick J. (2010) "FBI investigation of 2001 anthrax attacks concluded; U.S. releases details." *The Washington Post.* Website: http://www.washingtonpost.com/wp-dyn/content/article/2010/02/19/AR2010021902369.html

17. Khushwant Singh. (2010) "$82,000 profit from illicit cough mixture business." *The Straits Times.*

18. Source: Ministry of Health Singapore.

19. Carbamazepine is indicated for the treatment of epilepsy and other conditions such as diabetic neuropathy, trigeminal neuralgia, and bipolar disorders.

Fifty Years of Clinical Quality

Voo Yau Onn*

Regulation of Professional Standards

The Private Hospitals and Medical Clinics Act was enacted to provide for the licensing of healthcare facilities in order to safeguard patient interests and to ensure that practices met with stringent public health requirements. It ensured that healthcare facilities were properly managed and maintained, and were not used in a manner that was detrimental to public interests.

Its origins date back to the now-defunct Registration Ordinance of Maternity Homes and Nursing Homes, passed in 1959. The former legislation was enacted to address concerns associated with the proliferation of maternity and nursing homes, but when the problem receded by the time Singapore had gained her independence, the Ordinance was set aside.

With the emergence of new private hospitals, medical and dental clinics, as well as nursing homes over time, the need for new legislation to regulate such establishments began to resurface. After a long gestation period during which comparable legislation in other countries was thoroughly reviewed, a new Act was proposed to regulate the running of private hospitals, clinics, laboratories, and nursing homes. However, care was exercised to ensure that the Act did not encroach on professional liberties granted under the Medical Registration Act and the Dental Registration Act.

The Private Hospitals and Medical Clinics Act was passed in Parliament in 1980, but it underwent several further rounds of internal deliberation before it came into force in 1991. During this period, few hospitals were being built and clinics that were established relied mainly on the professional integrity and accountability of the

* Director, Clinical Quality & Safety Division, Ministry of Health, Singapore. Honorary Visiting Consultant, Medical Board (Quality), National University Hospital, Singapore.

physician leaders as registered medical practitioners under the Singapore Medical Council. As a statutory board set up under the Medical Registration Act of 1953, the Singapore Medical Council employs professional self-regulation to safeguard patient care, by ensuring that registered medical practitioners are competent and fit to practice, uphold standards of professionalism and maintain public confidence.

In the meantime, circumstances were changing since the Act was mooted. Concerns had been raised over whether the quality of professional care rendered by doctors and nurses was up to standard, whether general practitioners were giving adequate treatment, and whether laboratories were consistently giving accurate and reliable results. Several other emerging factors influenced the shape of the Act, including providing for the necessary establishment of a national blood bank with adequate controls over the blood donation and distribution system for quality and patient safety reasons; as well as the need for governance over new clinical practices such as *in vitro* fertilisation and other high-risk and high cost investigations and procedures.[1]

However, traditional medicine and their practitioners were excluded from the Act for the same reasons that they were exempted from the Medical Registration Act. The amendments to the Private Hospitals and Medical Clinics Act in 1999 provided flexibility for traditional and complementary medicine establishments to be regulated as deemed necessary. In cases like these, MOH decided to tread cautiously as many of these practices involved boundaries that were vague and claims were difficult to evaluate.[2]

Following the growth of the private medical sector, and with the corporatisation and privatisation of government health facilities beginning from 1985, the Private Hospitals and Medical Clinics Act began to take on an even greater significance as a regulatory instrument.

Quality Assurance Programmes

Clinical review of medical management has been an integral part of continuous improvement in hospital practice. These activities — which included teaching ward rounds, preoperative rounds, clinical tutorials and mortality conferences — became formalised as quality assurance activities among government hospitals in 1974, with the setting up of the Tissue Audit Committee and a Nosocomial Infection Control Programme.

In 1985, following a detailed MOH study, a two-tiered quality assurance system was established. All hospitals were required to maintain their own quality assurance

---

[1] Lee MH. (2004) *Evolution of the PHMC Act*, (a personal compilation from MOH archives).

[2] Hansard of the Parliamentary debate at the Second Reading of the Private Hospitals and Medical Clinics (Amendment) Bill, 1999.

programmes, which was reviewed by a central MOH Quality Assurance Committee. This Committee was a multi-disciplinary peer review body chaired by Dr. Chew Chin Hin, DDMS (Hospitals) and comprised senior clinicians from various specialties and hospitals, administrators, a forensic specialist and pathologist. The major quality assurance programmes at that time included the following:

(i) Medical Audit — In response to a complaint or alleged mismanagement or reviews of selected hospital inpatient care standards or procedures. The Committee monitored the hospitals' quality assurance programmes, audit and incident reports, and selected one or two areas of special focus for major review each year, e.g. maternal mortality.

(ii) Mortality Review — Conducted weekly at department level, in particular, to review cases of "unexpected" or "avoidable" deaths.

(iii) Infection Control — To monitor rates of hospital-acquired infections and to facilitate concerted and timely remedial action across hospitals in the event of an outbreak.

(iv) Nursing Quality Assurance — Chaired by the Principal Nursing Officer (now called Chief Nursing Officer), monitors issues related to nursing care and standards.

(v) Pharmacy & Therapeutics and Antibiotic Review Committees — To formulate drug-related policies in the hospital, recommend drugs to be included in the formulary, review drug utilisation and appropriateness of antibiotic prescribing practices, as well as medication related adverse events.

(vi) Blood Transfusion Committee — Work in conjunction with the Singapore Blood Transfusion Service to monitor the appropriateness and extent of usage of blood and blood components and adequacy of supply.

(vii) Utilisation Review Committee — Looks into the utilisation of facilities and investigations to maximise the benefits of limited resources.

However, as hospital restructuring continued, the voluntary submission of reports declined, and it became necessary to require hospitals to conduct quality assurance programmes as a licensing requirement. In 1991, the Medical Audit & Accreditation Unit was established "to set up basic standards for all healthcare institutions, monitor and safeguard professional standards for all aspects of care, and inspect, license, monitor and accreditate all hospitals, medical clinics, nursing homes and laboratories." By 1993, two years after the Private Hospitals and Medical Clinics Act came into force, all hospitals were required to implement quality assurance programmes as a licensing requirement.[3]

---

[3] Emmanuel S. (1991) *A Review of Quality Assurance & Medical Audit Programmes in Government and Restructured Hospitals 1974–1990.* Medical Audit & Accreditation Unit, Ministry of Health.

In 1999, when the Private Hospitals and Medical Clinics Act underwent its last major revision, details of the quality assurance programmes that hospitals were directed to implement included elements and stages that reflected the steps of a generic quality improvement cycle: "monitor and evaluate"; "identify and resolve problems"; "make recommendations to improve"; and "monitor the implementation of the recommendations made."[4]

Additionally, following the example of legislation enacted in the United States and in Australia to support quality assurance programmes in healthcare, the Private Hospitals and Medical Clinics Act was revised to incorporate similar revisions to prevent forced legal disclosure of quality assurance matters in hospitals and other healthcare establishments.

Under Section 11 of the Private Hospitals and Medical Clinics Act, hospitals are required to set up Quality Assurance Committees to facilitate the conduct of effective quality assurance programmes by reviewing "the quality and appropriateness of services provided and the practices and procedures carried out"[5] at the institution. In return, members of the Quality Assurance Committees are granted protection from personal liability, and their findings cannot be used as evidence that the service or practice was inadequate or inappropriate. Neither can they be compelled to disclose their findings before a court or tribunal.

Such protection was important as the quality assurance programmes were based on a peer review process, which require doctors to evaluate and pass judgment on each other's professional performance, and removal of the possible legal consequences of participation has helped to facilitate the current high levels of open sharing and trust among healthcare professionals and institutions, both in the public and private sectors.

Sentinel Events

Prior to 2002, hospitals routinely submitted Committee of Inquiry reports every six months and Tissue Audit figures as part of reporting obligations to MOH. The Committees of Inquiry comprised external committees convened by MOH or the hospitals to review critically serious clinical incidents "so as to identify procedures and processes in the clinical management that could be modified to minimise the occurrence of similar incidents in the future." Tissue Audit focused on the frequency of removal of tissues that were subsequently found to be normal on histological examination. It served as a means of detecting surgical operations that may not have been clinically justified.[6]

---

[4] *Private Hospitals and Medical Clinics Act*, s.11(1).
[5] *Private Hospitals and Medical Clinics Act*, s.11(1)(a).
[6] Ministry of Health Singapore. (1999) *Guidelines on Tissue Audit*.

With the advent of the Sentinel Event Reporting System in May 2002, Committee of Inquiry reports were no longer required. Whereas the old Committees of Inquiry tended to be convened by MOH and focused on identifying lapses on the part of a particular individual,[7] the new Sentinel Event Reporting System relied on Quality Assurance Committees appointed by the hospital which were convened to identify systems gaps and issues that needed to be addressed in order to prevent recurrence of similar events. The Quality Assurance Committee is typically multidisciplinary in composition, and the review process would follow a prescribed sequence and employ root cause analysis methodology. While the process is not focused on identifying individuals to blame, any identified disciplinary matter would be channelled for further consideration under the hospital's disciplinary inquiry mechanism. This system was superior to the old Committees of Inquiry in that members of the Quality Assurance Committees were legally protected, as discussed above.

Extensive roadshows were organised to introduce and explain the purpose of the new reporting system to the management and clinicians at each acute hospital in order to secure buy-in. As a result of the introduction of the new reporting system, which shifted the emphasis from reporting accountability to sharing lessons and the engagement process leading up to its implementation, the number of reports received nationally grew from an average of about six to seven a year[8] to about ten times that figure in the first few years of implementation, and now stands at about 250 reports annually.

Following the occurrence of a sentinel event — now renamed as a serious reportable event — a de-identified initial notification report would be sent to MOH, followed by a subsequent detailed root cause analysis report, and finally an update indicating whether a recommendation made by the Quality Assurance Committee has been implemented. MOH collates and analyses the reports and annually releases aggregate summaries and statistics back to the institutions. From the reports received, MOH may also discern significant trends that would require further investigation or flag out cautionary alerts to be issued promptly to all hospitals in order for them to take the necessary preventive action.

Clinical Audit

Continuing along the lines of the two-tiered quality assurance approach introduced in the 1980s, one of the major provisions of the revised Private Hospitals

---

[7] Smith R. (2000) "Elsewhere, doubts had also been raised about the unsatisfactory nature of many inquiries," cf *Inquiring into inquiries*, BMJ.

[8] Source: Medical Audit & Accreditation Unit, MOH. This figure had remained fairly constant since formal quality assurance activities were introduced in government hospitals in the mid 1980s, see Emmanuel *op cit*, p. 5.

and Medical Clinics Act was to enable more effective medical audits to be carried out by the Ministry. It was envisaged that this would help to ensure the delivery of higher levels of professional standards of care. Section 12 provides an authorised officer of MOH powers of access to patient medical records without having obtained prior consent as part of medical audit of treatment rendered for certain medical conditions in order to assess the quality and appropriateness of care given to patients. Typically, areas targeted for medical audit are found where there is a large number of patients and where the cost is high, or where there is potential for "errant practice." The objective is to study the quality of clinical management for a particular group of patients and not for the purposes of identification of an individual patient, which the Act itself safeguards against.

MOH was to then closely monitor the indicator trends and reports of incidents that were routinely submitted, and to conduct focused clinical audits in areas of concern. In the initial years from 2000 onwards, the types of clinical audits that were conducted to determine appropriateness would generally fall under one of the following:

- To assess the outcomes of specific procedures in relation to volume performed, or by the experience of the doctor using a specialised equipment,
- To identify instances of upcoding of simple procedures as complex ones,
- To assess whether a complex procedure that was carried out was indicated,
- To assess whether an admission for a particular category of patients was indicated,
- To compare the complications and outcomes between a new procedure against the conventional procedure.

Such audits were resource intensive and therefore expensive to conduct. The burden of proof necessary to arrive at a definitive conclusion of poor management was often stacked against the auditors, resulting in general recommendations based on observations on performance trends. Among the factors that could account for this result are: medicine is an inexact science, underlying patient factors may themselves result in poor outcomes, the lack of clearly established criteria for determining clinical appropriateness, and necessity for benefit of the doubt given the fact that the auditors would not have all the information at their disposal based on the available clinical documentation.

However, the other kind of audit conducted — investigating "errant practices" among general practitioners, such as those who prescribed liberal amounts of sleeping pills and/or slimming pills to their patients over prolonged durations — was relatively more successful. MOH had been monitoring this situation and working closely with the Central Narcotics Bureau and the Health Sciences Authority.

In 2005, the guidelines for treatment of opiate-dependence were formulated by a national workgroup involving the expert inputs of addiction specialists from the Institute of Mental Health. This led to the successful investigation of general medical practitioners for excessive prescription of these dependence causing drugs resulting in prosecution by the Singapore Medical Council.

Clinical Performance Indicators

MOH set out to monitor the clinical performance of hospitals using a set of dashboard indicators developed by the Maryland Hospital Association in the US, that a group of hospital administrators had several years earlier identified and found suitable for their use.[9] From this list of indicators, hospitals were required to monitor and submit a set of 8 hospital-wide clinical performance indicators to MOH at six-month intervals, which included unexpected mortality, perioperative deaths, unplanned readmissions and unplanned returns to the operating theatre. From April 2000, all hospitals were mandated to participate in the international clinical benchmarking programme with international and US hospitals under the Quality Indicator Project. This meant that Singapore hospitals as a group could now be benchmarked against comparably-sized institutions internationally.

In 1999, MOH had moved away from per diem subvention for public hospitals, based on 19 clinical specialties, to a new DRG Casemix subvention system introduced as part of overall measures to control the escalation of healthcare costs. The system chosen was based on the Australian National DRG (AN-DRG) classification system.

The Casemix Taskforce, which was set up to ensure smooth implementation of the new subvention system, also recommended that the Ministry monitor the quality of clinical care as a consequence of the switch to Casemix subvention and, in particular, to look out for possible deterioration in care as tracked by measures such as premature discharges. Accordingly, in October 1998, then Director of Medical Services, Dr. Chen Ai Ju, appointed a separate Committee on Quality of Care, led by Dr. Ong Bee Ping, "To advise MOH on the appropriate quality indicators and quality of care targets to be used in a Casemix environment, and the framework for implementation of these quality indicators."

As part of the Ministry's Casemix implementation plan, Clinical Classification Committees were formed to determine the relevance and applicability of the AN-DRG classification system to local practice. Separate Medical Specialist Workgroups were formed under each Clinical Classification Committee to develop DRG-based specialty specific indicators for the purpose of monitoring the quality of care following Casemix implementation. The Medical Specialist Workgroups

---

[9] Personal communication with Mr. Liak TL.

comprised a heterogeneous mix of specialists from several related specialities. Many of them had no prior experience with development of quality indicators, and were initially concerned that the indicators would be used as a tool by the Ministry to scrutinise the practice patterns of medical practitioners. The Committee on Quality of Care, nevertheless forged on and worked with them to select a set of suitable specialty-specific clinical indicators based on those developed for the Care Evaluation Programme by the Australian Council on Healthcare Standards (ACHS). This set of indicators were discussed with and accepted by the Specialist Training Committees before they were issued to supplement the set of hospital-wide clinical indicators already introduced earlier and benchmarked internationally with the set of measures selected from the Maryland Quality Indicator Project.

Following a critical review of the mandatory reporting of clinical performance indicators, the requirement to participate in the Quality Indicator Project for benchmarking was lifted from 1 January 2005, although hospitals were encouraged to continue monitoring and benchmarking relevant indicators, which were to be used as red flags for further drill-down and corrective action. The requirement to collect and report the specialty-specific clinical indicators were also subsequently reviewed and replaced from 1 July 2009 with indicators that were developed under the National Standards for Health Care from 2008.

Unlike the previous implementation model, the National Standards for Health Care provided a performance management framework, under which strategic targets, annual targets and workplans could be specified, negotiated and set. The framework was set against the Service Agreement between MOH and the clusters. MOH also provided support in the form of funding for Healthcare Performance Offices which was sited within the institutions to drive its implementation. This is expected to result in a more concerted series of actions towards clinical outcomes and performance improvement.

Decade of Learning

In 2000, the Institute of Medicine in the US released its landmark publication *To Err is Human*. This work created a burning platform that raised the awareness of the world to the impact of errors in medicine and healthcare in general. The report cited US studies that estimated the rates and impact of medical error, and recommended urgent attention to address deficiencies in the safety of healthcare in the US. Using the same methodology, similar studies were conducted elsewhere, in Australia, New Zealand, Canada, and the United Kingdom. Estimates of the incidence of medical error among hospital inpatient admissions were generally around 10%.

Soon, questions were raised in Singapore's local media and in Parliament as to the adequacy of safeguards that were in place to ensure high standards of medical practice. Reassurance was given in terms of the presence of effective regulation with specifications for quality assurance programmes, the achievement of comparable or better outcomes in major surgical procedures such as coronary artery bypass grafting and post-surgical infection rates through benchmarking, and in the comprehensive formative and in-service training programmes for healthcare professionals that had been developed.

Around that time, the media began to spotlight reports of medication and other healthcare related errors. Following an incident in 2003 in which a student in an Environmental Health Institute laboratory became infected with the SARS virus due to biosafety lapses, reactionary criticism was quickly levelled, with calls for punishing those responsible as though their actions were criminal. In an incisive piece written in response, Dr. Edison Liu remarked that "calls for vengeance as a form of judicial deterrence solve nothing and overlook the true meaning of the events. [...] The mature question is how to prevent such incidents from happening again."[10]

This has been the default national approach to patient safety and risk management over the past decade, and one which has in our assessment, served us well in building the trust that the amendments to the Private Hospitals and Medical Clinics Act sought to preserve and promote. It involves trying to identify systematic weaknesses through a thorough analysis of adverse events and incidents. It avoids jumping to premature conclusions or pinning blame on the person at the front line even if it is convenient to do so. Instead, it balances personal responsibility and individual accountability for patient safety in a just manner,[11] using a standardised and well-established decision tree for evaluating culpability for unsafe actions or behaviour.[12]

Another significant development that occurred around that time also helped cement the trust among the hospitals and the Ministry. Adopting specialty-specific clinical indicators led to a subsequent Memorandum of Understanding (MOU) between MOH and ACHS for the latter to provide consultation and training in quality improvement. The MOU was signed in Singapore in April 2000. Two months later, a study visit to the ACHS in Sydney was conducted. The visit was led by Dr. Tan Chor Hiang, DDMS (Health Regulation) and the 14-member delegation comprised 4 MOH officers and 10 senior representatives from public and private sector hospitals. The aim of the visit was to study the development and implementation of specialty-specific clinical performance indicators under the National

---

[10] Liu E. (2003) "What's just punishment for offence?" *The Straits Times.*

[11] See Marx D. (2001) *Patient safety and the 'just culture': A primer for healthcare executives.* New York, Columbia University.

[12] Reason J. (1997) *Decision Tree for Determining Culpability for Unsafe Acts: Managing the Risks of Organizational Accidents.* Ashgate Publishing.

Medical Audit Programme and to explore opportunities for further collaboration with ACHS, spread over five-days of meetings and hospital site visits organised by the ACHS. It culminated in the formal adoption of the specialty-specific clinical indicators which were benchmarked with Australian hospitals as a supplement to the hospital-wide Quality Indicator Project measures implemented earlier.

More than that, the visit proved to be pivotal in shaping the thinking and approach taken at MOH over the next decade, and cemented ties among the senior quality leaders in MOH and public and private hospitals that paved the way for the start of a national collaborative quality journey.

Institutional Initiatives, Clustering and Quality

When the Ministry announced its plans to reorganise the public healthcare providers into two vertically integrated delivery networks in November 1999, which became incorporated in early 2000, the networks were expected to provide more integrated and better quality healthcare services through more cooperation and collaboration amongst the various providers. This would minimise duplicating services, and ensure optimal development of clinical capabilities, as well as increased efforts in collaborating for improvement.

With the increased collaboration between MOH and the two clusters, the first international healthcare quality conference in Singapore was held in September 2002. The event was co-organised by the Institute for Healthcare Improvement (IHI) in the US and the BMJ Publishing Group in UK and drew almost 800 local and international participants from 27 countries. Keynote speakers for the event include such eminent healthcare quality experts as Dr. Don Berwick from IHI, Dr. Brent James from Intermountain Health Care and Dr. John Oldham from the National Primary Care Development Team of the National Health Service in UK.

Thereafter, the Ministry and the public hospitals continued to organise the Healthcare Quality Improvement Conference each year. Within the clusters and among the larger private hospital groups, parallel quality week events were held concurrently to the conference to celebrate successfully completed quality improvement projects and to reinforce thematic emphases related to patient safety and clinical quality improvement.

Since 2002, this annual event drew a steady stream of renowned experts in the field of healthcare quality and patient safety to Singapore each year, including, aside from the experts named above, Dr. Lucian Leape, Dr. Jim Bagian, Dr. Jerod Loeb, Dr. Mark Chassin, and Dr. Rene Amalberti, among many others.

There were a number of individuals who spent extended time coaching our quality champions and imparting knowledge and skills to those who currently may be considered "local faculty." Foremost among them would be Dr. Ross Wilson. An Australian intensivist who was instrumental in conducting the landmark Quality in Australian Healthcare Study, Dr. Wilson became a prominent figure in Singapore's quality journey when he served as a consultant first to the National Healthcare Group (NHG) of hospitals and later to the SingHealth (SHS) institutions. He introduced a framework for patient safety and quality that was adopted by NHG and later SHS institutions.

Hospitals in Singapore have pushed themselves relentlessly towards higher levels of achievement in every aspect of their service and have attained many international and local awards and certification, such as ISO[13] and Singapore HEALTH Award. MOH has encouraged this effort and continues to do so. Arising from the earlier MOU with the ACHS, training sessions were held in Singapore to develop local capability in quality improvement and patient safety. Meetings were also arranged with visiting officials from specific healthcare accreditation agencies including the ACHS, Trent Accreditation, Joint Commission International (JCI), and Accreditation Canada.

When NUH became the first Singapore hospital to achieve JCI accreditation in 2004 — coupled with increasing interest expressed by other hospitals — JCI accreditation presented yet another possibility for knowledge transfer and benchmarking in the hospital sector. In conjunction with EDB, MOH facilitated the setting up of JCI's Asia Pacific Office in Singapore in September 2006. MOH also co-organised the first annual JCI Singapore International Practicum on Quality Improvement and Accreditation, which was held in June 2006. The practicum enabled local hospitals to host mock accreditation surveys and benefit from fielding staff to interact directly with global experts. Without aligning with any particular international healthcare accrediting organisation, we were nevertheless able to harness accreditation as a path to achieving "universal quality health coverage"[14] in the country.

Finally, we took the effort to celebrate our achievements and ensure that the deserving are accorded due recognition. The National Medical Excellence Awards was established in 2008 to recognise clinical and research excellence in the biomedical sciences, clinical research and medicine. In 2010, in conjunction with the third excellence award, two new award categories — the National Outstanding Clinical Quality Activist Award and the National Clinical Quality Improvement Team Award — were added to recognise clinicians for their exemplary leadership in advancing clinical quality and patient safety. Multidisciplinary institutional teams

---

[13] ISO 9001, ISO 14001, OHSAS 18001 are among the categories relevant for healthcare institutions.

[14] Mate KS, et al. (2014) "Accreditation as a path to achieving universal quality health coverage." *Globalization and Health*. **10**: 68.

were also recognised for spearheading and spreading innovations and improvements in patient care across departments and institutions, respectively.

The winners of the National Outstanding Clinical Quality Activist Award were: Associate Professor Tan Kok Hian and Mrs. Nellie Yeo (2010), Adjunct Associate Professor Tai Hwei Yee (2012), Associate Professor Quek Swee Chye (2013), and Associate Professor Ong Biauw Chi (2014). These are the most prominent from among the many who have led the way to champion patient safety and clinical quality from within their institutions and across the healthcare system in Singapore. We look forward to many more who will come after them, but that will be for the next chapter over the next 50 years.

7 The Growth and Development of Healthcare Professionals

K. Satku* and Lee Chien Earn†

A critical element that drove Singapore's healthcare standards and achievements was its professional workforce. When the nation began self-government in 1959 and then gained independence in 1965, much of the infrastructure for healthcare professional training was already in place.

A medical school had been set up in 1905 to train doctors for both Malaya and Singapore. The school gained faculty status in 1949, when the University of Malaya was formed by the amalgamation of the school — by then known as the King Edward VII College of Medicine — and Raffles College. The University of Malaya was then located in Singapore. With Malaya's independence in 1957, the Malayan Government decided to build its own university, the University of Malaya, along with a medical school in Kuala Lumpur, Malaya. The University of Malaya in Singapore was renamed in 1962 as the University of Singapore, now the National University of Singapore (NUS).

The dental school began in 1929, as the Department of Dentistry in the medical school. It became a full-fledged faculty, with the establishment of the University of Singapore in 1962.

Pharmacy education began in 1905 in the medical school's Department of Pharmaceutics, which trained individuals to dispense medication. A diploma course was introduced with the founding of the University of Malaya in 1949. This was upgraded to a degree course in 1957 and a School of Pharmacy was established at the University of Singapore in 1965.

Nurses were initially trained on the job; it was not until 1956 that a formal school for training registered staff nurses was established on the grounds of the

*Professor, Department of Orthopaedic Surgery, National University Health System; former Director of Medical Services (2004–2013), Ministry of Health, Singapore.
†Chief Executive Officer, Changi General Hospital, Singapore.

General Hospital, now Singapore General Hospital. A school to train assistant nurses was established at the Thomson Road Hospital when it was built in 1959.

The school to train radiographers was set up in 1963[1] and schools to train other allied health professionals were set up after independence.

For postgraduate studies, healthcare professionals initially had to be sent overseas, mainly to the United Kingdom, but beginning in the 1960s, part of the studies could be completed locally. By the 1970s, all of the major post-graduate programmes were locally available.

At the time of independence in 1965, Singapore's population stood at 1,865,000 and was served by 988 doctors, 342 dentists, 126 pharmacists and 4272 nurses.[2] While there would have been some healthcare professionals who had their basic training abroad, the majority had been trained locally, either in the schools of nursing or the University. Most of the dentists and pharmacists, and almost half the doctors, were in private practice. However, the majority of nurses practised in the government hospitals. The above statistics and the ratio of healthcare professionals to population are shown in Table 7.1.

Within the public service, at the time of independence, there was a significant shortage of staff of all categories. Many senior expatriate staff, doctors and nurses in particular, had left under the Malayanisation programme, so several senior staff were recruited from Israel, Japan, and Australia to help manage the transition.[3]

By the early 1970s, Singapore had sufficient numbers of healthcare professionals for its needs. However, there have been two periods when the intake of medical and dental students was reduced. It was thought that too many doctors and dentists would create an artificial, supplier-induced demand for healthcare.

The demand for healthcare has grown steadily since the new millennium and with it, the demand for healthcare professionals. This demand has partially been met by increasing the intake of the various schools. However, for medical and nursing manpower, more schools have had to be built; Singapore has had to recruit international healthcare professionals as well.

Table 7.1.   The Distribution of Healthcare Professionals in 1965

	Registered Healthcare Professionals (1965)			
Healthcare Professionals	Doctor	Dentist	Nurse	Pharmacist
Public	519*(52%)	75 (22%)	3037 (71%)	37 (29%)
Private	469 (48%)	267 (78%)	1235 (29%)	89 (71%)
Total	988	342	4272	126
Professional to Population Ratio[†]	1:1888	1:5453	1:437	1:14,800

* Including 69 House Officers.
[†]Population in 1965 1,865,000.

Table 7.2.   The Distribution of Healthcare Professionals in 2013

Healthcare Professionals	Registered Healthcare Professionals (2013)			
	Doctor	Dentist	Nurse	Pharmacist
Public	7283 (64%)	396 (22%)	21707 (60%)	1082 (46%)
Private	4150 (36%)	1411 (78%)	8826 (25%)	1104 (47%)
Others (Not working or Other jobs)			5542 (15%)	190 (7%)
Total	11433	1807	36,075	2376
Ratio	1:470	1:2990	1:180	1:2270

Population: 5,399,000 (2013).

To meet the need for doctors, we now have three schools. For registered nurses (previously termed "staff nurses"), we also have three schools: two offering diploma programmes and one a degree programme; together they have an annual output of some 1600 registered nurses. There are two schools for enrolled nurses (previously termed assistant nurses) which together have an annual output of some 350 enrolled nurses.

The clinical training for both undergraduate and postgraduate studies is done almost exclusively in our public healthcare institutions and by the healthcare professionals working in them.

Table 7.2 shows the distribution and numbers of healthcare professionals in 2013.[4–8]

Policies and Philosophies that have Guided Manpower Development

A number of policies and philosophies have guided the development and distribution of healthcare professionals.

Professional Self-regulation

Almost all healthcare professionals working in Singapore — doctors, dentists, pharmacists, nurses, allied health professionals, optometrists and opticians — are regulated by a profession-specific Act of Parliament. Broadly, these Acts allow for self-regulation. The governing body has to ensure that individuals registered to practice are competent and are fit to practice their profession, uphold the standards of practice, and retain public confidence in the profession.

The Acts governing the medical and dental professions have mandated continuing professional development as a requirement for the renewal of practicing certificates.

Health Manpower Development Plan (HMDP) and Other Training Programmes

For a nation with no natural resources, the philosophy has been to optimise the capability and capacity of each and every individual. In this respect, many opportunities are provided for the staff of public healthcare institutions to improve themselves and to excel.

In the early years as a developing nation, Singapore benefitted from scholarships offered by World Health Organisation and foreign governments. These included the WHO Fellowships, the Colombo Plan Scholarships, and Commonwealth Government Scholarships. Their numbers were, however, limited.

In 1980, the Ministry of Health established the Health Manpower Development Plan (HMDP). It was initially meant for doctors and dentists, but was subsequently extended to all healthcare professionals.[9] Under this programme, resources have been set aside to: (i) sponsor healthcare professionals for further training at centres of excellence such as the Mayo clinic and Cleveland clinic so that we learn from the best and are able to provide a similar level of service for our patients; and (ii) bring experts in various fields to spend one or more weeks in Singapore to train and guide healthcare professionals.

The programme has also been extended to help senior staff upgrade themselves through short attachments of a few weeks or a few months. The HMDP has proven to be one of the best and most successful programmes for the training and the development of our healthcare professionals. It has allowed for excellent knowledge transfer, and has built international networks and contributed immensely to the wealth of expertise that now resides in Singapore's healthcare system.

There are also other sponsorships that staff can access to attend courses or conferences, both locally and abroad.

Service Obligation

A policy that was instituted in 1978, due to a significant shortage of doctors, has now become the norm for all graduates of our medical and dental schools. This is the requirement to serve a term of some years (duration depending on course of study and citizenship) as a service obligation, in view of the heavy subsidies that medical and dental graduates receive for their education. For the other healthcare professionals such as nurses, scholarships are readily available if they have secured a place in a nursing school, but these too come with a service obligation. There is also a service obligation for those who accept fellowships and train abroad under the Health Manpower Development Plan. This policy enables the public sector institutions to have sufficient manpower to manage the large volume of work that they undertake. The service obligation also ensures that the healthcare professionals have gathered sufficient experience for independent practice should they choose to practice in the private sector.

Limiting Intake of the Best Local Students

In 1980, Dr. Tony Tan, the then-Minister of Education, spoke at a faculty of Medicine dinner. He explained that while the medical profession could be "justifiably proud of its major role in the achievement" of accessible, high quality healthcare which allowed Singaporeans to gain a standard of health which had caught up with that in developed nations, there was concern for fields other than medicine, as the number of good students who chose to study medicine and dentistry was disproportionately high. As a result, Dr. Tan remarked that "government has had to take the unpopular but necessary step of limiting the admission of bright students to the Medicine/Dentistry course so as to obtain a better spread of talent among the university disciplines."[10] Coupled with limiting the intake into these two disciplines, top students were offered scholarships in other disciplines.

This policy currently continues. In view of our small resident population, looking out for the various professions needed in Singapore necessitates ensuring that a fair number of good students take up the relevant university courses.

International Healthcare Graduates

Recognising that needs may blindside even the best of healthcare planners, a system to facilitate entry of international graduates, from schools we recognise as excellent, has been put in place. These schools are listed on the schedule of the Acts governing a profession's practice. The process enables these graduates to be registered conditionally without the need to take examinations and to begin practising in institutions accredited as having a "learning environment." This accreditation is done by the profession's regulatory body on application by the institution. In this environment, the international healthcare professionals will be supervised, provided guidance, and their performance monitored. A multi-rater assessment is also done by peers. Once they have fulfilled the required duration of supervised practice satisfactorily, they are given full registration and may choose to work at any healthcare institution. Only about 1–2% of those recruited under this scheme do not get full registration at the completion of the period of conditional registration.

While many countries insist on examinations, we have chosen not to do so. We believe that many healthcare professionals recruited under this scheme can be trained to meet our needs. Also, we avoid regulatory capture by the profession who may make exams difficult, thereby denying the state's need to recruit health-care professionals.

This "dual tap" system of local and foreign supply has worked well and has helped Singapore to manage the demand for healthcare professionals and meet the numbers required, while at the same time ensuring that standards of practice are not compromised. The process has also brought in outstanding talent and has contributed to our success in healthcare. Approximately 25% of our doctors are international medical graduates; there is a similar proportion in the nursing profession.

International Students

In all our schools which train healthcare professionals, most of the places are kept for Singapore residents. However, we have also welcomed foreign students — a few of whom can always be found in each class. This "enriches intellectual life in the university" and some of these high achievers continue to live and work in Singapore, contributing to Singapore's success. In the 1980 speech, the then-Minister Tony Tan cited the example of the medical faculty at that time, where 30 persons out of 136 academic staff were born outside Singapore, but had taken their first degrees within the country and had stayed on to teach after obtaining higher qualifications.[10] This policy of infusing some foreign students into each cohort has been maintained. The service obligations for graduates and scholarship holders ensure that they work in Singapore for, at minimum, the required period and possibly longer.

Postgraduate Education and Recognition of Professional Advancement

An important driver for excellence is the recognition and career progression accorded to individuals who pursue further studies and advance their knowledge and skills.

Among doctors, dentists, pharmacists and nurses, a career structure has been developed which recognises those who have pursued professional advancements in the form of post-graduate education. Many of these post-graduate qualifications are recognised through formal regulations. Besides the register of medical practitioners, dentists, nurses, and pharmacists, additional registers accord recognition to those who have completed post-graduate studies. For the doctors, there is a Register of Specialists and a Register of Family Physicians. For the dentists, there is a Register of Dental Specialists. For the pharmacists, there is a Register of Pharmacist Specialists; and for nurses, there is a Register of Advance Practice Nurses.

The Future

Healthcare professionals in Singapore have done well and have delivered a high level of clinical care for the population at affordable prices. A natural progression of the pursuit of excellence is healthcare specialisation and then subspecialisation. All healthcare professions are headed in this direction. While this subspecialisation may be stimulating to pursue and advantageous to the healthcare professional's practice and to patients who need sub-specialised care, we need to be careful not to allow it to be practised in isolation of general specialisation. Otherwise, this will lead to fragmentation of care and suboptimal outcomes, which may harm patients and raise healthcare costs for both the individual and the healthcare system. The White Paper on Affordable Healthcare has set limits on the proportion of doctors who can specialise, and this has been adhered to. However, this alone is insufficient to contain the fragmentation of care. We need to also ensure that the generalists such as family physicians and broad-based specialists are encouraged, given due recognition, and are empowered to provide a high level of continuing holistic care in the community as well as in the hospital. This would best serve the patient's interest. Family physicians and general practitioners also play an important role as gate-keepers of the healthcare system, preventing unnecessary cost to the patient and to the healthcare system. This will be the challenge for the leaders of the profession during the course of the next lap.

References

1. *Singapore Ministry of Health Report 1963*. Singapore-Malaya Collection, National University of Singapore Medical Library.
2. *Singapore Ministry of Health Report 1965*. Singapore-Malaya Collection, National University of Singapore Medical Library.
3. *Singapore Ministry of Health Report 1959*. Singapore-Malaya Collection, National University of Singapore Medical Library.
4. Singapore Dental Council. *Annual Report 2013*.
5. Singapore Nursing Board. *Annual Report 2013*.
6. Singapore Medical Council. *Annual report 2013*.
7. Singapore Pharmacy Council. *Annual report 2013*.
8. Department of Statistics. *Population Trends 2014*. Ministry of Trade & Industry, Republic of Singapore. ISSN 1793–2424.
9. *Singapore Ministry of Health Report 1980*. Singapore-Malaya Collection, National University of Singapore Medical Library.
10. Information Division, Ministry of Culture Singapore. *Health — A crucial Concern, Excerpts from Ministerial Speeches on Health 1980–1982*. Singapore-Malaya Collection, National University of Singapore Medical Library.

7.1 Dental Manpower Development

Patrick Tseng,* Grace Ong† and Chew Chong Lin‡

Singaporeans in general enjoy good dental health. Factors that contribute to this include our water fluoridation policy and School Dental Health Services as well as dental services provided by both our public and private dentists.

To meet the demands for dental services of the population, including school children, Singapore has been training its own dentists as well as Dental Therapists (formerly known as School Dental Nurses) for more than 50 years.

Dental Manpower

The dental needs of the population are mainly provided by dentists registered with the Singapore Dental Council. As of December 2013, we have a dentist population of 1821, giving a dentist: population ratio of 1:2960. This includes a total of 309 dental specialists.

MOH projects demand for dental manpower to increase to between 2500 to 2860 by 2030. It expects to improve the dentist: population ratio from 1:2960 to between 1:2150 to 1:1890 by 2030.

Dental training started in 1929 with the establishment of the Department of Dentistry within the King Edward VII College of Medicine, with the Department of Dentistry having gained Faculty status in August 1966. Since then, more than 2000 dentists have graduated from our local University and sixty-eight percent (68%) of our dentists have been trained locally.

The Faculty of Dentistry is well-recognised for its high quality of undergraduate training. Our curriculum has been regularly reviewed and is comparable to

*Clinical Associate Professor, Chief Dental Officer, Ministry of Health, Singapore.
†Associate Professor, Dean Faculty of Dentistry, National University of Singapore.
‡Professor, Faculty of Dentistry, National University of Singapore.

international standards. In 1997, we moved from a traditional discipline-based curriculum to a competency-based one. The most recent review, which was completed in 2012, focused on the intent to teach less but learn more. In view of the rapidly ageing population, both locally and globally, a multidisciplinary module on Geriatric Dentistry was established. The collaborative teaching of Geriatric Dentistry will help the students acquire a more comprehensive and holistic approach to managing the geriatric oral health issues.

Students are also posted for community-based experiential learning platforms like hospices and nursing homes to interact with patients and residents to inculcate into them the values of care and compassion. They are also given the opportunity to go overseas to participate in dental welfare projects (Figs. 7.1.1 and 7.1.2).

The Faculty has also embarked on exposing the students to Dental Implantology through workshops and will increasingly be using IT for teaching. This includes CAD/CAM Dentistry and the use of IT for pre-clinical training (Fig. 7.1.3).

Dental Specialists

There are currently seven (7) recognised dental specialties in Singapore namely: Dental Public Health, Endodontics, Oral & Maxillofacial Surgery, Orthodontics, Paediatric Dentistry, Periodontics and Prosthodontics. Except for Dental Public Health and Paediatric Dentistry, training in the other five (5) specialties are available in Singapore.

In 2008, there were only seven (7) paediatric dentists registered with the Singapore Dental Council. This was far short of the recommended paediatric dentist: population ratio of 1:20,000.[1,2] There was also no dentist trained in Geriatric and

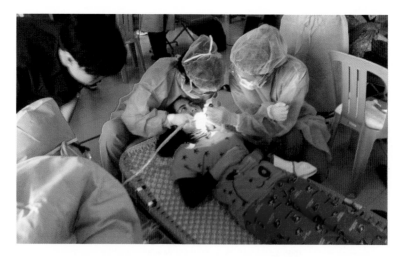

Fig. 7.1.1. Project Seam Reap in Cambodia.

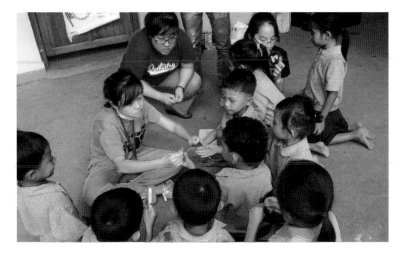

Fig. 7.1.2. Project Sabai in Cambodia.

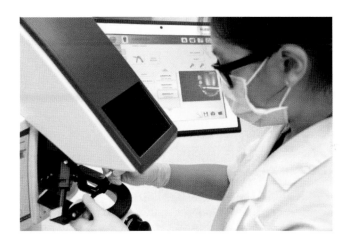

Fig. 7.1.3. The Moog simulator for preclinical training.

Special Needs Dentistry. To increase the number of specialists in paediatric dentistry and geriatric dentistry, MOH offered 18 Health Manpower Development Plan full training scholarships for graduate residency programmes in Paediatric Dentistry (9) as well as 9 for the Geriatric and Special Needs programme.

To date, we have a total of 312 dental specialists on our specialists register. The breakdown is shown in [Table 7.1.1].

Postgraduate dental education in Singapore has grown from strength to strength since the establishment of the School of Postgraduate Dental Studies in October

Table 7.1.1.   No. of Dental Specialists in Each Specialty

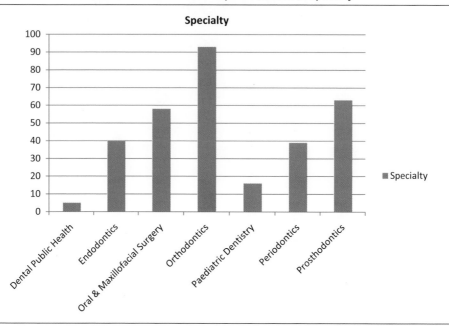

1970. To date, we have a total of 223 dentists with the Master of Dental Surgery (MDS) degrees.

Postgraduate training had moved from a non-structured to a structured 2-year programme since 1989. Subsequently, in 1999, all the five specialty programmes became 3-year structured programmes with a compulsory research component. To provide better recognition to our MDS qualifications, in view that our programmes were relatively new, we obtained agreement with Edinburgh College to conduct conjoint examinations in four (4) of the specialties except for Oral & Maxillofacial Surgery as their examination requirements are not similar to our requirements. We held the first conjoint examination in Orthodontics in 2000, Endodontics and Prosthodontics in 2001 and Periodontics in 2005. Candidates who passed the conjoint examinations were awarded the MDS from NUS and the Membership from Edinburgh University.

The MOH has also contributed to the continued development of our specialists by providing HMDP sponsorships. Over the years, 17 visiting experts have been invited to share their expertise with the profession. In addition, it continues to sponsor our trainees and specialists for overseas training.

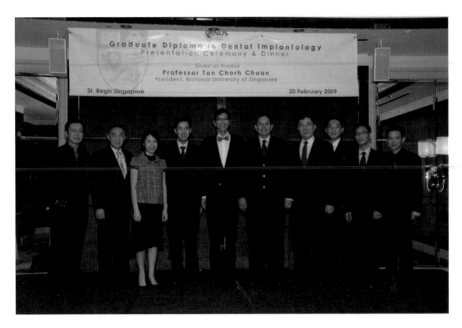

Fig. 7.1.4. First batch of graduate diploma in dental implantology students.

The Centre for Advanced Dental Education

In 2005, the Faculty set up the Centre for Advanced Dental Education to conduct training programmes to upgrade the clinical competency of our general dental practitioners. The Graduate Diploma in Dental Implantology was introduced as a 2-year part-time programme in 2007 (Fig. 7.1.4). To date, 34 dentists have graduated from this programme.

The Singapore Dental Council introduced compulsory Continuing Professional Development in October 2007 to ensure that dentists are up to date with the development in dentistry. The Centre supports this development by conducting continuing dental education courses on a regular basis.

Going forward, the Graduate Division will be starting the MDS (Paediatric Dentistry) and the Graduate Diploma in Advanced General Dentistry in July 2015 to help to meet the national demands.

Oral Health Therapists

The Oral Health Therapist training course was established in 2006. The Diploma training programme at the Nanyang Polytechnic prepares them to function both

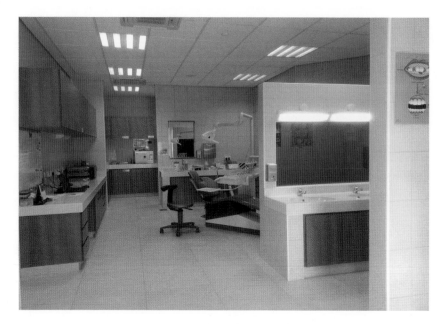

Fig. 7.1.5.   Modern school dental clinic.

as Dental Therapists and Hygienists enabling them to work in the School Dental Service and private sector. Their predecessors were the Dental Therapists and School Dental Nurses, the training of the latter started in 1962. All primary schools have a dental clinic in their premises (Fig. 7.1.5). There are a total of 364 Oral Health Therapists on our register.

The development of dental manpower is an ongoing process. In anticipation of our elderly population increasing by 2030, the MOH would need to work with institutions to do epidemiological studies to understand the dental needs of this population and plan the manpower needs accordingly.

References

1. European Academy of Paediatric Dentistry. *Newsletter,* Iss. 2, June 1997.
2. Consultants and Specialists in Paediatric Dentistry. *Publication.* Vol. 23. The British Society of Paediatric Dentistry.

7.2 Medical Manpower Development

K. Satku*

Much of the infrastructure to train physicians for the nation's needs was already in place when the nation gained independence in 1965. The medical school (now the Faculty of Medicine, National University of Singapore (NUS)) founded in 1905, had been operating for 60 years and had sufficient expertise to continue to train doctors.

In the initial years after independence, the school was still serving the needs of both Malaya and Singapore (the University of Malaya, with its medical school, in Kuala Lumpur, was only started in 1962) and of the approximately 80 graduates annually, many returned to Malaya. It was only after the introduction of the service obligation in 1978 that the graduates had to serve in Singapore[1] (see Chapter 7).

The intake of medical students varied according to the projected needs of the nation. When it was estimated that there would be too many doctors and that this could drive demand for healthcare, the intake of medical students was reduced. When the estimates fell short of the nation's needs, intake of medical students was increased. To address the needs during the intervening period (until the new intake of students graduated), the list of medical schools on the Second Schedule of the Medical Registration Act (MRA), i.e. those schools whose medical degrees are recognised in Singapore, was expanded so that the country could recruit more international medical graduates.

The current framework in place enables these international medical graduates to be conditionally registered without the need to take examinations, so that they may begin practising in institutions accredited as having a "learning environment." This accreditation is done by the Singapore Medical Council on application by the

*Chairman, Health Sciences Authority, Singapore. Professor, Department of Orthopaedic Surgery, National University Health System, Singapore. Professor of Health Policy, Saw Swee Hock School of Public Health, National University of Singapore. Former Director of Medical Services (2004–2013), Ministry of Health, Singapore.

institution. In this environment, the international medical graduates are supervised, provided guidance, and their performance is monitored. A multi-rater assessment is also done by peers. Once they have fulfilled the required duration of supervised practice satisfactorily, these doctors are given full medical registration and may choose to work in any healthcare institution.

Since 2004, the estimated number of doctors required has been increased substantially in anticipation of the needs of an ageing population. Thus, the intake of students to our medical schools has increased. The current intake is about 400 students annually. The number of schools on the Schedule has also increased, with 159 schools from 28 countries on the Schedule.

The increased number of schools on this Schedule also allows Singaporeans who have not been able to enter the local medical schools and who wish to return to practise medicine in Singapore, to apply to any of the schools on the Second Schedule to study medicine. In recent years, the state has offered grants for the later years of study for Singaporeans studying abroad in the schools on the Schedule. This grant is tied with the service obligation which brings the Singaporeans back to work in Singapore.

With the growth of the biomedical sector and recognising the demand for clinician scientists, the Duke-NUS School of Medicine (a graduate entry programme) was set up in 2005 through a collaboration with Duke University, Durham, USA. Duke-NUS's current annual intake is approximately 70 students and remains focussed on producing clinician scientists.

A collaboration with Imperial College, London began in 2009 for a third medical school. The Lee Kong Chian School of Medicine (LKC SoM), an Advanced-level/International Baccalaureate entry programme, to train doctors for service, opened its doors in 2013. LKC SoM is expected to increase its intake to about 150 to 200 students annually. We can expect about 500 to 600 doctors to graduate annually from our 3 medical schools from about the early 2020s.

Clinical teaching for the three medical schools is carried out almost exclusively in the public healthcare institutions. Figure 7.2.1 shows the Yong Loo Lin School of Medicine, NUS, the oldest and largest medical school in Singapore.

Through the Medical Registration Ordinance in the initial years and later the Medical Registration Act (1970), the privilege to practice medicine is limited to those with recognised qualifications registered with the Singapore Medical Council (SMC). The Medical Registration Act enables the profession to self-regulate with the stated objective of protecting the health and safety of the public by providing for mechanisms to:

a. Ensure that registered medical practitioners are competent and fit to practise medicine;
b. Uphold standards of practice within the medical profession; and
c. Maintain public confidence in the medical profession.

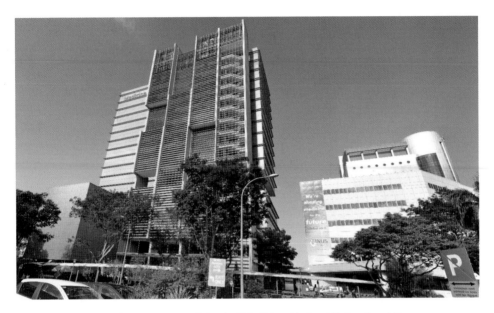

Fig. 7.2.1. The Yong Loo Lin School of Medicine, National University of Singapore.

The population of physicians has grown significantly over the years. In 1965 there was a total of 988 physicians (including 69 house officers) for Singapore's resident population of 1.8 million — 1 doctor for every 1900 people.[2]

With a resident population of 5.4 million in 2013, the number of physicians was 11,433 (including 480 house officers). This gives a ratio of 1 doctor for every 470 people.[3,4] [See Table 7.2.1]

The population has grown three-fold over the last five decades and the doctor population 11-fold. Approximately 60% of our doctors are locally trained.

Postgraduate Education

The path to specialisation began before Singapore's independence. In the early years doctors had to go abroad, in particular to the UK, to be trained and pass the Royal College exams to be certified as specialists. Because substantial periods had to be spent in training in the UK, the numbers of specialists that we could train was small. Between 1946 and 1960, 40 local doctors obtained postgraduate qualifications.[5]

However when Singapore began to have a sufficient number of qualified staff to train specialists, we began part of the training locally. In 1961, a Committee on Post Graduate Medical Studies was formed, with representatives from the major professional organisations such as the Faculty of Medicine and the Ministry of Health.[6] Significant help was obtained from the Royal Australian Colleges. The Committee organised full-time courses in basic medical sciences leading to the primary Fellowship of the

Table 7.2.1. Number of Medical Practitioners by Residential Status, Place of Training and Employment Sector

Registration Type	Public Sector							Private Sector							Grand Total
	Singapore Residents				Non-Residents		Public Sector Total	Singapore Residents				Non-Residents		Private Sector Total	
	Singapore Citizens Local Trained	Singapore Citizens Foreign Trained	Singapore Permanent Residents Local Trained	Singapore Permanent Residents Foreign Trained	Non-Residents Local Trained	Non-Residents Foreign Trained		Singapore Citizens Local Trained	Singapore Citizens Foreign Trained	Singapore Permanent Residents Local Trained	Singapore Permanent Residents Foreign Trained	Non-Residents Local Trained	Non-Residents Foreign Trained		
Full Registration	3281	493	214	421	72	341	4822	2788	655	188	266	16	72	3985	8807
Conditional Registration	26	281	4	217	7	1074	1609	—	15	—	29	—	100	144	1753
Provisional Registration	262	69	13	6	23	107	480	—	—	—	—	—	—	—	480
Temporary Registration (Service)	—	5	—	32	—	335	372	—	—	—	6	—	15	21	393
Grand Total	3569	848	231	676	102	1857	7283	2788	670	188	301	16	187	4150	11433

Royal Australian College of Surgeons (FRACS) examinations and courses for the written examinations for Fellowship of the Royal Australian College of Physicians (FRACP). Instructors were guest lecturers from Australia and local teachers. The Colleges accredited the local hospitals as training sites so that the trainees' initial training in Singapore could be recognised and contribute to the required training duration for qualifying to sit the Royal Australian Colleges' examinations. By special arrangements with the Royal Australian Colleges, candidates who passed the written examinations could do further training in Australia and sit the final examinations in Australia.[6] The next 10 years saw the certification of 86 doctors as specialists.[5]

By 1970, it was acknowledged that we were ready for our own postgraduate training school as there were enough specialists and there was a core of experienced teachers within the country. The School of Postgraduate Medical Studies was set up, independent of the Faculty of Medicine, under a board comprising members from the Faculty of Medicine, the Academy of Medicine and the Ministry of Health. The early programmes were for the Master of Medicine in Internal Medicine, Paediatrics, Surgery, and Obstetrics and Gynaecology, with Anaesthesia and Public Health added later. The Master of Medicine conferred by the School for Public Health was later changed to a MSc Public Health.[5]

Rigorous standards were set and candidates had to fulfil training requirements before they could sit the examinations. This emphasis to fulfil training was increased by selection of the doctors as trainees for specialist training. To guard against isolation and self-satisfaction that could lead to obsolescence, course teachers from abroad were enlisted and both internal as well as external examiners were appointed. Over the next 12 years 391 doctors were certified as having completed their postgraduate examinations.[5] Despite an increase in the number of specialists leaving for private practice, the public sector had a sufficient number of specialists.

The training programme and examinations for the various specialties have not progressed in a uniform manner. The training for all specialties is now conducted locally. While Singapore has gained much from the British system of undergraduate medical education and specialist training, the prevailing system of postgraduate education based on an apprenticeship style of training was reviewed in 2006. A decision was made to adapt the US system of residency training, contextualised to our needs, for our postgraduate training. This was implemented in phases starting in 2010.

The key features of the system include a well-defined curriculum, a system of assessments including regular formative assessment, dedicated faculty with protected time, and a rigorous system of accreditation of the training institutions.

The summative assessments are still designed very much in the UK style with intermediate and exit examinations. While some specialties such as anaesthesia and public health have been conducting the examinations locally for years, other specialties have developed conjoint examinations with the UK Royal Colleges in the spirit of the initial years. With the switch to a "residency style" of training, the opportunity to develop collaborations with the American Board of Medical Specialties was taken to enable Singapore to develop intermediate or exit examinations. These collaborations are ongoing and it is hoped that we will be able to make some progress with respect to developing our own postgraduate examinations.

Specialist Certification

In the early years, the Ministry of Health was entirely responsible for certifying individuals as specialists. In the 1970s and 1980s this function was done together with the Academy of Medicine and the School of Graduate Medical Studies at the NUS.

In 1998 the Medical Registration Act (MRA) was amended and a Statutory Body, known as the Specialist Accreditation Board (SAB), was set up under the provisions of the Act and was given the responsibility to oversee specialist accreditation. The pathway to accreditation was subsequently established by the SAB for local trainees. Although specialist qualifications from the UK, Australia, US, Canada, and the European Union were recognised, specialists were accredited on a case-by-case basis after review of their training. In 2005 the SAB formalised a framework for specialists trained abroad. They are subject to the same supervisory framework as international medical graduates; and are accorded conditional registration and are required to be under supervision for two years.

In an attempt to contain fragmentation and the growing trend to sub-specialise, the SAB in 2012 permitted dual accreditation and also introduced five subspecialties. We now have 4124 specialists registered for practice in Singapore. Of this number, 274 are either doubly accredited in another specialty or are also accredited in a subspecialty.

A White Paper on sustainable healthcare in 1993 set a limit of 40% for the proportion of specialists within the healthcare system and this has not been exceeded.[7]

The Table 7.2.2 below lists the specialties and subspecialties.

Approximately 37% of all specialists are in private practice while about 63% are in our public healthcare institutions.

In 2010 the MRA was amended to recognise general practitioners who had obtained further qualifications, to be registered as Family Physicians. Today, 1400 of the some 2000 general practitioners in Singapore have been accredited as Family Physicians. The majority of the Family Physicians are in private practice. Less than 300 are in public healthcare institutions. The Family Physicians in the public sector have a career track similar to specialists. If enough family physicians can be retained in the public sector as in the case of specialists, the public sector may play a larger role in primary care services than it has hitherto done.

Table 7.2.2.   Number of Specialists by Specialities as at 31 December 2013

Registered Specialty	Public Sector		Private Sector		Total
	Number	%	Number	%	
Anaesthesiology	230	61.3	145	38.7	375
Cardiology	113	62.4	68 (1)	37.6	181 (1)
Cardiothoracic Surgery	30	69.0	13	30.2	43
Dermatology	57	57.0	43	43.0	100
Diagnostic Radiology	181	70.0	77	29.8	258
Emergency Medicine	111	94.1	7	5.9	118
Endocrinology	68 (1)	73.9	24 (1)	26.1	92 (2)
Gastroenterology	64 (3)	62.7	38	37.3	102 (3)
General Surgery	143	53.4	125	46.5	268
Geriatric Medicine	65 (2)	89.0	8	11.0	73 (2)
Haematology	39 (1)	75.0	13	25.0	52 (1)
Hand Surgery	21	72.4	8	27.6	29
Infectious Diseases	39 (2)	76.5	12	23.5	51 (2)
Internal Medicine	70 (1)	69.3	31	30.7	101 (1)
Medical Oncology	56	59.6	38 (1)	40.4	94 (1)
Neurology	57	74.0	20	26.0	77
Neurosurgery	24	61.5	15	38.5	39
Nuclear Medicine	12	57.1	9	42.9	21
Obstetrics & Gynaecology	89	29.3	215	70.7	304
Occupational Medicine	17	45.9	20	54.1	37
Ophthalmology	128	62.7	76	37.3	204
Orthopaedic Surgery	112	60.9	72	39.1	184
Otorhinolaryngology	55	53.9	47	46.1	102
Paediatric Medicine	178	55.3	144	44.7	322
Paediatric Surgery	15	78.9	4	21.1	19
Pathology	112	81.8	25	18.2	137
Plastic Surgery	29	52.7	26	47.3	55
Psychiatry	130	69.5	57	30.5	187
Public Health	59	56.7	45	43.3	104
Radiation Oncology	38	86.4	6	13.6	44
Rehabilitation Medicine	28	90.3	3	9.7	31
Renal Medicine	53	74.6	18	25.4	71
Respiratory Medicine	70	72.9	26 (1)	27.1	96 (1)

(*Continued*)

Table 7.2.2.   (Continued)

Registered Specialty	Public Sector		Private Sector		Total
	Number	%	Number	%	
Rheumatology	37 (3)	78.7	10 (1)	21.3	47 (4)
Urology	42	55.3	34	44.7	76
Sub Total	**2572 (13)**	**62.8**	**1522 (5)**	**37.2**	4094 (18)
Sub-Specialties (4)					
Intensive Care Medicine	1 (99)	100.0	(69)	0.0	1 (168)
Neonatology	1 (29)	100.0	(24)	0.0	1 (53)
Palliative Medicine	8 (21)	53.3	7 (5)	46.7	15 (26)
Sports Medicine	7 (4)	53.8	6 (6)	46.2	13 (10)
Sub Total	17 (153)	56.7	13 (104)	43.3	30 (257)
Grand Total	2589 (166)	62.8	1535 (108)	37.2	4124 (274[8])

Conclusion

The investments in professional development have created a medical workforce that has contributed significantly to the transformation of the health of the population. The profession is deeply rooted in its values and has pursued goals primarily for the benefit of the patients it serves. The free market environment and emerging trends such as healthcare as a business threaten this paradigm. Much responsibility rests on the Singapore Medical Council, which as the profession's regulatory body, has to steer the profession and chart its future.

References

1. Service obligation SMOH report (1975).
2. *Singapore Ministry of Health Report* (1965) Singapore-Malaya Collection, National University of Singapore Medical Library.
3. Singapore Medical Council. *Annual Report 2013.*
4. Department of Statistics, Ministry of Trade & Industry. *Population Trends 2014.* Republic of Singapore ISSN, pp. 1793–2424.
5. HB Wong. (1982) "Postgraduate medical education in Singapore." *Annals of the Academy of Medicine* **11**(3): 473–477.
6. Seah CS. (1982) "Medical Progress in Singapore — A review of the last three decades 1951–1980." *Annals of the Academy of Medicine.* **11**(3): 309–312.
7. Ministry of Health. (1993) *Affordable Health Care — A White Paper.* Published by SNP Pte Limited. ISBN 9971-88-390-2.
8. Singapore Medical Council Annual Report 2013.

7.3 Pharmacy Manpower Development

Lita Chew* and Azah Subari†

Pharmacy in Singapore has undergone metamorphic changes over the last five decades. The pharmacy practice model has both evolved slowly and changed rapidly, keeping in pace with the growth of Singapore's medical and healthcare sectors.

From the early 1950s to the early 1980s, pharmacy practice focused heavily on small-scale manufacturing and distribution of medications. Medicines for government hospitals and outpatient dispensaries were manufactured and supplied by the Government Pharmaceutical Laboratory and Store. Hospitals also carried out small-scale manufacturing activities for lotions, ointments, creams, and other extemporaneous preparations. Public sector pharmacists performed various pre-packaging activities from the bulk supplied by the government manufactory. Pharmacists spent most of their time in the pharmacy and patient records were paper records, and were not readily accessible to the pharmacist.

The study of pharmacy began to take shape in the 1950s, with a two-year diploma course introduced in 1951, followed by a degree course in 1957. Pre-registration pupillage or training, which had been in place as early as 1910, was shortened to one year after the introduction of the degree course. In 1970, the Bachelor of Pharmacy degree was replaced with the Bachelor of Science (Pharmacy) degree to mainly reflect the increasing scientific content of the course.

The law for pharmacist registration was first gazetted as the Straits Settlement Registration of Pharmacists Ordinance in 1903. In 1935, Pharmacists Ordinance was passed, resulting in the establishment of a Pharmacy Board with statutory powers

*Chief Pharmacist, Ministry of Health; Assistant Professor, Pharmacy Department, National University of Singapore; Head, Pharmacy Department, National Cancer Centre, Singapore.
†Senior Manager, Chief Pharmacist office, Ministry of Health, Singapore.

over the registration, discipline, and training of pharmacists. In 1979, the Pharmacists Registration Act was passed in Parliament and replaced the Pharmacists Ordinance, which allowed the pharmacy profession to be self-governing by altering the composition of the Pharmacy Board to comprise members of the profession only. The revised Act came into force in January 1981.

The 1980s saw significant changes as the role of the pharmacists evolved from one that was drug-oriented to one that was patient-oriented. Manufacturing activities in the former Pharmaceutical Department at the Ministry of Health ceased in 1987. Pharmacy facilities were upgraded, machines were brought in for repackaging, and a computer system was introduced in government hospitals and primary health-care pharmacies to label and charge for medications. There was greater focus on the pharmacists as part of the healthcare team, with pharmacists playing a bigger role in patient counselling and offering drug information to both the public and to healthcare professionals.

In the 1990s, the transformation in pharmacy practice towards a patient-centric model gained great momentum. Pharmacists in hospitals, working in inpatient wards and outpatient specialist clinics, were getting more involved in improving the outcome of drug treatment by providing clinical pharmacy services on therapeutic drug monitoring and dose adjustment, as well as specialised medication counselling for asthma, diabetes, hypertension, and oncology.

In 1997, the pharmacy course was extended to four years to provide for more training of patient-oriented skills to support a pharmaceutical care model of the future. A 12-week Pharmacy Practice Preceptorship Programme was incorporated into the course to allow students to imbibe professional ethics and practices under the tutelage of experienced practitioners.

Since 2004, pharmacist preceptors have been trained through workshops to mentor, coach, and lead pre-registration pharmacists. The skills of clinical preceptors have also been upgraded in order to support the development of structured local pharmacy residency training programmes. The Medical Education Unit of the Yong Loo Lin School of Medicine, and the American College of Clinical Pharmacy have been engaged to conduct workshops for clinical assessment and learning.

In 2006, a competency standards framework was developed to strengthen the professional excellence of pharmacists practising in Singapore. It states the minimum competency standards for entry to practice, the desired outcomes of pre-registration training, and the exit criteria to enter the Singapore Register of Pharmacists. The Pharmacist's Pledge was adopted in 2008, embodying the values, ethics, vision and professionalism to remind pharmacists of their duties and responsibilities to their patients, to their colleagues, and to the public.

With the aim to help raise the practice standards of pharmacists and ensure that the laws remain relevant to the practice of pharmacy, the Pharmacists Registration Act was revised in 2007 and came into effect on 1 September 2008. The Singapore Pharmacy Council (SPC) was established as a statutory board, with enhanced powers to enable it to perform its regulatory functions more effectively. In addition to full registration, conditional and temporary registrations of pharmacists were also introduced under the SPC. Compulsory continuing professional education for pharmacists was also implemented so that pharmacists will continually upgrade themselves and keep abreast of the latest developments in the field of pharmacy.

Biotechnology, genomics, proteomics, and nanotechnology, have contributed to the increasing number of therapeutic entities and the complexity of treatments. Pharmacists with specialised expertise are increasingly required, for example, in pharmacotherapy, oncology, critical care, and geriatrics, to ensure safe, evidence-based and cost-effective use of medicines for better patient outcomes. Responding to this, as well as a growing number of pharmacists with specialised qualifications, provisions for a separate register for specialist pharmacists and the registration of such specialists has been put in place. In February 2012, the Specialists Accreditation Board for Pharmacy (PSAB) was appointed by the Minister for Health to define pharmacy specialities and to determine the requirements for specialist registration. Specialist pharmacist accreditation and registration commenced in October 2012. Twenty-eight specialist pharmacists were accredited by the PSAB as of 30 September 2013.

Since 2008, the MOH has set aside funding for scholarships to equip pharmacists in the public sector with the right skills and advanced knowledge to meet the healthcare needs of the population. These scholarships would enable pharmacists to pursue postgraduate education and overseas pharmacy residency training in specialised practice. In 2009, National University of Singapore (NUS) started the Doctor in Pharmacy (PharmD) program to train pharmacy practitioners in clinical leadership to assume expanded responsibilities in the care of patients and be at the forefront of the pharmacy profession and healthcare.

In response to training needs, pharmacy residency training programmes were developed by NUS and local institutions to provide structured postgraduate training for advanced-level clinical practice. In 2008, Singapore General Hospital (SGH) commenced the Infectious Disease Pharmacotherapy Residency programme (PGY2). NUS Department of Pharmacy commenced a clinical pharmacy residency in Haematology/Oncology (PGY2) in 2010, in collaboration with the National Cancer Centre Singapore, NUH and SGH. In 2012, NUH commenced a broad-based clinical pharmacotherapy programme (PGY1) intended as a foundation for advanced-level or specialised clinical practice. In 2014, NUS Department of Pharmacy commenced the

Postgraduate Year Two (PGY2) Ambulatory Care Pharmacy Residency in conjunction with Tan Tock Seng Hospital and National Healthcare Group Polyclinic Pharmacy.

In retrospect, comparing the practice model and human resources that we have had in the past to the one that we have today, the pharmacy profession has indeed witnessed metamorphic changes. The profession's movement towards patient-centric practice which started in the 1990s, continues to be moving in tandem with emerging practice trends and patient care needs. A unified philosophy that clearly identifies the patient as the primary beneficiary of the profession and pharmacy services will continue to be the invisible force that moves the profession as a body to meet the rising demands on the healthcare system and changes in the delivery of healthcare.

References

1. Ministry of Health, Singapore. (2002) *Pharmacy in Singapore — A Journey through the Years.*
2. Department of Pharmacy. (2012) "NUS Pharmacy — The Pharmily History." National University of Singapore. www.pharmacy.nus.edu.sg/about/history.html. Accessed on 8 Dec 2014.
3. Pharmaceutical Society of Singapore. (2012) www.pss.org.sg/about-pss. Accessed on 8 Dec 2014.

7.4 Allied Health Professionals

Lau Hong Choon*, Elaine Teo[†],
Celia Tan Ia Choo[‡], Lau Cheng Mun[§],
Lim Hua Beng[¶], Melissa Chua[||], Gary Tan**,
Jasper Tong[††] and Gladys Wong[‡‡]

The Allied Health Professions in Singapore — An Overview

The Allied Health Professions are a diverse yet common group of healthcare professionals providing care to patients. Although there is no international consensus on the healthcare professions under the umbrella of "allied health" professions, it is used in Singapore to refer to healthcare professions who work alongside the

*Director, Manpower Standards and Development Division, Ministry of Health, 16 College Road, Singapore 169854.

[†]Deputy Director, Manpower Standards and Development Division, Ministry of Health, 16 College Road, Singapore 169854.

[‡]Group Director, Allied Health, Singapore Health Services, 168 Jalan Bukit Merah #03-02 Surbana One S(150168).

[§]Director, Allied Health, Nanyang Polytechnic, School of Health Sciences, 180 Ang Mo Kio Ave 8, Singapore 569830.

[¶]Manager, Occupational Therapy, Nanyang Polytechnic, School of Health Sciences, 180 Ang Mo Kio Ave 8, Singapore 569830.

[||]Head, Speech Therapy, Singapore General Hospital, Speech Therapy Department, Outram Road, Singapore 169608.

**Manager, Diagnostic Radiology, Singapore General Hospital, Outram Road, Singapore 169608.

[††] Deputy Group Director, Allied Health (Service Integration), Singapore Health Services, 168 Jalan Bukit Merah #03-02 Surbana One S(150168).

[‡‡]Chief Dietitian, Khoo Teck Puat Hospital, Department of Nutrition and Dietetics, 90 Yishun Central S768828.

doctors and nurses in the public healthcare system; for example, radiographers, physiotherapists, occupational therapists, clinical psychologists, speech therapists, podiatrists, audiologists, medical social workers, and dieticians, amongst others. In healthcare, allied health professionals are integral members of various multi-disciplinary healthcare teams. Many of the allied health professions also offer essential services in the social services and special education sectors in Singapore.

In hospitals, occupational therapists provide rehabilitation from injury or diseases, such as hand therapy, driving assessment, burns and plastics rehabilitation, and oncology rehabilitation, to name a few. In the special schools and disability services, occupational therapists work with children and young adults with development disorders, or physical disabilities to help them to achieve maximum independence in self-care, play, school perfomance or work, and living in the community despite their disabilities.

Prior to the more common use of the term "allied health" in recent years, these professions were also referred to in the past as "paramedical professions," "professions supplementary to medicine," or "health sciences professions." This may erroneously give the impression that the allied health professions held largely technical and/or subordinate roles to the medical doctors in healthcare when, in fact, the allied health professions have emerged to meet distinct patient needs alongside the developments in technology, medical science, public health, and health systems.

Podiatry had its humble beginnings at TTSH in 1993. At that time, the first podiatrist worked in the Artificial Limbs Centre to provide wound care for patients suffering from diabetic foot ulcers. Today, there are podiatrists in every restructured hospital, providing services such as clinical gait analysis, orthotic therapy, and nail surgery under local anaesthesia.

Over time, the allied health professions have developed a core body of knowledge, skills, and expertise in their specific disciplines. Some of these professions, such as physiotherapy, speech therapy, and podiatry, have developed the tools and capability to assess and provide interventions within their specialised areas of practice. Education and training levels required for entry-to-practice evolved over time to commensurate with the increasing complexity of their jobs, along with the need for such professionals to make independent decisions in their practice and care of patients. Tertiary education at the degree level typifies the preparatory training for entry-to-practice in the various allied health professions. In some countries, the training has evolved to Masters or Clinical Doctorates.

Development of the Allied Health Professions in Singapore

The larger groups of allied health professions, such as radiographers, physiotherapists and occupational therapists, were first introduced to Singapore by the British in the early 20th Century. At that time, qualified radiographers, physiotherapists, and occupational therapists were all expatriates and were supported in their work by hospital attendants and nurses. By the mid-1950s, the government started to send Singaporeans to be trained overseas in the various allied health disciplines through the Colombo Plan Scholarships to build local capability in healthcare. Subsequently, Singapore government scholarships were established by the Public Service Commission to attract talent into these allied health services for the public sector.

Demand for allied health services in Singapore were spurred by the various public health issues of the time. In the post-World War II period and early years of Singapore's development in the 1950s and 1960s, the high incidence of polio and post-war injuries drove the demand for physiotherapists and occupational therapists for the rehabilitation of the patients. With the prevalence of tuberculosis then, there was also a high demand for radiographers to perform X-rays and physiotherapists to improve lung function through chest percussion and drainage. Similarly, malnutrition and food safety issues drove the demand for nutritionists, and they worked closely with public health practitioners to roll out national programmes to improve nutrition for children in schools and for pregnant mothers.

As Singapore developed, new public health issues emerged with longer life spans and affluence. Cancers and chronic diseases, such as diabetes, hypertension, heart disease, stroke, and mental health issues became more prevalent. The demographic shift to an older population with more chronic disabilities expanded the demand for allied health services from the management and rehabilitation of acute conditions and diseases in hospitals to rehabilitation services in the community and long-term care sector.

Training and Education of Allied Health Professionals

With rising demand for the various allied health services, the overseas scholarships could not produce enough numbers to meet the growing need, so local allied health education and training was developed. The School of Radiography in the

Outram Campus was set up in 1963, and was helmed by the returned Colombo Plan scholars to train diagnostic radiographers. The School of Radiography introduced the Diploma programme in Therapeutic Radiography in 1975.

Although there were plans to increase the number of occupational therapists and physiotherapists to support Singapore's rehabilitation needs in the 1980s, the start of these plans for local education in the allied health professions was unfortunately not ready in time to avert a crisis in physiotherapy services by 1988. Four out of six government hospitals had to close outpatient physiotherapy services at that time due to an acute shortage of physiotherapists from attrition and inadequate supply. Local diploma programmes in physiotherapy and occupational therapy were eventually set up in 1992 in the the newly established Nanyang Polytechnic in collaboration with the University of Sydney (UOS) with a team from UOS headed by Associate Professor Ron McCartney. The Nanyang Polytechnic School of Health Sciences started in Outram Campus before moving to the new Ang Mo Kio campus in 1998. At that time, the School of Radiography (which started in 1963) and the Radiation Therapy programme (which started in 1975 at the School of Radiography) were transferred to Nanyang Polytechnic as well.

Over time, other local allied health degree programmes were introduced. These included the Masters in Speech and Language Pathology set up at the National University of Singapore in 2007; and the Masters in Psychology (Clinical) in 2009, and the Masters of Science in Audiology in 2013. Local degree-conversion programmes were set up in 2012 for physiotherapy and occupational therapy at the newly established Singapore Institute of Technology, and degree-conversion programmes in radiography and radiation therapy were introduced in 2014 with a view to develop full degree programmes in these professions over time to meet Singapore's needs for these allied health professionals. There is great anticipation amongst the allied health professionals for the launch of the full 4-year local degree programmes in the Singapore Institute of Technology planned for 2016.

For smaller allied health professions, such as podiatry and orthoptics, which do not have the scale or intakes to support local training, overseas training and education will remain the mainstay. Postgraduate training of allied health professionals through the Health Manpower Development Plan is also supported through overseas attachments and through the visiting experts programme.

Regulation of the Allied Health Professions

Regulation of the various allied health professions evolved with the development of the professions in Singapore. Many of the allied health professions established professional associations and societies to promote the profession's development. The associations and societies exercise a limited measure of self-regulation amongst its members to maintain professional standards. As the numbers in these professions grew and services expanded, developments in these professions raised several concerns for the associations and societies. These ranged from those masquerading as bona fide professionals to others with dubious professional conduct and competence. As membership in the associations and societies were voluntary, and these professional bodies did not have any statutory powers, self-regulation through these bodies were ineffective.

The Allied Health professional community worked with the Ministry of Health to establish the Allied Health Professions (AHP) Act and the Allied Health Professions Council in 2011 to regulate the allied health professionals' conduct, ethics, and practice. The primary purpose of the law and the regulator was to protect public interest through mandating registration and regulation for specific groups of allied health professions. The occupational therapists (OT), physiotherapists (PT), and speech therapists (ST), were registered in the first phase of implementation in 2013. Statutory registration and regulation for other groups in the Act will be implemented in phases over time.

References

1. Chng, Yi Hong, Ler, Marvin Bor Lin. (2008) *Celebrating 50 Years of Illuminating Lives: Singapore Society of Radiographers, Golden Jubilee, 1958–2008*. Singapore Society of Radiographers.
2. Wong WP. (2008) *Celebrating the Past, Advancing into the Future, Physiotherapy at Singapore General Hospital*. Department of Physiotherapy, Singapore General Hospital. Armour Publishing.

Nursing Manpower Development

Ang Wei Kiat* and Pauline C.J. Tan†

Nursing as a profession started in Singapore in 1885 and has since touched the lives of many sick and infirmed. Today, 130 years later, nurses form the backbone of the public healthcare system, comprising more than 60% of the healthcare workforce. Nurses journey with patients through various life stages — from conception, to child health, to school health, to adulthood, and to end-of-life or palliative care. This chapter will look at how nursing started in Singapore and how, over time, it envisioned its role for the future as it continued to play a vital role in Singapore's healthcare system.

Early Beginnings

In the early years of Singapore's history after becoming a British colony, the rapidly expanding population accentuated the need for proper healthcare facilities. Care was inadequate and was provided by medical subordinates, dressers, orderlies, and patients' themselves. In 1885, French nuns answered the call to care for the sick. Although untrained, they performed limited simple nursing duties such as cleaning and cooking with selfless dedication, which brought much comfort to patients.

Strong public support for proper nursing training led to the arrival of trained English nurses in 1900. At that time, high infant mortality rate plagued Singapore (269 per 1000 live births). Mrs. Blundell, a Municipal nurse, was tasked with the responsibility of instructing non-European mothers in the proper care of their infants. In 1910, the Maternal and Child Health Services was established and training of pupil midwives was set up.

*Nurse Manager, Nursing Service, Tan Tock Seng Hospital.
†Chief Executive Officer, Yishun Community Hospital, Alexandra Health System & Immediate past Chief Nursing Officer (2007–2014), Ministry of Health, Singapore.

As demand for nurses grew, a structured nursing programme was instituted. In 1916, General Nurse Training commenced at St. Andrew's hospital (Picture 1 of Annex). Eight years later in 1924, a four-year nursing training programme based on the medical model started at the General Hospital. In 1929, the first local Health Nurse, Mrs. ME Perera was hired by St. Andrew's Mission Hospital. In 1937, she became the first locally appointed Nursing Sister and in 1952, was promoted to Public Health Matron. By 1962, the highest nursing positions in Singapore were held by local nurses — Miss KN Lim, who was Principal Matron, and Miss HL Ling, who became Senior Tutor. Both were designated as Chief Nursing Officer and Principal Nursing Officer (Tutor), respectively in 1974.

Public Health Nursing

In the 1920s, with more emphasis on public health, the School Health Service was introduced and local midwives provided smallpox vaccinations. In 1927, Singapore's first Public Health nurse, Miss Ida Mabel Murray Simmons, was appointed to extend child health services to the rural areas (Picture 2 of Annex). She made use of a mobile dispensary to make routine visits to monitor the development of new-borns in their first year of life. She also educated mothers on infant feeding methods, maternal and infant nutrition and basic infant care. She trained local nurses and midwives, who formed the core team of staff manning the rural welfare centres. Their efforts paid off. In 1938, there was significant reduction in infant mortality rate to 86 per 1000 babies. Miss Simmons would eventually establish a rural healthcare service that comprised 17 rural maternity and child health centres operated by a team of local nurses (Picture 3 of Annex).

The school health nurse assisted the school female doctor during medical inspection; treating and following up on malnutrition, sores, head lice and worm infection in children. She also "rounded up" and sent school children to dental clinics for treatment. School nurses in the "travelling dispensary" conducted regular home visits and used deworming drugs, tonics, skin lotions and other medications to treat children (Picture 4 of Annex).

In 1924, the Pauper Hospital for Women and Children in Kandang Kerbau was established to provide maternity care and training for medical students and pupil midwives in an attempt to reduce mortality rates. In 1938, half of the 11,206 babies born in Singapore were delivered at KKH.

The outbreak of World War II in 1942 disrupted nursing development in Singapore as nurses were allowed to return home or leave Singapore and those who stayed were transferred to the Mental Hospital. During this chaotic and difficult time, nurses continued to care for their patients. Anecdotal records reported that the nurses packed essential drugs into urinals and smuggled them from the General Hospital to the Mental Hospital against the orders of the Japanese soldiers.

Drugs became so scarce that the staff stretched the stocks for $3\frac{1}{2}$ years, relying on good nursing, and only turning to medicine as a last resort. After the war ended in 1945, local nurses continued to make rapid strides in areas of career development, autonomy, recognition, and education.

Nursing and midwifery greatly expanded after the war to cater to the needs of the rising population (Picture 5 of Annex). To combat malnutrition and Tuberculosis (TB) among school children, nurses were mobilised to perform Mantoux testing and made regular home visits to ensure treatment compliance as well as distributing cod liver oil and "soup mix powder" (Picture 6 of Annex). They also provided invaluable advice to the community on diet and hygiene. The Domiciliary After-Care service was introduced in 1952 to alleviate the demand for maternity hospital beds. In addition to the 24-hour home delivery service and ante-natal care, District Midwives provided essential care and health education to mothers discharged from the hospital 24–36 hours after delivery. In 1955, Singapore was awarded the Kettering Shield for having the best Maternal and Child Health Service in the Commonwealth (Picture 7 of Annex). District Nursing Service was also introduced in 1958 to provide home nursing care.

Working Conditions

The working conditions for nurses back then were far from ideal. There was shortage of nurses to manage the wards and nurses often had to work long hours. Post-war, two Staff Nurses (SN) and two Assistant Nurses (AN) or Student Nurses cared for 40 to 60 patients on a typical day shift. They had to work seven continuous night shifts every two to three weeks. Nurses' involvement with unionism was fostered. The formation of the Amalgamated Union of Public Employees in 1960s served as an official bargaining power for collective agreement on the scheme of service. In 1963, unionised nurses in government hospitals staged a five-day strike that resulted in improvement of their pay and work conditions (Picture 8 of Annex).

Team nursing was introduced in the 1980s, with SNs as the team leaders, supported by ANs and Student Nurses. Together, the team looked after a specific number of patients. SNs had autonomy to coordinate care according to the needs of the patients (Picture 9 of Annex). In 1983, the "Nursing Process" was piloted in Singapore General Hospital where nurses adopted a systematic and holistic approach in patient-centred care. Gradually, this was modified and adopted by other hospitals. Nurses now continue to assess, plan, implement and evaluate patient care (Picture 10 of Annex). Patient and family education was embedded into mainstream practice to help patients and caregivers understand the nature of illness, treatment and progress. They were encouraged to be responsible for their own health as far as their condition permitted. To bring decision-making closer to patients, nurse managers were given more autonomy and accountability for their units' operations, budgeting and staffing.

Expansion of Community and Home Nursing

After Singapore's independence, the Maternal and Child Health nursing service expanded to include family planning programmes to manage overpopulation. In 1975, the Nurse Practitioner (NP) Scheme was initiated at outpatient clinics to provide treatment (including prescription) for patients with minor ailments such as coughs and colds. NPs also managed chronic patients with diabetes, asthma, and high blood pressure. The School NP scheme was introduced in 1977 to include vision and audio testing, height and weight screening, and administration of immunisations in schools.

To promote affordable home-nursing and community care, the Home Nursing Foundation (HNF) was established in 1976. HNF nurses played a big role to help frail, semi-ambulant and non-ambulant elderly in the community and actively mobilised patients and their caregivers to participate in self-care (Picture 11 of Annex). They also coordinated with public and private agencies to integrate care. The District Nursing Service and Maternal and Child Health nursing staff were subsequently amalgamated for economies of scale. Community Psychiatric Nursing Service was set up in 1988 to care for the mentally ill beyond the confines of the "brick and mortar." Nurses were equipped with specialised psychiatric nursing training to independently manage discharged patients and their caregivers in their homes and community (Picture 12 of Annex).

Nurses and midwives in the polyclinics also grew over time and played pivotal roles in the prevention and early detection of diseases. They also performed immunisation, antenatal and postnatal care, as well as screened women for cervical and breast cancers. Nurse midwives empowered mothers to engage in active breastfeeding and care of their newborns. Today, nurse-midwives can also perform epidural infusion top-up, artificial rupture of membranes, foetal scalp insertion, and episiotomy repair.

Professional Regulation

The rapid development of nursing also provided nurses with more autonomy and decision-making. Self-regulation was necessary to protect public safety. The Nurses Registration Ordinance was passed in 1949, requiring nurses to be registered for practice in Singapore. The Nurses and Midwives Act (Act) was enacted in 1975 to establish the Singapore Nursing Board (SNB) to regulate the scope and standards of nursing education and practice. In 2005, the Act was amended to provide for the regulation and certification of Advanced Practice Nurses (APNs) to take on extended nursing roles to manage patients with complex health problems. The amendment also made provision for SNB to appoint a nurse as Chairman of the Board and for the Director of Medical Services or his representative to be a member of the Board. This paved the way for the first nurse to be appointed as Chairman of SNB in 2006.

Nurses continued to develop, adapt, and adopt innovative ways to enhance system and process optimisation. In 1985, MOH Nursing Service spearheaded a Nursing Standards and Quality Assurance Committee to set nursing care standards for the different specialities. In 1995, the Nursing Research Committee was formed to encourage nurses to conduct or utilise research to improve care delivery. The same year, a Nursing Ethics Committee was established to facilitate a culture of ethical practice for the nursing community in an increasingly complex healthcare landscape.

The profession recognised that it needed to be connected to the international community to stay relevant and engaged. The formation of the Singapore Trained Nurses' Association in 1957 played a significant role in promoting professionalism among nurses. Singapore became a full member of the International Council of Nurses in 1961 (Picture 13 of Annex), changing its name to the Singapore Nurses Association in 1990 to include nursing students. The Association now has sixteen Specialty Chapters which gives nurses opportunities to enhance their knowledge and practice through seminars, courses, and professional exchanges.

Nursing Education

After the war in 1945, a generous public wanting to show their appreciation for nurses offered scholarships for local nurses to pursue specialised nursing training overseas. This greatly impacted nursing education. Qualified nursing tutors developed a nursing curriculum to meet national needs. In 1951, the Block system of nursing education was introduced. The AN Training Course in TB Nursing commenced at Tan Tock Seng Hospital and midwifery training began in 1952, using the British model. In 1956, the senior Cambridge certificate became an academic requirement for entry to General Nursing. The School of Nursing (SON) was built to provide nursing education in Singapore (Picture 14 of Annex).

Education was not confined to formal basic and post-basic courses. The year 1959 saw the first Nursing seminar being held in SON for all trained staff in Government institutions, with some nurses from private hospitals. These seminars continued annually. Senior nurses went on field trips, and attended lectures on administration, psychology and advances in medicine and nursing in Singapore.

Nursing training continued to keep up with the changing healthcare trends. In March 1963, the AN training programme was revised to include Medical Surgical, Paediatric, and Psychiatric Nursing. General Nurse training was also revised to offer trainees wider clinical experience while also adding Psychiatry and Community Health Care. With successful family planning and the declining birth rates in the Republic, Midwifery training was ceased in 1977.

Direct entry into the three-year General Nursing Course was discontinued in 1977. The change in policy was a major setback for the profession. Applicants need to enrol in the two-year AN Training Course before progressing to the Student Nurse course. This led to a longer qualification time to become a Staff Nurse regardless of the entrants' entry academic qualification. Not surprising, the number of applications dropped and in 1982, the direct entry of school leavers into the three-year General Nursing Course was reintroduced to encourage more to take up nursing as a career.

The General Nursing Course curriculum was revamped in 1986. Using a nursing model as a framework, the revised curriculum integrated the physical, biological, behavioural sciences, and nursing studies. Nursing Process was emphasised as the tool for systematic nursing care planning. At the same time, the number of post-basic nursing specialty courses was increased to meet the expansion of the health services. Before 1969, there were no formal cardiac specialty nursing courses. With assistance from the World Health Organisation (WHO), post-registration specialty nursing was introduced at the School of Nursing (SON). Cardiac nurses subsequently joined the intensive care nursing course.

Nurses were also awarded scholarships by World Health Organisation, the Australian International Foundation, and the Health Manpower Development Programme (funded by the Local Ministry of Health) to pursue degree and post-graduate courses aboard. Nurses could major in specific clinical specialties, nursing administration, or nursing education. For instance, two nurses from National Skin Centre were sent to the United Kingdom and returned to set up Nurse-led phototherapy services. Another breakthrough in nursing education was achieved in 1988 when the government offered A-level students Public Service Commission scholarships to pursue nursing degree courses overseas.

In 1992, nursing education moved from certificate to diploma level at Nanyang Polytechnic (NYP) School of Health Sciences, under the purview of the Ministry of Education. The NYP three-year Diploma in Nursing equipped graduates with critical thinking skills and to proactively respond to a dynamic healthcare environment. Students were exposed to board-based knowledge in nursing, biological and behavioural sciences, computer studies, research methods, and statistics. Such academic rigour fostered better problem-solving and decision-making abilities. Bursaries were offered by MOH and various hospitals and the first cohort of NYP diplomats graduated in 1995. In 2005, Ngee Ann Polytechnic (NP) became the second school to offer Diploma in Nursing. Most of the post-basic specialty courses, formerly conducted at SON, were upgraded to Advanced Diploma courses at NYP, NP and Parkway College (a private nursing education provider).

Opportunities abound for nurses to pursue higher learning and degree upgrading, either through the NUS Alice Lee School of Nursing or through post-registration upgrading pathway via the seven accredited SNB-accredited courses (Picture 15 of Annex). Masters and PhD nursing programmes were also introduced in 2003 and 2010 respectively, at NUS to enable RNs to further expand their capabilities. Today, around 40% of local nurses in the public sector have a degree.

New Career Pathways

As nursing services expanded, new career paths were developed to assist nurses fulfil their career aspirations. In July 2000, a new nursing career structure was introduced, which allowed nurses to progress in clinical, educational, management positions. The RN workforce profile was set at 5% RNs at Level 3 (senior management), 25% at Level 2 (middle management), and 70% at Level 1 (rank and file staff nurses). Over time, clinical nurses developed special expertise in tandem with medical advancement. For instance, the Nurse Clinician (NC) for Diabetic Care collaborates with doctors, pharmacists, and dieticians to manage diabetic patients requiring specialised support (Picture 16 of Annex). NCs are also developed for Infection Control, Stoma Care, Breast Care, Pain Management, Head and Neck Care, Bone Marrow Transplant Care, Neuroscience, Cardiothoracic Care, Lactation Care, and Continence Care. Specialisations such as Fall Care, Oncology Care, and Home Ventilation and Respiratory Support Services were developed to address the challenges of our shifting healthcare trends.

As part of a national initiative to upscale nurses in 2007, senior Enrolled Nurses (ENs) were able to upgrade to become the Principal ENs. This expanded role allowed PENs to assist in nursing assessment and plan of care, venepuncture, basic ECG interpretation, preceptorship, and clinical education (Picture 17 of Annex).

In 2006, the first cohort of Advanced Practice Nurses (APNs) — RNs who have a Master degree in clinical nursing — was formally certified by the Singapore Nursing Board. They are trained in the diagnosis and management of common medical conditions, including chronic illnesses. APNs work independently and collaboratively with the healthcare team to improve patients' clinical outcomes. They also influenced the development of nursing, health practice, and policy through evidence-based practice (Picture 18 of Annex). As of 2013, there are 117 APNs in Singapore who provided expert clinical nursing in medical-surgical, acute care, mental health, and community areas.

The New Paradigm

In December 2012, MOH set up a National Nursing Taskforce (NNT) to review and recommend ways to enhance career development, autonomy, recognition, and education for nurses in the public healthcare sector. A slew of 15 recommendations were articulated and in August 2014, Minister for Health, Mr. Gan Kim Yong, accepted the

Taskforce's recommendations. These recommendations are currently in the various stages of implementation. Notable areas included enabling ENs to pursue their Diploma in Nursing without relying solely on GPA scores. Instead, recognition of working experience (minimum of three years) and a testimonial provided by the employer would be used. A new tier of Assistant Nurse Clinician was created to recognise experienced nurses for their clinical expertise to lead the nursing unit in direct patient care settings. A dual portfolio would also be offered for experienced nurses to widen their organisational role, yet contribute to inter-institutional learning. For example, a nurse could be an NC in a direct patient care role and concurrently serving as an adjunct lecturer at the academia.

Plans are underway to expand Nurse-managed rehabilitation wards, Nurse-managed clinics and Nurse-initiated referrals. APNs and experienced senior nurses would be granted authority to make protocol-based diagnoses and investigations for certain disease profiles and order treatment. They would also be able to prescribe, review, titrate, and discontinue medications. Where patient care needs are relatively simple and routine, support care staff will be up-skilled to take on higher roles delegated by nurses.

The advanced diploma nursing courses are under revision. For instance, the new Advanced Clinical Education (ACE) framework would have an added focus on broad-based modules and community nursing to equip nurses to better case manage and integrate care across the spectrum of acuity and needs. The ACE would be a mandatory pre-requisite for the Master of Nursing course. Additionally, APN interns would enjoy a standardised internship process to assure quality of professional nursing development nationally. An inter-ministry and inter-agency National Council of Nursing Education would be set up to oversee nursing training and development for the nationally re-defined roles.

Nursing Technology

A cross-cluster National Nursing Technology workgroup is being formalised to use technology to drive productivity and decision support. Nurses are key proponents of using Information technology (IT) and have, over time, launched several worthwhile initiatives with productivity, cost, and care-effectiveness considerations. For instance, Tan Tock Seng Hospital initiated the SmartSense Vital Signs monitoring system in 2008 that used radio frequency identification (RFID) to monitor body temperatures, track patients' locations, and upload the readings to an electronic clinical chart (Picture 19 of Annex). The Medical Device Interface (MDI), launched in 2012 to automatically upload and document vital signs readings, radically reduced the average amount of time nurses spent per patient on vital signs documentation by half.

National University Hospital embarked on an e-rostering system project where nurses could bid for preferred work shifts in advance. Implemented in 2005, the time spent by nurse managers on workforce management-related activities has been reduced by over 70%.

CGH developed an iPad "patient care communicator" application to mitigate the frustration of patients admitted to the intensive care unit who were unable to speak. The application contained features in four languages that patients could use to communicate with the medical team (Picture 20 of Annex).

Besides clinical nursing, IT has also benefited nursing education, management, and research. Some nurses had gone on to specialise in IT and are contributing their expertise to the larger healthcare system.

Recognition

Nurses' Week celebrations were introduced in 1965 and included graduation ceremonies for nurses and midwives, concerts, exhibitions, blood donation drives, and charity fundraising projects. Nurses Week was changed to Nurses' Day in the 1980s. Since 1990, the President opened the Istana to nurses on Nurses' Day as a mark of appreciation for their contributions to the health and well-being of the nation (Picture 21 of Annex). The Minister for Health, Mr. Yong Nyuk Lin, when speaking at the 1964 Graduation ceremony said:

> *"We want the people of Singapore to get to know more of the excellent and hard work performed by our nurses and midwives. We want our secondary school children to be inspired to become nurses and midwives, not just as any other job but as a vocation and a calling."*
>
> — *Minister of Health, Mr. Yong Nyuk Lin,*
> *speaking at the 1964 Graduation ceremony*

The annual Nurses' Merit Award was started in 1976 by MOH to acknowledge outstanding nurses for their exemplary work performance and dedication. Awardees receive a medal to be worn as part of their nurses' uniform and $200, which was revised upwards to $1000 in 2014.

The annual President's Award for Nurses (PAN) established in 1999 is the highest accolade to be given to the country's most outstanding RNs who had distinguished themselves in patient care, education, leadership, research, and administration (Picture 22 of Annex). Awardees receive this prestigious Award (a trophy, certificate and $6000 to be used for their professional development) from the President at the Istana, which is attended by about 650 nurses and guests from the healthcare family. In 2014, along with the NNT recommendations, the award was increased to $10000.

The Tan Chin Tuan Nursing Award was started in 2006 to recognise exemplary Enrolled Nurses for their dedication to their patients, demonstrated excellence, and significant contributions in advancing the nursing profession. Awardees receive a gold medallion and cash to be used for their professional development. The first three winners receive $3500, $3000 and $2000 respectively; followed by $800 for the 4th to 10th place winners.

The Next Lap

Skilled nurses form the backbone of the healthcare industry. The evolution of nursing had imbued a culture that is progressive, inquisitive, and daring, in the profession. With nine percent (9%) of the population above 65 today, which is expected to triple by the year 2030, Singapore faces the challenge of an ageing population. As life expectancy increases, so will multiple chronic diseases. These issues will shape the future nursing landscape dramatically (Picture 23 of Annex). The nation must have an ample number of quality, dedicated nurses. Driven by the NNT's broad audacious transformation strategies, the nursing profession will take the next leap of faith to make an even greater impact on Singapore healthcare system going forward.

Annex

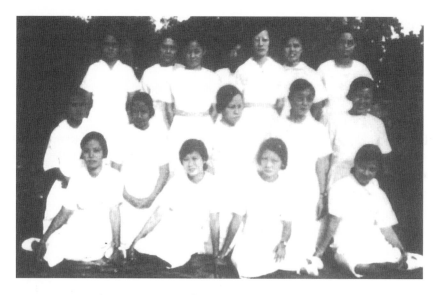

Picture 1.   The untiring nurses of St. Andrew's Mission Hospital in the thirties.

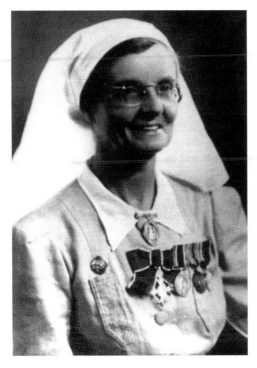

Picture 2. The first Public Health Nurse, Miss I.M.M. Simmons, made significant contributions to child health services.

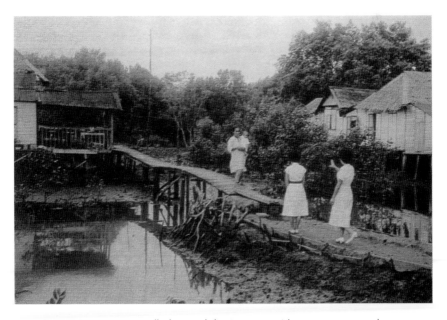

Picture 3. Nurses travelled to rural districts to provide proper post-natal care.

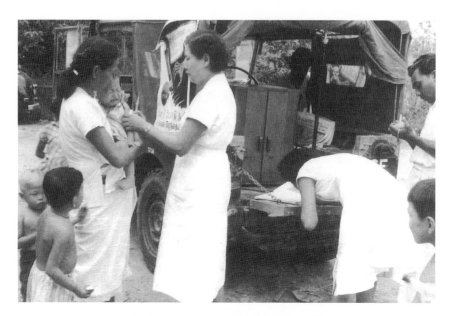

Picture 4.   Nurses on wheels brought care and relief to patients living in the rural areas.

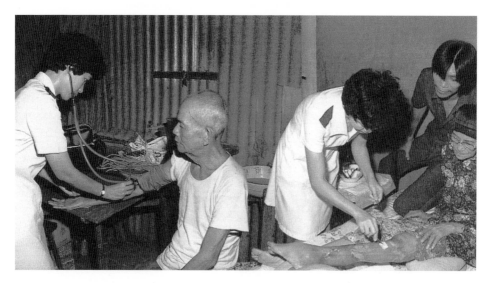

Picture 5.   Despite working under tremendous stress and strain in the public health arena, nurses persevered in providing nursing care, treatment, and health education to the public.

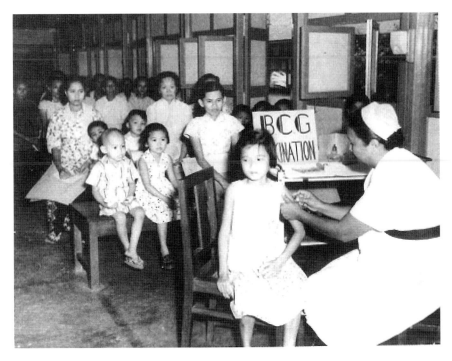

Picture 6. BCG vaccination was administered in the battle against tuberculosis.

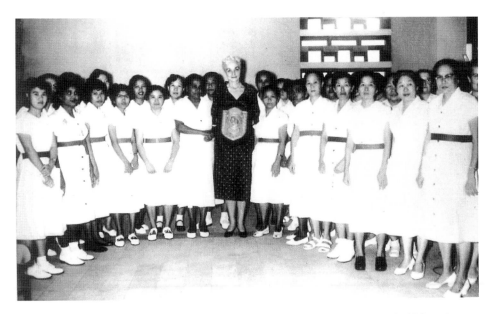

Picture 7. A memorable day for nurses. Singapore was awarded the Kettering Shield for achieving the best Maternal and Child Service in the Commonwealth.

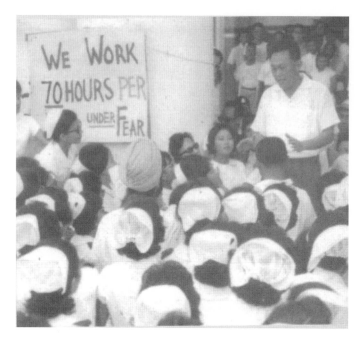

Picture 8.   Prime Minister Lee Kuan Yew (1963) addressing the concerns of nurses on strike.

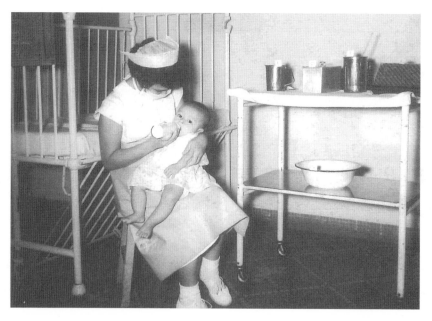

Picture 9.   Before Team Nursing, patient care was fragmented and nursing was functional. Here a "Feed Nurse" is seen in action.

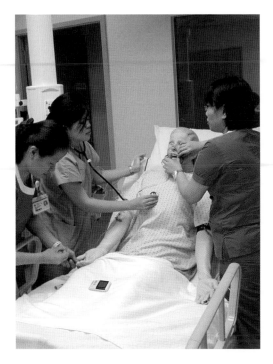

Picture 10.   Nurses now able to assess, plan, implement, and evaluate patient care in collaborative simulations.

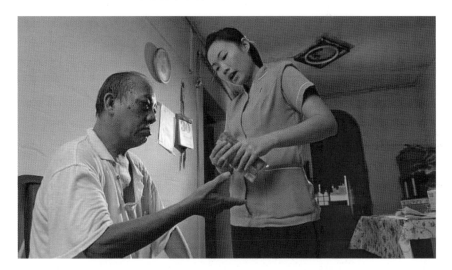

Picture 11.   Home Nursing Foundation's nurse sorting out the medication for her patient. She visits him at home once every two weeks to ensure he is taking the right dosage — (*Source:* Straits Times *photo: DESMOND WEE*)

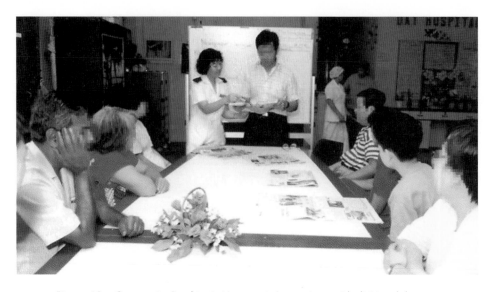

Picture 12.   Community Psychiatric Nurse assisting patients with divisional therapy.

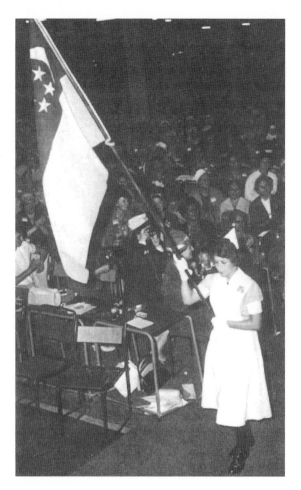

Picture 13.   The Singapore flag flying high in Melbourne, Australia, at the ICN Conference (1961).

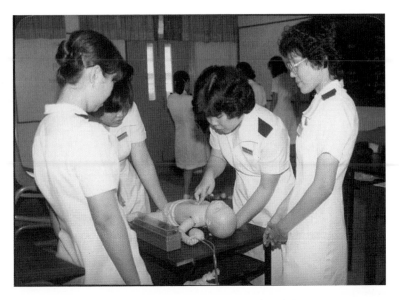

Picture 14. A lesson in SON on infant CPR.

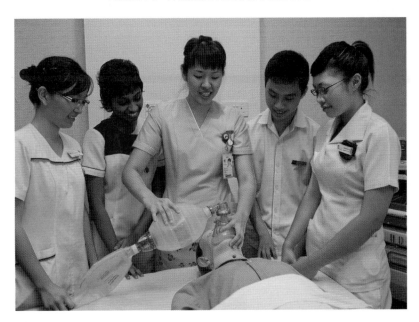

Picture 15. Acquiring clinical compentency.

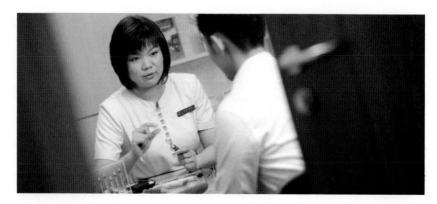

Picture 16.   The Nurse Clinician (Diabetes Care) giving education on insulin and its administration.

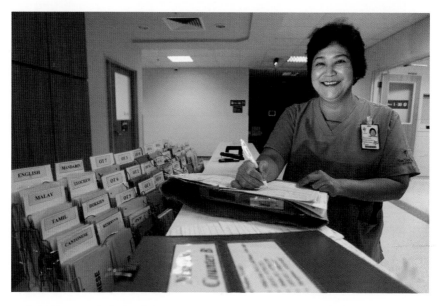

Picture 17.   The expanded role of the Principal Assistant Nurse opens up a career opportunity for an Enrolled Nurse.

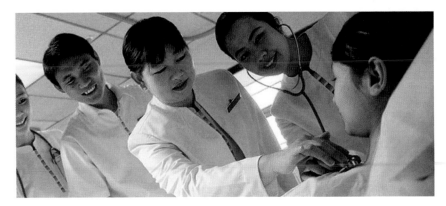

Picture 18. With their unique education and training, the Advanced Practice Nurse possesses the best of both worlds and bridge the gap between nurses and doctors.

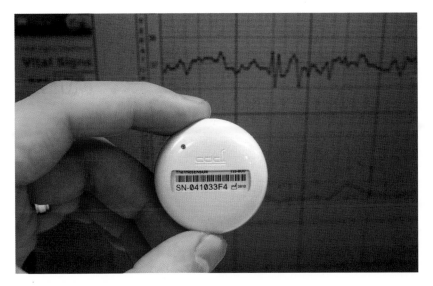

Picture 19. Using Radio Frequency Identification (RFID) technology, nurses could better monitor patients' temperature, track their locations, and keep electronic records of their vital signs.

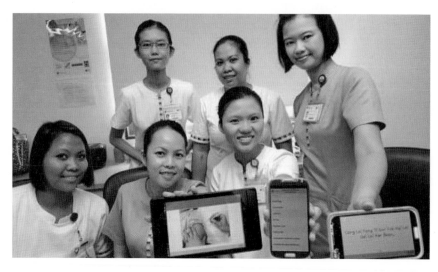

Picture 20.　The "patient care communicator" application allows nurses to communicate more effectively with their patients.

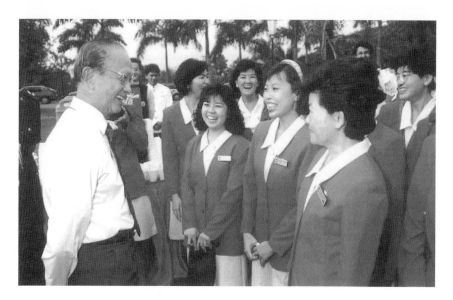

Picture 21.　Meeting the President, the late Mr. Wee Kim Wee (1991), at Istana for Nurses' Day.

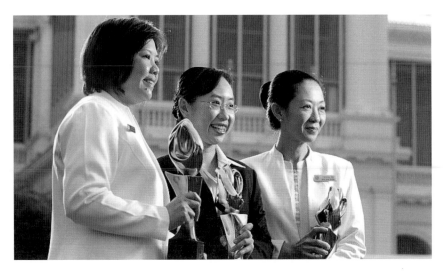

Picture 22.   The deserving recipients of the President's Award for Nurses at the Nurses' Day Istana Reception on July 24, 2012.

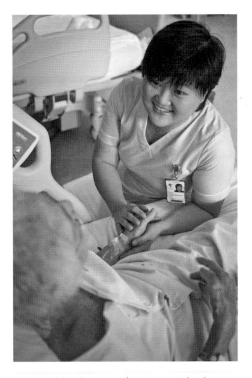

Picture 23.   Bringing about care with a heart.

References

KK Women's and Children's Hospital. (2014) *Hospital Milestones*. Available online: http://www.kkh.com.sg/AboutUs/Overview/HospitalMilestones/Pages/Home.aspx

Ministry of Health. (1997) *More than a Calling: Nursing in Singapore since 1885*. Singapore: Ministry of Health.

Ministry of Health Singapore. (2014) *Health Manpower*. Available online: https://www.moh.gov.sg/content/moh_web/home/statistics/Health_Facts_Singapore/Health_Manpower.html

Ministry of Health Singapore. (2014) *National Nursing Taskforce Recommends New "Care" Package to Enhance Growth, Professional Development and Recognition of Nurses.* Available online: http://www.moh.gov.sg/content/moh_web/home/pressRoom/highlights/2014/care-for-nurses.html

Mudeliar V, Nair CRS, Norris RP (ed). (1976) *Development of Hospital Care and Nursing in Singapore*. Singapore: Ministry of Health.

National Archives of Singapore. (2014) *Family Planning*. Available online: http://www.nas.gov.sg/archivesonline/article/family-planning

National Library Board Singapore. (2014) *Ida Simmons — Singapore's First Public Health Nurse*. Available online: http://eresources.nlb.gov.sg/history/events/6df003cc-1236-4a8b-b953-73c2c2e373fd

School Health Service. (1970) *SHS File Records*. Singapore: School Health Service.

Tan Tock Seng Hospital. (1994) *150 Years of Caring — The Legacy of Tan Tock Seng Hospital*. Singapore: Tan Tock Seng Hospital.

Tan Tock Seng Hospital. (2013) *Practising the Profession: The Choice Institution for Great Nursing*. Singapore: Tan Tock Seng Hospital.

9 Health Promotion — Our Journey

Chew Ling,* Jeanne Tan,* Jael Lim,*
Lyn James,† Derrick Heng† and Chew Suok Kai†

Introduction

"Singaporeans are living longer. Moving forward, the next question to ask really is, 'Are we also enjoying a better quality of life with this longer lifespan?'"

— *Healthy Living Master Plan*[1]

The healthcare system in Singapore is considered by many to be world-class and is credited for the current state of health that Singaporeans enjoyed. Its state-of-the-art technology and well-qualified health workers mean that Singaporeans enjoy high standards of healthcare from infancy to old age, earning Singapore its place as one of the world's healthiest countries.[2,3]

Over the years, the Singapore government has put quality health services in place which are both accessible and affordable to the general population. The country's healthcare spending is expected to grow to $12 (SGD) billion by 2020, up from $4 billion in 2011.[4] In 2011, about $160 million was allocated to health promotion[5] signifying government's commitment in this area. This spending in the health system is complemented by further government investments in an effective public health system such as the provision of clean drinking water, good sanitation, enforced food safety standards, and pollution control.

These factors have helped to make Singaporeans one of the longest living people in the world today. The 2014 World Health Organisation's (WHO) World

*Health Promotion Board, Singapore.
†Ministry of Health, Singapore.

Health Statistics showed that the female life expectancy at birth in Singapore is 85.1 years, fourth longest in the world; while that of male is 80.1 years old — the fifth ranked longest expected lifespan in world.[6]

Challenges to the Health System

Singapore now faces two key challenges when it comes to ensuring that Singaporeans stay healthy.

First, Singapore is facing demographic changes brought about by rapid population growth. The population exceeded five million for the first time in 2010. At the same time, the number of Singaporeans aged 65 years and above is projected to grow from 405,000 to 900,000 by 2030.[7]

Secondly, like many fast moving, knowledge-based economies, Singaporeans are increasingly engaged in sedentary type of work while relying on technology for greater convenience in their daily lives. National surveys show that in 2010 almost 40% of adult Singaporeans, aged 18 to 69 years,[8] do not have sufficient total physical activity compared to 18% in 2007.[9] The surveys also showed that 60% of Singaporeans frequently eat out of their homes and a similar proportion consumed more calories daily than the recommended daily caloric intake.[10]

The Singapore Burden of Disease Study 2010[11] showed that approximately 70% of the burden of deaths and ill-health in the population were caused by non-communicable diseases (NCD) such as heart diseases and stroke, cancer, diabetes, mental disorders, and chronic respiratory diseases. This burden of disease had increased from 2004, due to ageing and population growth.

Many of the NCDs have common lifestyle risk factors, namely unhealthy diets, low physical activity levels, smoking, and poor mental health. Tackling these risk factors well would contribute to a significant reduction in the burden of disease. Health promotion has played a significant role in raising health awareness and literacy through public education. To continue keeping Singaporeans healthy, especially in the light of the challenges, there is a need to shift from creating awareness to changing the context to enable the individual to make the healthier choice despite the many competing priorities he or she faces.

The Early Years (From 1950s–1960s) — Getting the Basics Right

> "Health education ... used to be simpler telling people about hygiene, e.g. boiling water before consumption or to wash their hands and to take nutritious food."

> — Dr. Chen Ai Ju
> Director of Medical Services, 1996–2000[12]

The early years of preventive health were about setting the foundation for health. In the 1950s, after the second World War, Singapore was in a state of disrepair. Many of the civilian population was severely malnourished and diseases such as beri-beri, malaria, cholera, and tuberculosis, were then widespread. At the same time, Singapore had to deal with the strain on healthcare resources brought about by a post-war baby boom.

The then-rudimentary health system centred around three main hospitals — the General Hospital, Tan Tock Seng Hospital, and Kandang Kerbau Maternity Hospital. A primary medical care system including a chain of maternal and child health clinics and travelling dispensaries was set up in 1951 to reach out to the largely rural population in whatever way it could. Through this network of services, the population was educated on basic hygiene, proper child nutrition, and the importance of taking preventive measures such as immunisations. The early community health workers often had to struggle with limited resources to convince the largely uneducated population to take on preventive measures, which are now readily practised in Singapore.[12]

In 1955, the Health Education Council was created to provide all educational materials, training, and coordination among different governmental bodies regarding sanitation and general health. Health education, mainly through campaigns such as the Diphtheria Immunisation Campaign, Tuberculosis X-ray Campaign, and other campaigns on nutrition, childcare, and food hygiene were carried out to enable the population to understand the importance of preventive health.

The year 1959 was a pivotal point in Singapore's history. The People's Action Party (PAP) won the General Election that year, with Mr. Lee Kuan Yew becoming the first Prime Minister of Singapore. For the first time in history, Singapore had an independent government and one of its main priorities was to re-organise the country's health services for better coordination of health policies and services.

In 1960, the Health Education Council was abolished and all local medical services came under the Public Health Division of the newly created Ministry of Health. The Health Education Training and Special Assignment Branch was then formed to take over all the health education activities of the country, with one basic mission — to provide health education and training in health promotion. The Branch was also tasked with promoting and educating the nation on family planning to curb the then-high birth rate.

One key service that continued ceaselessly throughout this period was the School Health Service (SHS). This Service was established in 1921 to safeguard children's health in the colony on the premise that a good and healthy start was crucial to their good health later in life. The SHS remains a key feature in Singapore's health promotion efforts today.[13]

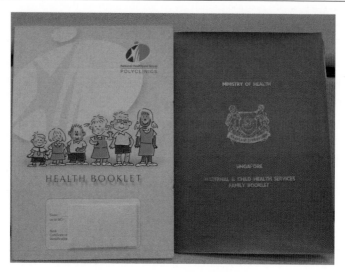

Health Booklet circa 2005 (*left*) and Health Booklet circa 1978 (*right*).

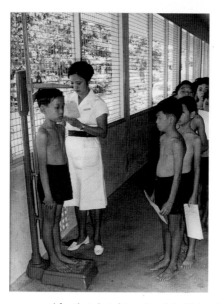

School children being measured for their height and weight (School Health Service in the 1960s).

The year 1921 saw the birth of the School Health Service. Many generations of Singaporeans will remember the no-nonsense nurses who conducted examinations on eyes, ears, and spines. In screening every child, the School Health Service played a critical preventive role in detecting and managing medical issues before they became serious.

School Health Service

Following the end of the Japanese Occupation, there were more demands on the service as more children started attending school and a vast majority were found to have serious health issues. Malnutrition was a major problem. To address this, free and subsidised meals were given in schools. To ensure comprehensive coverage, schools were divided into zones and were annually visited by a team of doctors and nurses. By 1958, the SHS had a permanent home at the Institute of Health on Outram Road.

Besides early detection of childhood developmental conditions, the SHS also played a key role in the National Childhood Immunisation Programme. Since the introduction of the Programme in the 1960s, the SHS had consistently ensured high coverage (more than 95%) for herd immunity for infectious diseases such as diphtheria and measles for each school-going age cohort year after year.[14,15] Several doctors had contributed significantly at the SHS to ensure the good health of successive cohorts of school children. They included Drs. Connie Lim, Uma Rajan, and Rose Vaithinathan.

School Dental Service

Besides taking care of the general health of children, it was also necessary to ensure good oral hygiene habits from young. During the 1960s, dental hygiene standards were low. Half of the population did not yet know how to brush their teeth properly, while half of all school children did not even have toothbrushes. Having toothbrushes also did not necessarily lead to better dental health, as these children were also not brushing regularly or correctly.

To develop good dental hygiene habits, dental care education was introduced to ten primary schools in 1968. Through the joint efforts of the Ministry of Health and the Ministry of Education, this programme reached all Primary One to Three classes by 1969. At that point in time, Singapore was the first country in the region to carry out a dental health education programme on such a scale.

Each child was given a set of toothbrush and plastic mug. The set, which was paid for by the schools, cost 25 cents each, a significant sum then. A total of 367,000 children from 439 primary schools participated in the Programme and an estimated 1.5 million toothbrushes were sold in two years alone from 1969 to 1970.[16] Riding on this success, the programme went to all kindergartens in 1973. When the Health Promotion Board was set up in 2001, dental services were extended to all secondary schools.

School children had compulsory tooth-brushing sessions, usually during recess, and lessons on the techniques of tooth-brushing.

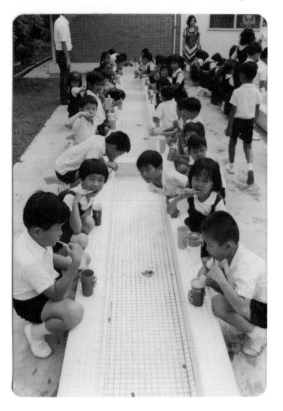

School children brushing their teeth during recess in the 1970s.

The impact of the Programme on the oral hygiene status was strong. The index for oral health, "Decayed, Filled, Missing Teeth" or DFMT index for a 12-year-old child, was 1.39 in 1989 and has remained below 1 since the mid 1990s.[17] The benchmark set by the WHO was DMFT index of 2 at 12-years old in 2010.

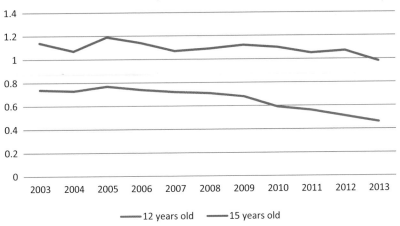

Oral Health Status
DMFT Trends for 12 years and 15 years old from 2003-2013

12 years old   15 years old

Source: Health Promotion Board

The Formative Years (From 1970s–1990s) — Creating Awareness Through Public Education and Use of Legislation

"With the current disease profile, the main thrust of such approaches must lie in health promotion and disease prevention... We firmly believe that this should be the basic philosophy to Singapore's healthcare policies."

— *Review Committee on National Health Policy 1991*[18]

Why do people eat, live, or play the way we do? What motivates us? These are a few of the questions that the people who are in the business of health promotion ask in order to help everyone live healthy lifestyles. Healthy living goes beyond being free from diseases; rather, "healthy living" is to reach a state of complete physical, mental, and social well-being so that the individual can realise aspirations, satisfy his needs, and cope with his environment.[19]

To this end, the pioneers in health promotion have worked tirelessly to create awareness of the need for healthy living, and to inculcate the motivation to adopt healthy lifestyles in Singaporeans through public education continuing with the government's strategy of nationwide campaigns which started in 1960s. The period between 1970s and 1990s saw a slew of disease prevention and health promotion programmes. This included expanded immunisation programme reaching out to all children and regular health examinations for infants and children up to 16 years old, complemented by sustained health education programmes through the media and print materials, as well as regular large scale campaigns against smoking and unhealthy eating habits, along with promoting exercise.

This period also coincided with the rapid economic development and rising affluence among Singaporeans. By the 1990s, Singapore had developed into a modern and vibrant metropolis. But moving from Third World to First also meant that Singapore was facing health issues of the developed nations. An affluent lifestyle gave Singaporeans access to a wider variety of foods, but it did not mean that these foods were healthier. People were increasingly sedentary as more moved into professional, managerial, and executive occupations. Better infrastructure and connectivity in transport links also led to people walking less and sitting more. And with a much faster pace of life, Singaporeans were facing greater mental stress.

National Healthy Lifestyle Programme

In 1991, Singapore's health promotion efforts were given further impetus following the release of the recommendations of the Review Committee on National Health Policies.[16] The Committee had found that Singaporeans were increasingly succumbing to "lifestyle" diseases. Obesity was becoming an issue of significance among children and the adults, along with obesity-related diseases such as heart disease and diabetes. The two main causes of obesity were attributed to a largely sedentary lifestyle and poor dietary habits.

The Report recognised that, "[T]he Ministry of Health's efforts must be supplemented by other government departments, health providers in the private sector, employers and unions as well as community organisations and voluntary associations," and that the "strategies for health promotion must be broad-based, and the voluntary commitment of the public to healthy living must be secured for long term effectiveness." The role of the individual in taking responsibility and ownership of his/her health was also emphasised.

One way to prevent an increasing population of unhealthy Singaporeans down the road was to target risk factors such as obesity, lack of physical activity, smoking, and high cholesterol from poor diets. Tackling these "lifestyle" related issues became the focus of the government over the next decade. Health promotion moved upstream, with greater emphasis on the prevention of diseases and educating the public on the modifiable risk factors.

The National Healthy Lifestyle Programme was set up in 1991. Spearheaded by the Ministry of Health, this Programme involved different sectors of the government

The National Healthy Lifestyle Campaign made it to the Guinness Book of Records in 1993 for having 26,107 people exercising simultaneously in the Great Singapore Workout.

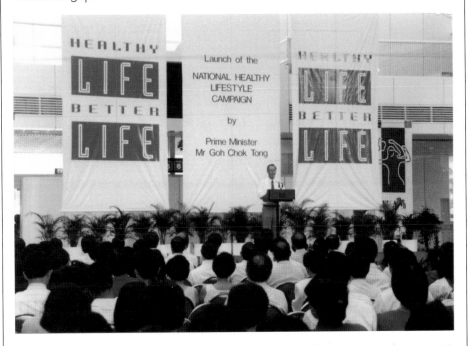

Launch of the first National Healthy Lifestyle Campaign in 1993.

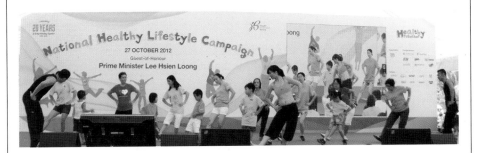

Launch of National Healthy Lifestyle Campaign (2012).

including education, defence, public service division, and labour, each bringing to the table their plans to promote a healthier lifestyle within their sector.[20]

That year, an ambitious National Health Fair was organised. HealthLand '92 covered 8578 sq. metres of the former World Trade Centre Hall 3 (now the HarbourFront

Centre). With a theme-park approach, it had 15 pavilions, some of which provided screenings for cholesterol, blood sugar, and blood pressure. More than half a million people attended the two-week long event.[21]

In 1993, the inaugural National Healthy Lifestyle Campaign (NHLC) was launched to promote healthy lifestyles among Singaporeans by the then-Prime Minister, Mr Goh Chok Tong. The NHLC targeted groups such as children, employees, and national servicemen with targeted programmes such as the All Children Exercising Simultaneously (ACES) Day and the Workplace Healthy Lifestyle Programme in the civil sector. ACES Day aimed to promote physical activity and fitness by getting pupils to participate together in an enjoyable and non-competitive activity.

But no matter who it targeted or what form it took, the aim of the Campaign has always stayed the same since its inception — to get Singaporeans interested and actively involved in their own health. This Campaign also received the highest political support in that the Prime Minister or his deputy would grace the occasion consistently to show their unwavering support for healthy living.

This flagship health campaign celebrated its 20th anniversary in 2012 at the Gardens by the Bay, drawing more than 20,000 visitors to learn how healthier choices have been made accessible and affordable to all Singaporeans through their communities.

National Nutrition Campaigns

An awareness of good diet and nutrition has always been a key focus in the government's drive to promote a healthy lifestyle among Singaporeans. As early as the 1970s, there was already an awareness of the need to educate Singaporeans in managing their nutrition.

To address this, Ministry of Health organised campaigns such as "Better Food, Better Health" and Nutrition Week to raise the public's awareness of the importance of good nutrition for health.

In 1990, the Ministry of Health established the Food and Nutrition Department to promote healthy eating and to monitor the eating habits of Singaporeans. Nutrition campaigns such as the "Healthy Meals, Healthy Family," "Ask For," and "Eat Healthy" Campaigns were organised to promote healthy eating to the public. To deal with increasing obesity among the young, the government's nutrition campaigns also reached out to school children and school canteen vendors.[22] A Food Consumption Study to understand Singaporeans' eating patterns was carried out in 1993. This was later replaced by the National Nutrition Survey distributed every six years starting in 1998.[23]

The Ask For Healthier Food campaign aimed to get Singaporeans to ask for less oil, less salt and more vegetables when ordering food from hawker centres or food courts. In 1999, about 5800 hawker stalls and 86 restaurants participated in this campaign.

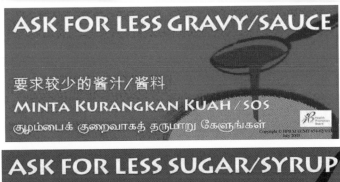

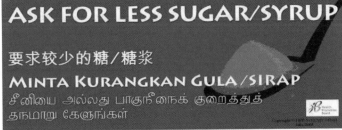

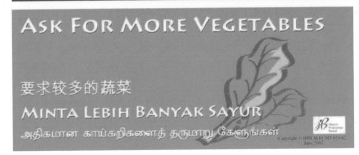

Some of the labels used during the "Ask For" Campaign to get Singaporeans to eat healthily.

Anti-Smoking Campaign

Today, Singapore has one of the lowest smoking prevalence in the world. This achievement was a result of a committed public administration that was persuaded by the evidence from Wynder *et al.* and Doll *et al.* in the 1950s that smoking was major risk factor for many chronic diseases.[24]

Singapore saw a rise in the number of smokers and smoking-related deaths from 1950 to the 1980s, in tandem with a spike in cigarette sale from 3.6 million kg in 1973 to peak at 4.4 million in 1983. From 30 deaths due to cancer in 1950, the numbers peaked at around 100 deaths in 1984. Similarly, the number of deaths due to heart diseases rose from a little over 50 deaths in 1950 to more than 110 deaths in 1984.[25]

Singapore was one of the earliest countries in the world to introduce a slew of legislative and fiscal measures against smoking, such as the control of marketing, the sale of tobacco products, the prohibition of smoking in public spaces, and the enforcement of heavy tobacco taxes starting from 1970. Stringent enforcement of these measures was complemented with educational outreach and smoking cessation services. In 1986, the National Smoking Control Programme was launched to consolidate the smoking control efforts of the country.[26]

> The Anti-Smoking Campaign was inaugurated by the Minister for Health, Dr. Richard Hu at a ceremony held at the Public Utilities Board Auditorium on 1 December 1986. On the same day, 42 public and private organisations put up "No Smoking" signs on their premises to discourage staff from lighting up.

The impact of the Programme was tremendous. Smoking prevalence rate among adults in the country steadily dropped from 26% in the 1970s to 13.8% in 2010. In the same period, lung cancer incidence rates, particularly among the males, dropped from 63 per 100,000 in the period 1978–1982 to 40.8 per 100,000 in 2003–2007.[27]

The anti-smoking campaigns in the earlier years focused on the diseases that a smoker might succumb to. "Scare tactics" which used graphic pictures of diseased lungs and health ravages of the effects of smoking were common. By the mid-1990s, the focus shifted away from highlighting smoking-related diseases to emphasising the health benefits of not smoking. For example, young people were informed how smoking affected their looks, pockets, and relationships. Services to help smokers quit were made easily available and peer support became a central part of the programme to help fellow smokers kick the habit.[2,4]

In 1990, these efforts to create a smoke-free lifestyle for the population were recognised by the WHO which awarded the Ministry of Health with the World No-Tobacco Day medal. Singapore was again recognised in 1999, when the then-Ministry of the Environment received the same award for its work to establish smoke-free public places in Singapore.[2,4]

2000s — The Expansion Years — From Public Education to Influencing Choices to Achieve Better Health for Singaporeans

"Each of us is responsible for our own health. The first thing we need to tackle is our own behaviour.... We aim to catalyse a whole-of-Singapore effort, in which healthy living becomes a shared vision."

— Gan Kim Yong, Minister for Health 2013[28]

By the turn of the millennium, Singapore was a developed nation, with world-class health facilities and an educated workforce. Results of the National Health Surveys were used as indicators of health promotion efforts, showing that until 2004, many of the behavioural risk factors were well under control. This success was due in part to the effective raising of health awareness and literacy through public education and national campaigns. However, chronic diseases continued to trend upwards. Coupled with an ageing population, a dedicated approach was required to drive health promotion efforts to the next level.

Formation of the Health Promotion Board

In 2001, the Health Promotion Board (HPB), a new statutory board, was set up by MOH to drive Singapore's national health promotion and disease prevention programmes. The HPB's approach to health promotion was to drive behavioural modification through the awareness, adoption, and sustaining of healthy behaviours.

The HPB started with five divisions and 730 staff, many drawn from the Primary Health Division in the Ministry of Health — School Health, School Dental, National Health Education, and Food and Nutrition Departments. The early divisions were Youth Health, Adult Health, Corporate Marketing and Communications, Research and Information Management, and Corporate Services. A decade later, two new divisions, Healthy Ageing and Community Partnerships, were added on to the corporate structure, reflecting the increasing emphasis in these emerging areas. By then, the staff strength had grown to about 850 people, with the majority still involved in preventive care for school children. This growth in capacity reflected the increasing emphasis on health promotion by the government.

The HPB's first Chief Executive Officer (CEO), Dr. Lam Sian Lian, an accomplished public health physician, continued the momentum of health promotion work that was started by the Ministry of Health. One major area of work remained: school health and school dental services. Public education to raise awareness about the causes of specific diseases such as osteoporosis, impact of unhealthy lifestyle habits such as unhealthy diets, smoking, and sedentary lifestyles, and campaigning continued to be the main tactic adopted. Programmes such as myopia screening for preschoolers and mental wellness promotion were also added on.

The HPB expanded its approach to promote a supportive environment to make "healthier choice the easier choice." It increasingly adopted a targeted approach to reach the different segments of the population — the healthy, those at-risk of getting diseases, and those with existing health conditions — at various life stages and through various settings such as the school, workplace, and community.[29]

This was complemented by the development of health promotion policies and guidelines (e.g. Healthier Choice guidelines), and introduction of grants and recognition awards for health promoting workplaces and schools. Training to build capacity on health promotion were targeted at healthcare professionals, healthy lifestyle advocates, community leaders, and care-givers, through programmes delivered through schools, the workplaces and the community, in addition to running public education campaigns.

By the time Dr. Lam retired in 2005, it had become apparent that there was a need for additional strategies to help Singaporeans adopt and sustain healthy habits. Mr. Lam Pin Woon, her successor, was an experienced marketer in fast-moving consumer goods (FMCG) products, having worked in several food and health supplement multinationals. Under his term, the HPB made forays into engaging the private sector, mainly the food industry, to initiate the development of healthier products at their source. As a result of this engagement, the growth of Healthier Choice products accelerated during this period. More than 2600 Stock Keeping Units (SKUs) across more than 60 food product categories were made available in the local market by 2014.

During this period, the HPB expanded its outreach to the masses beyond public education. HealthLine, a toll-free telephone information service by trained nurse advisors who provided personal advice and counselling on health matters was scaled up. It proved to be an effective direct communication channel as the HealthLine handled more than 4000 calls on average per month by 2014.[30]

Similarly, in the mainstream media, media strategies for this campaign evolved. Riding on the popularity of reality programmes, the HPB commissioned the production of a four-episode reality television series on a weight management bootcamp programme, "Lose to Win," which attracted 450,000 viewers over a month. By the seventh season in 2014, more than 4000 participants had passed through the programme with 6 in 10 losing an average of 3 kg.[31]

To reach out to an increasingly tech-savvy population whose main source of information were social media platforms, the HPB expanded its online engagement efforts through its presence on popular social media platforms such as Facebook, Twitter, and Instagram.

Towards the end of first decade in the new millennium, it was clear to the HPB that it needed to intensify its efforts beyond public education and campaigns. The few decades of health promotion campaigns had led to a higher level of health awareness and literacy among Singaporeans. Many of the HPB publicity campaigns also won prestigious marketing awards.[32,33] However, these did not mean that Singaporeans were practising what they knew.

In 2011, under the guidance of its third CEO, Mr. Ang Hak Seng, the HPB moved into a ground up approach in health promotion. Mr. Ang who was from the Singapore Police Force, had extensive experience in community engagement. The HPB embarked on a strategy of touch points to create an integrated health promotion ecosystem and shifted into a phase of co-creation of solutions with the community which were then deployed within the community.

To support the shift to community engagement, the HPB's volunteer programme was expanded. The Health Ambassador Network (HAN) was launched in October 2011 with 1000 volunteers, on the premise that behavioural change could be driven through role modelling and inspiring others to take up healthy lifestyles. By 2014, HAN had grown to over 7000 members.[34]

In the meantime, health authorities worldwide increasingly recognised that lifestyles were influenced by a myriad of social and environmental factors which often did not fall entirely under the ambit of the health sector. At the 8th Global Conference on Health Promotion in June 2013, Dr. Margaret Chan, Director-General of the WHO, spoke about these trends and challenges of health promotion:

> "Instead of diseases vanishing as living conditions improve, socioeconomic progress is actually creating the conditions that favour the rise of non-communicable diseases. Economic growth, modernisation, and urbanisation have opened wide the entry point for the spread of unhealthy lifestyles."[35]

Effective health promotion thus required the concerted and synergistic collaboration of a wide range of health and non-health stakeholders across the public, private, and people-oriented sectors.

The HPB needed to take a more integrated approach to achieve its vision of a healthy citizenry. It also needed to focus on various stakeholder engagement and finding trigger points to change human behaviour so that Singaporeans would take ownership of their own healthy lifestyles. Sufficient number of healthy choices e.g. healthier foods and physical activity amenities needed to exist in order to impact behaviour change for the healthier across the population. To do so, the HPB needed to mobilise partners who had the reach crucial to making a large enough environmental shift to influence consumer choices.

> "Singaporeans agree more can be done to improve their health, particularly in the areas of physical activity and regular health screening. However, such awareness has not yet prompted Singaporeans to proactively adopt a healthier lifestyle."
>
> — AIA 2013
> Healthy Living Index Survey

Under Mr. Zee Yoong Kang, its fourth CEO who assumed the role in 2013 and had extensive experience in engaging diverse stakeholders, the HPB focused on "tilting the market" by working with public and private sectors partners to make healthier choices more accessible and affordable. The HPB also began to use behavioural economics to nudge and incentivise individual decisions towards healthier choices. On a group and community level, gamification and the regional health network were leveraged to motivate Singaporeans towards healthier choices. Several large scale programmes such as the "Million Kilogram Challenge" for healthy weight management and the iQuit Campaign calling on peer and family support to motivate the smoker to quit received positive responses.

> Amongst the many issues raised during the Our Singapore Conversations held from 2012 to 2013, healthcare surfaced as one of the top concerns. At the same time, many also shared that they knew these concerns could be mitigated by leading a healthy lifestyle.

Healthy Living Master Plan — A Blueprint for Health Promotion

Singaporeans aspire to lead healthy lives. To do so, the adoption of healthy lifestyles becomes an important dimension in ensuring that Singaporeans continue to enjoy a good quality of life as we age. It is about enabling Singaporeans to live long and to live well.

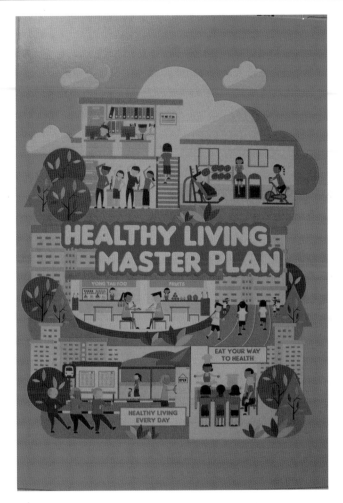

Cover of *Healthy Living Master Plan Report*, released April 2014.

To make this happen, it would require the efforts of the whole-of-government and whole-of-society to be integrated to enable healthy living options to span seamlessly across the settings where the population live, work, and play.

This was the main recommendation from the Healthy Living Master Plan Taskforce chaired by Associate Professor Muhammad Faishal Ibrahim, Parliamentary Secretary (Health). The resulting Healthy Living Master Plan, released in April 2014, focused on three key thrusts that would enable healthy living to become natural and effortless for Singaporeans. Besides increasing accessibility and affordability of healthy food choices through inter-agency and industry partnerships, the third key thrust was to build a social movement to normalise healthy behaviours. The common thread among these three thrusts was the use of behavioural insights or "nudges" to encourage people to take on healthy behaviours.

The vision of the Master Plan was simple: "Healthy Living Every Day." What this meant was that Singaporeans were to have easy access to healthy living. By 2020, one in two Singaporeans can look forward to having access to at least three healthy living options at the doorstep of their home, office, and school so that they can embrace healthy living as a part of their everyday routine. About one million employees will work in a health-promoting workplace and more than 90% of Singaporean students from pre-schools to junior colleges will be enjoying healthier meals in their schools. This vision will drive the country's efforts in the next lap of health promotion.

Conclusion

Singapore has come a long way in its health promotion efforts, from a developing country in the 1950s to the developed city state that it is today. As the world evolves, the challenges to healthy living will also evolve. Singapore's health authorities thus need to constantly innovate and look for new solutions to keep Singaporeans healthy even while being a sustainable steward of the nation's health promotion policies and programmes that protect all Singaporeans.

Acknowledgements

We would like to thank Mr. Zee Yoong Kang (Chief Executive Officer, HPB) for his guidance in the writing of this chapter. Our appreciation also goes to the colleagues in the various divisions and teams, who generously shared their experiences and photographs with us.

References

1. Ministry of Health & Health Promotion Board, Singapore. *Healthy Living Master Plan 2104*. Available: http://www.moh.gov.sg/healthylivingmasterplan
2. Cheshire, Sara. (2014) "The CNN 10 healthiest Cities: Singapore — Care that costs less." *CNN*. http://edition.cnn.com/interactive/2014/09/health/cnn10-healthiest-cities/?hpt=hp_c4
3. "Bloomberg Ranks the World's Most Efficient Healthcare Systems" http://www.advisory.com/daily-3briefing/2013/08/28/bloomberg-ranks-the-worlds-most-efficient-health-care-systems, 28 Aug 2013.

4. Singapore Budget 2014: http://www.singaporebudget.gov.sg/budget 2014
5. Health Promotion Board Annual Report 2011/2012.
6. WHO Health Statistics 2014. http://www.who.int/mediacentre/news/releases/2014/world-health-statistics-2014/en/
7. Prime Minister's Office, National Population & Talent Division. (2013) "A Sustainable Population for a Dynamic Singapore: Population White Paper."
8. Ministry of Health, Singapore. (2010) *National Health Survey.*
9. Ministry of Health, Singapore. (2007) *National Health Surveillance Survey.*
10. Health Promotion Board, Singapore. (2010) *National Nutrition Survey.*
11. Ministry of Health, Singapore. (2010) *Singapore Burden of Disease Study.*
12. National Healthcare Group Polyclinics. (2002) *A Legacy in Health: A Photo Journey Through the History of Primary Healthcare in Singapore.* National Healthcare Group Polyclinics.
13. Health Promotion Board, Singapore. (2011) "10 Years of Inspiring Healthy Living."
14. Goh KT. (1985) "The national childhood immunisation programmes in Singapore." *Singapore Med J.* **26**: 225–242.
15. Liew F, Ang WL, Cutter J, *et al.* (2010) "Evaluation on the effectiveness of the national childhood immunisation programme in Singapore, 1982–2007." *Ann Acad Med Singapore.* **39**: 532–541.
16. National Library Board Singapore. (2008) "Dental Health Programme." *Singapore Infopedia, National Library Board.* Accessible at: http://eresources.nlb.gov.sg/infopedia/articles/SIP_1177_2008-12-05.html
17. Health Promotion Board, School Dental Service. Unpublished data.
18. Ministry of Health, Singapore. (1991) "Healthy Family, Healthy Nation: Report of the Review Committee on National Health Policies."
19. World Health Organisation. (1986) "First International Conference on Health Promotion, Ottawa." *Ottawa Charter for Health Promotion.* http://www.who.int/healthpromotion/conferences/previous/ottawa. Date accessed: 25 Oct 2014.
20. Ministry of Health, Singapore. (1993) *Healthy Lifestyle Unit Annual Report.*
21. Ministry of Health, Singapore. (1993) *Training & Health Education Annual Report.*
22. Ministry of Health, Singapore. "Food & Nutrition Department 1990–1993."
23. Health Promotion Board, Singapore. (2010) "National Nutrition Survey."
24. Chew L, Lee HP. (2013) "Live it up without lighting up." Editorial. *Ann Acad Med Singapore.*
25. Thulaja NR. (2004) "National Smoking Control Programme." *Singapore Infopedia.* National Library Board Singapore. http://eresources.nlb.gov.sg/infopedia/articles/SIP_373_2004-12-23.html
26. Tan ASL, Arulanandam S, Chng CY, Vaithinathan. (2000) "Overview of legislation and tobacco control in Singapore." *Int J Tuberc Lung Dis.* **4**(11): 1002–1008.
27. National Registry of Diseases Office. Singapore. (2010) "Trends in cancer incidence in Singapore, 1968–2007." *The Singapore Cancer Registry Report.* Iss. No. 7.
28. Committee of Supply, 2013. Speech by Minister for Health Gan Kim Yong, "Better Health for All" (Part 1 of 2). http://www.gov.sg/content/moh_web/home/pressRoom/

speeches_d/2013/COS2013SpeechBetterHealthForAllPart1of2.html. Date accessed: 1 Nov 2013.

29. Health Promotion Board, Singapore. *Annual Reports 2002–2005*.

30. Health Promotion Board, Singapore. *HealthLine 2013–14*; unpublished data.

31. Health Promotion Board, Singapore. "Lose-to-Win 2009–2013." unpublished data.

32. "Gold Effie to DDB Group Singapore for the Health Promotion Board's demential campaign." *Campaign Brief Asia*. Published 10 June 2014. Accessible at: http://www. campaignbriefasia.com/asia/2014/06/gold-effie-to-ddb-group-singap.html.

33. DDB Group Singapore. (2011) "Hall of Fame." *Catchfire Awards*. http://www.ddb. com.sg/?page_id=766

34. Health Promotion Board, Singapore. Health Ambassador Network, unpublished data.

35. Dr. Margaret Chan, Director-General of WHO. "Opening Address at the 8th Global Conference on Health Promotion," Helsinki, Finland, 10 June 2013. Accessible at: http://www.who.int/healthpromotion/conferences/8gchp.

10 Primary Care

Lim Wei* and Adrian Ee†

The Early Years — Before 1965

Primary healthcare in Singapore can be traced back to as early as 1819, where Sir Thomas Pandergast, a Sub-Assistant Surgeon, set foot on Singapore soil with Sir Stamford Raffles. Health conditions then were poor and much was needed to be done. Sir Thomas introduced Western medicine to Singapore[1] and initiated the beginning of Singapore's healthcare journey.

In the 1830s, the first Rural Health Officer was appointed, a measure of starting organised public health services in Singapore, where one of the biggest challenges then was bringing healthcare to the country's rural areas.

The population was largely formed by immigrants from China, India, the Malay Archipelago and beyond.[2] Although Western medicine was introduced, the population was inclined to seek medical help within their ethnic groups. In 1867, a group of migrants from China established Thong Chai Yee Say, currently known as Thong Chai Medical Institution, at a shop house in Upper Pickering Street, where they provided free medical consultation and herbal medicine to all people, irrespective of race, religion, and status.[3]

In 1884, the first outdoor dispensary was opened in the Maternity Hospital at Victoria Street and created a demand for healthcare workers, especially trained nurses.

*Executive, Corporate Communications, SingHealth Polyclinics, Singapore.
†Chief Executive Officer, SingHealth Polyclinics. Adjunct Assistant Professor, Duke-NUS, Singapore.
[1] National Healthcare Group Polyclinics. *A Legacy in Health: A Photo-Journey Through the History of Primary Healthcare in Singapore.*
[2] Your Singapore. (2014). "Our History." Retrieved October 31, 2014, from *Your Singapore.* Accessed at: http://www.yoursingapore.com/about-singapore/singapore-history.html
[3] Singapore Thong Chai Medical Institution. (2012) "Our History." Retrieved October 31, 2014, from Singapore Thong Chai Medical Institution. Accessed at: http://www.stcmi.org.sg/history.asp

The lack of proper training limited the scope of care provided by nurses. It was only in May 1900 that the first batch of trained English nurses took over nursing duties from the French nuns in Singapore. By November 1900, there were one Head Sister, seven Sisters, and five student nurses to provide proper care.

Initial Efforts Developing Primary Healthcare

The high infant mortality rate across the island was a key concern. In 1910, Mrs. Blundell, a Municipal Nurse, was appointed to investigate the conditions of early infant life and advise mothers on proper childcare. This led to the launch of the Maternal and Child Health (MCH) Services in Singapore. Mrs. Blundell hired local women to be trained as midwives. In the same year, the first city Outpatient Dispensary (OPD) was established at South Canal Road. The MCH and OPD are now recognised as the early core components of the public sector primary healthcare.

As the demand for nurses grew, a structured nursing programme was started in 1916 for local nurses at St. Andrew's Hospital.

The first rural OPD was opened in Paya Lebar in 1923. In the same year, the first MCH Clinic was also set up in a vaccination centre at Prinsep Street and in an old rickshaw station in Chinatown the following year in 1924. Miss I.M.M. Simmons was appointed as the first Public Health Nurse in 1927, to provide child health services to the rural areas. Based on her recommendation, a Travelling Dispensary was also introduced. Nurses travelled to rural areas to attend to the sick, especially children who suffered from debilitating diseases.

In January 1929, the first local Health Nurse, Mrs. M.E. Perera, was employed. With more nurses on board, public health services continued to expand and in 1931, the Joo Chiat MCH was built. The Public Health Act and Midwives' Act were also passed in 1936. However, Singapore's primary healthcare efforts were disrupted during World War II (1942–1945).

After the war ended, healthcare services were reorganised to meet community needs.

Post-War Challenges: Rebuilding and Consolidating

The war took a toll on Singapore. People were severely undernourished and diseases such as tuberculosis and malaria were prevalent. More than 50% of school children were malnourished. Great efforts were made to provide medical services. Clinic sessions were held in make-shift locations such as shop houses, coolie quarters, and police posts.

To alleviate the dire state of healthcare, Dr. W.J. Vickers, then the Director of Medical Services, drew up a Ten-Year Medical Plan, which advocated that the

Singaporean Government needed to accept full responsibility for medical care for people within her borders. The plan stressed the importance of primary healthcare and called for a chain of MCH clinics to be built throughout the island.

As tuberculosis ran rampant among school children in 1948, nurses carried out large-scale Mantoux tests on children. In the same year, a polio epidemic resulted in schools having to close for three months.

The MCH Service was expanded to meet the needs of the post-war baby boom. By 1951, ten Maternal and Child Welfare Centres were built and staffed by nurses and midwives. School nurses in the travelling dispensary provided medication such as deworming drugs, tonics, and other medication to school children.

The 1950s was also the period of health campaigns as the population continued to be threatened by diseases such as diphtheria, polio, and smallpox. Of these, diphtheria claimed the most lives, prompting the launch of the Anti-Diphtheria Campaign in 1952, followed by the Diphtheria Immunisation Campaign in 1957. In 1961, an ordinance was put in place that required vaccination of all children up to the age of seven.

In 1952, the Domiciliary After-Care (DAC) Service was introduced to relieve the demand for maternity beds. In addition, District Midwives provided nursing care and health education to mothers and newborns who were discharged from the hospitals, 24- to 36-hours after delivery.

In 1958, the District Nursing Service was introduced under the Outpatient Service of the Ministry of Health (MOH). Operating from six decentralised clinics, with the General Hospital acting as the control centre, the District Nursing Service provided home nursing care and rehabilitation for patients of all ages following their discharge from hospital. Thirteen new Rural Clinics were also established. The ten Maternal and Child Welfare Centres and 13 Rural Clinics looked after mothers and newborns. The MCH Service was awarded the Kettering Shield in 1958 by the National Baby Council, London, for outstanding work in the field of maternal and child health.

In the 1960s, the Maternal and Child Welfare Centres and Rural Clinics were reorganised to form seven large Rural Health Centres at Nee Soon, Holland Road, Thomson Road, Serangoon Road, Yio Chu Kang Road, Ama Keng, and Buona Vista. Soon after in 1963, the first two combined OPD and MCH Clinics were built in Queenstown and Still Road. Although physically co-located, both the OPD and MCH operated independently.

Post-War General Practice

In the public sector, nurses continued to anchor primary healthcare in the post-war era, but what about general practice? "During the colonial days when the British settled in Singapore, a number of their family physicians took over the healthcare in Singapore, outside the hospitals," shared Dr. Lee Suan Yew, former President of Singapore Medical Council, "Very little history in writing however, is available." There were General Practitioner (GP) groups like Trythall, Hoy and Partners, and Bains and Partners in the city area. There were also local GPs and GP groups like Clifford Dispensary who started their practices in town as well.

There were also local GPs who started their practices within small communities and kampong areas like Jurong Kechil and Ama Keng. The number of GPs practising in the neighbourhood communities grew in tandem with the growth of the nation as kampongs made way for housing estates. The early ones were in Tiong Bahru, Kallang, and Toa Payoh.

A New Beginning — The Road after Independence

Looking back, primary care took leaps and bounds over the last 50 years to keep pace with the growth of modern day medicine. Primary healthcare continued to change; the growing affluence of the people brought about new needs to be met. Not only was there growth in medical and nursing care; with the growth of services, administration of facilities became a sizeable service too. In terms of growth, today's epidemics take on a more threatening form due to accessibility of air travel. Hence, pandemic preparedness has become a new primary care role.

Nursing, the Stalwarts of Care

Post-independence brought about new roles for the nursing profession. The Domiciliary (Home) Delivery Service was phased out in 1966 due to increasing preference for deliveries in hospitals. The DAC Services were stopped in 1992 due to low demand.

The 1970s saw rising affluence in Singapore and with it, an increase in prevalence of chronic diseases such as hypertension and diabetes. Nurses in Outpatient Clinics were trained to review, educate, and manage patients whose hypertension or diabetes was stable. Such trained nurses were known as Nurse Practitioners. The main focus of Nurse Practitioners was on health counselling and public health education. This continues to be one of the key roles for senior nurses today.

Since 1989, Staff Nurses in polyclinics were trained to use the modified Denver Developmental Screening Test (DDST, Singapore) for screening cognitive and behavioural problems in preschool children. Nurses have also taken over Diabetic Retinal Photography (DRP) for patients with diabetes. These new responsibilities expanded the nurses' capability in providing care for patients.

Today, nurses in polyclinics (see Primary Healthcare Infrastructure & Administration) play an important role in the prevention and early detection of diseases through immunisation, screening programmes, and health education programmes targeted at both adults and children. While ante-natal and post-natal care for mothers are still provided by midwives in polyclinics, nurses also run the Well-Women Clinics in polyclinics. They assist in screening for breast and cervical cancer, and take on the roles of health educator and family planning counsellor.

From General Practitioners to Family Physicians

In 1971, a group of GPs saw the gap and need to promote the values and ideals of primary healthcare,[4] and they formed the College of General Practitioners Singapore.

Following the inauguration of the College, the first examination for diplomate membership, the MCGP (Membership of the College of General Practitioners Singapore), was held in 1972 — the first of its kind for Family Medicine in Singapore. The MCGP was recognised by the Singapore Medical Council as a post-graduate medical qualification. In 1974, Dr. Benjamin A. Sheares, the late President of Singapore, became a Patron of the College.

The leaders of the Singapore College of the day felt it would be invaluable for the College to host one of the triennial world conferences of family doctors — to bring the world's thought leaders of Family Medicine to Singapore. The result was the 10th World Organization of National Colleges, Academies, and Academic Associations of General Practitioners/Family Physicians (WONCA) World Conference on Family Medicine in Singapore in 1983.

The World Conference was a great success and it also helped to set the foundation toward postgraduate training in General Practice. As a follow-up, Singapore organised the World Conference a second time round, in 2007, 24 years later. Singapore benefitted much from these two world conferences in Family Medicine. Following that, Singapore also hosted the 2nd and 4th Asia Pacific Primary Care Research Conference (APPCRC) in 2010 and 2014 respectively to spur primary care research.

The Journey to Recognition for Family Medicine

The first development towards recognition of Family Medicine as a discipline was the change in name of the Department of Social Medicine and Public Health

---

[4] College of Family Physicians. (1999) "College Mission." Retrieved October 23, 2014, from College of Family Physicians. Accessed at: http://www.cfps.org.sg/about-us/college-mission/

(SMPH) of the then-Faculty of Medicine, National University of Singapore to the Department of Community, Occupational and Family Medicine (COFM) in 1987. This change was made possible through the intervention of the then Minister of Health, Mr. Howe Yoon Chong, and the College members. The duration of the under-graduate programme was increased from 2 weeks to 8 weeks. The Undergraduate Teaching Committee of the College worked closely with the Department in teaching Family Medicine at the School. In the two other medical schools that have been set up since in Singapore, namely the Duke-NUS and the Lee Kong Chian School of Medicine, Family Medicine is also taught in the undergraduate years.

Setting up the postgraduate Family Medicine programme was another milestone in the development of Family Medicine. A key development was the formation of the Steering Committee on Family Medicine Training in 1988. This was a tripart-ite body comprising the College, MOH, and the COFM. Several memorandums were proposed to undertake and develop a more holistic training and recognition for Family Medicine. The training programme leading to the award of the post-graduate Family Medicine degree — the Master of Medicine in Family Medicine (MMed FM) — was approved by the Senate of NUS in 1991.

In 1993, the College was appointed by the Singapore Medical Council to admin-ister the Singapore Medical Council-Continuing Medical Education Programme, to ensure continual training for non-specialists. In the same year, the first Master of Medicine in Family Medicine (MMed FM) examination was held, previously known as Programme A. This programme further enhanced the knowledge and skills of Family Physicians in Singapore. Shortly thereafter, on 17 November 1993, the name of the College of General Practitioners Singapore was officially changed to "College of Family Physicians Singapore" (CFPS).

In 1998, the Fellowship of the CFPS (FCFP) by assessment was inaugurated to provide Advanced Family Medicine Training to Family Physicians holding the MMed FM. Subsequently, in 2000 the first batch of eight family physicians was conferred Fellowship of the College.

In 2000, CFPS launched the Graduate Diploma in Family Medicine (GDFM), a commitment to further upgrade Family Physicians. To further enhance the efforts in training, the Institute of Family Medicine (IFM) was formed in 2001.

In 2011, the Residency training for Family Medicine was started in Singapore. The Family Physicians Register (FPR) was introduced in 2012 by Family Physician Accreditation Board (FPAB), so that practices in care settings that were consistent with the broader definition of Family Medicine were recognised too. Family Phys-icians are practising not only in polyclinics and GP clinics, but also in restructured hospitals, community hospitals, nursing homes, home care services, and even in palliative care facilities.[5]

The growing significance of Family Physicians in providing holistic care to the population enabled the CFPS to organise Singapore's first World Family Doctors' Day (WFDD) celebration in 2014.

Dr. Lim Shih Hui, Master, Academy of Medicine, proposed that a Chapter of Family Physicians be formed in the College of Physicians of the Academy; this has been duly adopted by the Academy and the College of Family Physicians. The first batch of Family Medicine Physicians was inducted as Fellows of the Academy of Medicine (Chapter of Family Medicine Physicians), Singapore, on 25 October 2014 — a significant milestone in the recognition of Family Medicine as a distinct specialty of Medicine.

The Enlarging Demand on Public Sector Primary Care

The post-war baby boom posed great stress on the nation's healthcare system. Families were large with 6 to 8 children and mothers were often at risk of health issues. In 1966, the Government launched the National Family Planning Programme to manage population growth, so as not to outpace economic growth and infrastructure support. The MCH Clinics were instrumental in disseminating information and initiating family planning programmes. These clinics provided free consultation, pregnancy tests, and sterilisation. On top of these services, the clinics also provided contraceptives at nominal charges.

MCH Service introduced the first Family Health Booklet in 1975, which included the antenatal records for three pregnancies and the records of 3 children from birth to 6 years old. It also recorded significant illness, infectious diseases, hospital referrals, and children's growth charts. Later, a Baby's Discharge Record was incorporated in the Booklet. When a child reached school-going age, this record was to be detached and forwarded to School Health Service for immediate follow-up.

In 1976, after a reorganisation at MOH, the Primary Healthcare Division was set up. The Division planned the development of polyclinics within the community for greater access to primary healthcare services, in both urban and rural areas.

---

[5] Kheng Hock L, Pak Yean C, Lee Gan G. (2012) "The College Mirror." Retrieved October 26, 2014, from College of Family Physicians Singapore: http://cfps.org.sg/publications/the-college-mirror/download/12

The first official polyclinic was built in 1978 at Toa Payoh Central. The success of this new care delivery model brought about the reorganisation and combination of 41 OPDs and MCH Clinics in the 1980s to form 16 polyclinics. The polyclinics had up-to-date facilities, well-planned consultation and treatment rooms as well as waiting areas. They provided a comprehensive range of services such as outpatient medical care, maternal and child healthcare, psychiatric care, dental services, rehabilitation, and health screening for the elderly.

It was also in 1984, Dr. Uma Rajan, then-Director for School Health Services, together with her team, devised a "Child Health Booklet" to replace the Family Health Booklet created in 1975 and medical cards for school-going children so that parents could keep track on their children's medical conditions.[6]

The Polyclinics Refined: Bigger and Better to Meet Modernised Demands

In 1988, the first "new-generation polyclinic" was opened at Toa Payoh Lorong 8. It was also the first polyclinic that used Information Technology (IT) — Polyclinic Patient Management System (PPMS) for greater efficiency in operations such as patient master index, appointment scheduling, patient call-up, and generation of reminders and account, and a management reporting system.

By 1992, Kallang OPD, Macpherson OPD, Still Road Polyclinic, and Aljunied MCH Clinic were combined as Geylang Polyclinic. Tampines Polyclinic, built in March 1990, was also the first polyclinic with X-ray facilities.

On 1 July 1992, Community Health Service (formerly Outpatient Service) and Maternal and Child Health Service were merged to form the Family Health Service (FHS). The FHS was part of the Primary Health Services, together with School Health Services, Training and Health Education Department, Healthy Lifestyle Unit, and Food and Nutrition Department.

In order to give greater personnel and financial flexibilities to the polyclinic system, Tampines and Toa Payoh Polyclinics piloted the concept of Autonomous Agencies in 1996 where the polyclinics had the autonomy to administer the service cost and financial performance.

Yishun Polyclinic was the last polyclinic officially opened in 1998 before the healthcare clustering started in 2000. The Healthcare Services underwent major

---

[6]Ming En, S. (2014) "Pioneers contributed ideas to the nation that still endure." Retrieved October 20, 2014, from Today: http://www.todayonline.com/singapore/pioneers-contributed-ideas-nation-still-endure

restructuring on 1 October 2000 and was reorganised into two clusters — National Healthcare Group (NHG) and Singapore Health Services (SingHealth). The polyclinics were also reorganised to be managed by National Healthcare Group Polyclinics (NHGP) and SingHealth Polyclinics (SHP). This clustering and reorganisation provided a platform for consolidation and integration in order to bring about better health outcomes and greater efficiency.

Two new polyclinics were opened in Pasir Ris (2002) and Sengkang (2005) respectively, to provide care for new and younger communities in the newly developed estates. Queenstown Polyclinic was also relocated from Margaret Drive to Stirling Road in 2009. Older polyclinics such as Ang Mo Kio, Clementi, Geylang, Marine Parade, and Tampines Polyclinics underwent major renovations to meet the needs of the community they served. Hardcopy medical records in both polyclinic clusters were migrated to electronic medical records for easier access to patients' medical history by polyclinic doctors and enhanced by clinical decision support tools.

To help reshape the primary healthcare landscape for the nation and support the development of GPs, a Primary Care Master Plan was developed in 2011 by MOH in consultation with more than 350 GPs. The plan covered three main areas — financing, infrastructure, and model of care.[7] In the same year, the National Electronic Health Record (NEHR) was implemented in phases for public and selected private healthcare providers, to provide a robust system that enables access for healthcare providers to shared medical data and improve clinical decisions for better care.

Staying Resilient — Primary Healthcare Challenges

In the early years, Singapore faced and successfully curbed diseases such as tuberculosis, smallpox, diphtheria, and polio. By 1978, the last case of polio was reported in Singapore. This was reflected in the book, "A legacy in Health: A Photo-Journey through the History of Primary Healthcare in Singapore" by NHGP. Today's primary healthcare challenges are in the prevention and management of chronic diseases; care of the growing numbers of the elderly; and care of the increasing Singapore population which is estimated to reach 6.9 million in 2030. Primary healthcare undertakes a key surveillance role in monitoring and detecting emerging infectious diseases, and primary healthcare pandemic preparedness is critical to ensuring community health.

---

[7] Ministry of Health, Singapore. (2011). "Transforming the primary care landscape: Engaging the GP community and our stakeholders in the journey." Retrieved October 28, 2014, from Ministry of Health, Singapore. Accessed at: https://www.moh.gov.sg/content/moh_web/home/pressRoom/pressRoomItem-Release/2011/transforming_theprimarycarelandscapeengagingthegpcommunityandour.html

Rise of HIV and AIDS

When the first HIV-positive case in Singapore was reported in May 1985, the Advisory Committee on AIDS was formed in the same year. In 1988, the government invested in a nationwide AIDS campaign, which included an educational blitz via radio and television advertisements. The government also lifted its ban on condom advertisements. The charges for AIDS testing were reduced and HIV testing centres were introduced at Bedok, Bukit Merah, Ang Mo Kio, Clementi, and Kelantan Polyclinics, the Kallang Outpatient Dispensary and Maxwell Road OPD. In addition, an AIDS Counselling Centre at Rochor OPD and AIDS helplines for information and counselling were also introduced.[8]

A Hazy Situation

The nation experienced its first haze risk as early as 1972, where the island was shrouded in a thick layer of haze and primary healthcare was at the forefront of the nation's swift response. One of the worst and unexpected episodes was in 1997 — when the Pollutant Standard Index (PSI) hit 226 in September 1997.

In 2013, the haze returned with an alarming PSI reading of 401 on 21 June 2013.[9] Both polyclinics and GPs attended to large crowds with respiratory and haze-related ailments. Many staff had to brave the hazy conditions and wore masks while working outdoors or in non-air-conditioned environment. The triage system was set up for the high-risk groups of patients such as pregnant women, infants, and patients with respiratory conditions. Air purifiers and portable air-conditioners were supplied by MOH at selected polyclinics that were non-air-conditioned for better air quality.

Fighting the Unknown — Severe Acute Respiratory Syndrome (SARS)

It was the Severe Acute Respiratory Syndrome (SARS) that shook the nation in 2003. A total of 238 cases were reported and there were 33 deaths,[10] including

---

[8] Thulaja NR. (2004). "National AIDS Control Programme." Retrieved October 28, 2014, from Singapore Infopedia, MOH, Singapore. Accessed at: http://eresources.nlb.gov.sg/infopedia/articles/SIP_372_2004-12-23.html

[9] Jaime K, Stephanie H. (2013). "Haze pollution." Retrieved October 28, 2014, from Singapore Infopedia, MOH, Singapore. Accessed at: http://eresources.nlb.gov.sg/infopedia/articles/SIP_2013-08-30_185150.html

[10] World Health Organisation. (2003). "Summary of probable SARS cases with onset of illness from 1 November 2002 to 31 July 2003." Retrieved October 26, 2014, from World Health Organisation: http://www.who.int/csr/sars/country/table2004_04_21/en/

healthcare workers. The three-month episode not only brought the nation together, but it also put the primary healthcare professionals to the test. As the polyclinics and GPs were usually the first point of contact, they were on high alert in identifying probable cases. At some polyclinics, outdoor tents were built to better manage the fever cases and to contain potential risk of spread. Staff from the various healthcare providers were deployed to all air, sea, and land checkpoints to screen inbound and outbound passengers for fever.

Traveller screening at Changi Airport was implemented and primary healthcare nurses were deployed to the airport.[11] Ms. Lee Yoke Yin, former Assistant Director for Nursing in SingHealth Polyclinics recalled, "My previous experiences gained from Changi Airport screening deployment gave me the knowledge and confidence during the SARS period at Changi Airport in 2003, where I oversaw the manpower deployment, rostering nurses from SingHealth Polyclinics, National Healthcare Group Polyclinics, School Health Service, and School Dental Service. Nurses were stationed at the departure and immigration to conduct the SARS fever screening among inbound travellers."

When the SARS risk finally abated, healthcare institutions focused on pandemic preparedness and staff training. A disease surveillance system and Influenza Pandemic Preparedness Plan was created to better manage such outbreaks, known as the Disease Outbreak Response System (DORS) — a five-colour alert system that progresses from Green to Yellow, Orange, Red, and Black.[12]

New Wave — Influenza A (H1N1) and What's Next?

When Singapore faced another infectious disease outbreak in 2009 — the Influenza A (H1N1) or Swine Flu, Singapore was prepared. The GPs and polyclinics were organised and equipped to set up Pandemic Preparedness Clinics. Triaging and segregation of patients with influenza symptoms were promptly carried out. Support was provided on ways to better manage the increased numbers of flu cases, scale-up flu vaccinations, and the supply of Personal Protection Equipment (PPE) if needed.

In September 2009, the final fatality occurred, bringing the total number of lives claimed to 18. More than 1.3 million vaccines were made available island-wide.

---

[11] *The New Paper.* (2013). "SARS Timeline." Retrieved October 26, 2014, from AsiaOne. Accessed at: http://yourhealth.asiaone.com/content/sars-timeline/

[12] Sara P. (2010) "Influenza A (H1N1-2009) outbreak." Retrieved October 26, 2014, from *Singapore Infopedia,* MOH Singapore. Accessed at: http://eresources.nlb.gov.sg/infopedia/articles/SIP_1759_2011-01-28.html

An estimated 400,000 people in Singapore were infected with the H1N1 virus and more than 420,000 local residents had received the H1N1 vaccination.

Health conditions and infections are evolving; what used to be deadly in the past may not be an issue now. Diseases are more communicable across the globe due to connectivity and accessibility brought about by the advancement in transportation technology. Therefore, primary healthcare providers, being the first contact points, play an important role in the nation's health.

Great Opportunities Ahead for Primary Healthcare

Primary healthcare has always been the first line of care and forms the foundation for our healthcare system. With a rapidly ageing society and a higher prevalence of chronic diseases (even amongst the younger population), the focus as outlined in the MOH Primary Care Master Plan released in 2011, is to develop and strengthen primary healthcare so that Specialist Outpatient Centres (SOCs) can focus on complex cases that require specialist care.

Primary Care Master Plan — Changing the Care Delivery

Under the Primary Care Master Plan 2011, the Primary Care Partnership Scheme (PCPS), was enhanced to the Community Health Assist Scheme (CHAS). It provided greater subsidies and included lower to middle-income patients. They were eligible for subsidised treatment at GP clinics, as well as for dental care at private dentists. Community Health Centres (CHCs) were also built to support GPs in chronic disease management. The CHCs provide services such as DRP, Diabetic Foot Screening (DFS), and health counselling for patients with diabetes. Family Medicine Clinics (FMCs) were also piloted. This new model of care is a collaborative effort between public and private sectors, where a group of GPs forms a clinic, coupled with services for chronic conditions, pharmacy, and laboratory.[13] In his speech, Minister Gan also shared plans to build more polyclinics by 2030.

However, to build up the capacity in primary healthcare for the future, more needs to be done to attract talent (doctors, nurses, and allied health professionals),

---

[13] Kim Yong G. (2013). "COS Speech By Minister for Health Gan Kim Yong — Better Health for All." Retrieved October 28, 2014, from Ministry of Health, Singapore. Accessed at: https://www.moh.gov.sg/content/moh_web/home/pressRoom/speeches_d/2013/COS2013SpeechBetterHealthforAllPart1of2.html

to Family Medicine. Dr. Ling Sing Lin, former Director for Family Health Service, opined that, "Healthcare costs can be effectively brought down without any loss in the quality of care," and therefore the role of primary healthcare needs to be profiled strongly within the context of the regional health systems for better integration.

Vision for the Future

The quality of primary healthcare is often measured using the six domains established by the 1978 Alma-Ata Declaration[14] — first contact, longitudinally, comprehensiveness, coordination, person or family-centeredness, and community orientation. For primary healthcare providers, the active involvement of the community, residents, families, and the patients is important in the next paradigm shift towards population care management.

"Everyone has a part to play, including the patients themselves. There should be more emphasis on primary healthcare," shared A/Prof. Cheong Pak Yean, former President for College of Family Physicians Singapore. "Perhaps there is a need to revisit the subsidy system so that patients receive the necessary aid and this could help patients receive more timely care within the community."

Ultimately, what matters most is the person, family, and community-centeredness of care; and this must always be the cornerstone of primary healthcare. "The right-siting of stabilised patients with chronic diseases back to the GP clinics is important," echoed Dr. Shanta Emmanuel, former CEO for National Healthcare Group Polyclinics, "as it can help transfer the patient crowd from many subsidised Specialist Outpatient Clinics (SOCs) in the public sector hospitals, but it can only be done if the drugs provided at the GP clinics are of the equivalent price as in the subsidised SOCs."

> "Polyclinics and GPs will complement each other to provide good primary care to Singaporeans, even as we build more hospitals and medical centres. By leveraging on each other's strengths, we will build a vibrant ecosystem that promotes health and enables seamless holistic care."
>
> — Mr. Gan Kim Yong, Minister for Health, 29 August 2014

---

[14] World Health Organization. (1978). "Declaration of Alma-Ata." *International Conference on Primary Health Care, Alma-Ata, USSR, 6–12 September 1978.* WHO. Retrieved December 3, 2014, from World Health Organization. Accessed at: http://www.who.int/publications/almaata_declaration_en.pdf?ua=1

Acknowledgement

This chapter cannot be completed if not for the following esteemed contributors:
[In alphabetical order]

A/Prof. Cheong Pak Yean

A/Prof. Goh Lee Gan

Dr. Henry Yeo Peng Hock

Dr. Lam Sian Lian

Dr. Lee Suan Yew

Dr. Lim Hai Chiew

Dr. Ling Sing Lin

Dr. Meenakshi Sundararaman

Dr. Paul Goh Soo Chye

Dr. Shanta Emmanuel

Dr. Swah Teck Sin

Dr. Uma Rajan

Lee Yoke Yin

National Healthcare Group Polyclinics

SingHealth Polyclinics

Bibliography

College of Family Physicians. (1999). *College Mission*. Retrieved 23 October 2014, from College of Family Physicians: http://www.cfps.org.sg/about-us/college-mission/

Cheong PY. (2014) "Education and training in family medicine: Looking ahead." *Singapore Med J.* **55**(3): 124–125. PubMed PMID: 24664376.

Goh LG, Ong CP. (2014) "Education and training in family medicine: Progress and a proposed national vision for 2030." *Singapore Med J.* 55(3):117–123. PubMed PMID: 24664375.

Jaime K, Stephanie H. (2013) *Haze pollution*. Retrieved 28 October 2014, from Singapore Infopedia, MOH: http://eresources.nlb.gov.sg/infopedia/articles/SIP_2013-08-30_185150.html

Kheng Hock L, Pak Yean C, Lee Gan G. (2012). *The College Mirror*. Retrieved 26 October 2014, from College of Family Physicians Singapore: http://cfps.org.sg/publications/the-college-mirror/download/12

Kim Yong G. (2013) *COS Speech by Minister for Health Gan Kim Yong — Better Health for All*. Retrieved 28 October 2014, from Ministry of Health, Singapore: https://www.moh.gov.sg/content/moh_web/home/pressRoom/speeches_d/2013/COS2013SpeechBetterHealthforAllPart1of2.html

Kim Yong G. (2014). *Speech by Minister for Health*. Retrieved 20 October 2014, from Ministry of Health, Singapore: http://www.moh.gov.sg/content/moh_web/home/pressRoom/speeches_d/2014/speech-by-minister-for-health--mr-gan-kim-yong--attribute-to-he.html

Kim Yong, G. (2014) *Speech by Mr Gan Kim Yong, Minister for Health, at Groundbuilding Ceremony for Changi General Hospital Medical Centre, 29 Aug 2014*. Retrieved December 3, 2014, from Ministry of Health, Singapore: https://www.moh.gov.sg/content/moh_web/home/pressRoom/speeches_d/2014/speech-by-mr-gan-kim-yong--minister-for-health--groundbuilding-c.html

Ming En S. (2014) *Pioneers contributed ideas to the nation that still endure*. Retrieved October 20, 2014, from Today: http://www.todayonline.com/singapore/pioneers-contributed-ideas-nation-still-endure

Ministry of Health. (1997) *More Than A Calling*. Singapore: Grace Communications Pte Ltd.

Ministry of Health, Singapore. (2011) *Transforming the Primary Care Landscape: Engaging the GP Community and our Stakeholders in the Journey*. Retrieved October 28, 2014, from Ministry of Health, Singapore: https://www.moh.gov.sg/content/moh_web/home/pressRoom/pressRoomItemRelease/2011/transforming_theprimarycarelandscapeengagingthegpcommunityandour.html

National Healthcare Group Polyclinics. (n.d.) *A Legacy in Health: A Photo-Journey Through the History of Primary Healthcare in Singapore*.

Sara P. (2010). *Influenza A (H1N1-2009) outbreak*. Retrieved 26 October 2014, from Singapore Infopedia: http://eresources.nlb.gov.sg/infopedia/articles/SIP_1759_2011-01-28.html

Singapore Thong Chai Medical Institution. (2012). *Our History*. Retrieved 31 October 2014, from Singapore Thong Chai Medical Institution: http://www.stcmi.org.sg/history.asp

The New Paper. (2013) *SARS Timeline*. Retrieved 26 October 2014, from *AsiaOne*: http://yourhealth.asiaone.com/content/sars-timeline/

Thulaja NR. (2004) *National AIDS Control Programme*. Retrieved 28 October 2014, from Singapore Infopedia, MOH: http://eresources.nlb.gov.sg/infopedia/articles/SIP_372_2004-12-23.html

World Health Organisation. (2003) *Summary of probable SARS cases with onset of illness from 1 November 2002 to 31 July 2003*. Retrieved 26 October 2014, from World Health Organisation: http://www.who.int/csr/sars/country/table2004_04_21/en/

World Health Organization. (1978) *Declaration of Alma-Ata*. Retrieved December 3, 2014, from World Health Organization: http://www.who.int/publications/almaata_declaration_en.pdf?ua=1

Your Singapore. (2014) *Our History*. Retrieved October 31, 2014, from Your Singapore: http://www.yoursingapore.com/about-singapore/singapore-history.html

11 Singapore's Hospitals — Introduction

Lee Chien Earn*

Hospitals are a key resource and also the key consumer of resources in health systems around the world. The role of hospitals extend beyond the care of patients include the fields of education and research. Singapore has a hybrid healthcare delivery system. The State continues, from the very early years, to play a dominant role, currently providing close to 80% of all acute care hospital services with the private sector providing the remaining 20%.

The development of hospitals in Singapore is a microcosm of the development of Singapore. From modest beginnings, our hospitals today are comparable with those in developed countries serving not just the local population, but also especially in the private sector foreign patients attracted by the reputation of our medical services. The public sector which had just two general hospitals for acute illness — the General Hospital at Outram Road and the Thomson Road General Hospital (TRGH) — now has six acute general hospitals with state of the art facilities and staffed by healthcare professionals drawn from around the world.

The governance of public hospitals has evolved over the years starting out as departments under the Ministry of Health (where hospital staff are civil servants) to private limited companies (wholly owned by government) with flexibility in human resources (e.g. hiring and promoting staff) and finances (e.g. setting of fees) taking policy guidance from MOH. Currently public hospitals are grouped into one of six regional systems to facilitate continuity of care.

The role of hospitals has also changed through the years in response to changing demographics, epidemiology and environmental factors. For example, our hospitals at independence are now seeing an increasing number of patients with multiple acute and chronic conditions compared to infections diseases at Singapore's

---

*Chief Executive Officer, Changi General Hospital, Singapore.

independence. As the role and priorities of hospitals evolve, some would argue that the system's pace of change needs to be hastened to be transformative in order to remain relevant to the needs of our population.

In this chapter the leadership of public and private hospitals share the historical development and vision for their respective institutions.

11.1 Singapore General Hospital

Ang Chong Lye*

With a history of nearly 200 years, Singapore General Hospital (SGH) arguably has had a head-start in advancing medicine and healthcare. However, staying at the forefront of medicine was not pre-destined — nor did it happen by chance.

SGH has remained in the minds of Singaporeans as "the People's Hospital" because we have stayed relevant. SGH anticipated the changing needs of Singaporeans — and in turn has adapted and evolved.

Since the 1980s when SGH and other public hospitals were given autonomy to operate as corporations in order to be more efficient, SGH has taken the path of specialisation. Several specialty departments were spun off into national centres: the Singapore National Eye Centre (SNEC), the National Heart Centre of Singapore (NHCS), the National Dental Centre of Singapore (NDCS), and the National Cancer Centre of Singapore (NCCS), which are all located on the SGH campus.

By the turn of the 21st century, our national centres have themselves matured and given their specialities distinct leadership positions that extend beyond the shores of Singapore.

Not content to rest on our laurels, we have embarked on a master plan that will thoroughly transform the entire campus in the coming decades. Work began with the completion of the Academia in 2013 and the NHCS in 2014. The Academia, which includes cutting-edge technology in pathological services, will help us realise our ambitions in research and training, while the new NHCS is now better able to provide a seamless and expanded service to heart patients. A new community hospital for post-acute care is in the works. It will create tremendous value as our Nation's healthcare transits into a more integrated model of care for the citizens.

*Chief Executive Officer, Singapore General Hospital; Deputy Group Chief Executive Officer (Clinical Services and Informatics), Singapore Health Services.

Meanwhile, our collaboration with the Duke-NUS Graduate Medical School, which also sits on the grounds of the SGH Campus, adds another dimension to SGH. As a teaching hospital, SGH doctors train medical students from Duke-NUS and the NUS Yong Loo Lin School of Medicine. SGH has always been the training ground for nursing and allied health students as well.

To serve Singaporeans in the years ahead, SGH is re-organising itself as a single service. Specialists from our various centres are coming together to offer patients an integrated service for any major condition. Combining different but related disciplines make seeing a condition easier for patients. Doing so also enhances the care we deliver to our patients. For example, the Head and Neck Centre brings the combined skills of surgeons and clinicians from various specialities together — from general surgery, plastic surgery, and ENT (ear, nose, and throat) surgery to oral and maxillofacial surgery. The Breast Centre groups the complementary skill sets of surgeons from both SGH and the KK Women's and Children's Hospital.

SGH is not simply grouping related disciplines, but it is also optimising and upgrading the skills of its nursing and allied health professionals who play a crucial role in supporting their clinical healthcare colleagues. For instance, nurses and pharmacists who have been trained in specific areas run clinics and see patients in stable conditions. They also play a role in counselling and educating patients, a task that is important in patient recovery.

Like other public hospitals, SGH is also extending its community outreach, working with a network of family physicians, polyclinics, and long-term care providers to offer the same level of care to patients with chronic disease.

This transformation in care delivery will hopefully ease the heavy patient load that puts significant stress on our resources. The SGH Campus receives over 1 million patient visits a year. The 1800 beds at SGH, including the 185 for NHCS patients, account for a quarter of the acute care bed space in public hospitals (see Table 11.1.1).

Table 11.1.1. SGH Campus' Market Share within Public Acute Sector in 2014

	Specialist Outpatient Clinic Attendances	Total Number of Surgeries	Admissions	Inpatient Discharges	Patient Days
Total workload in Public Acute sector (excluding Institute of Mental Health)	4,375,653	445,069	368,379	372,661	2,191,637
Workload by institutions on SGH Campus	1,239,054	146,486	88,404	88,413	525,659
SGH Campus market share in public acute sector	**28.3%**	**32.9%**	**24.0%**	**23.7%**	**24.0%**

Source: MOH Annual Statistics (Health Service Utilisation) 2014.

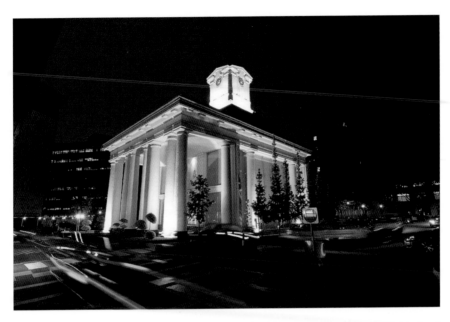

Opened in 1926, the iconic Bowyer Block which houses the SGH Museum is now a designated national monument. (Courtesy of Kwek Leng Beng.)

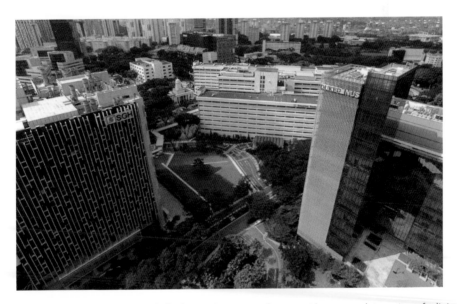

The SGH Campus is a vibrant hub for patient-centred care with a complete suite of clinical specialities that offers solutions to all our patient's clinical problems.

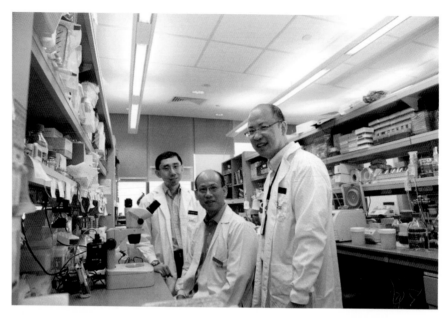

A commitment to improve care and a passion to find new treatment brings together doctors and scientists to translate research from the lab to the patient's. (*From left*: Dr. Charles Chuah, A; Prof. Ong Sin Tiong and Dr. Darren Lim found a mutation in a gene that makes some cancer drugs less effective for Asians, as well as a solution to tackle this problem).

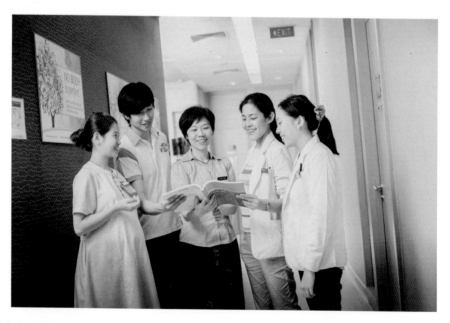

Multidisciplinary collaborations are critical, especially in tertiary academic medicine where doctors, nurses, and allied health professionals provide our patients with integrated care.

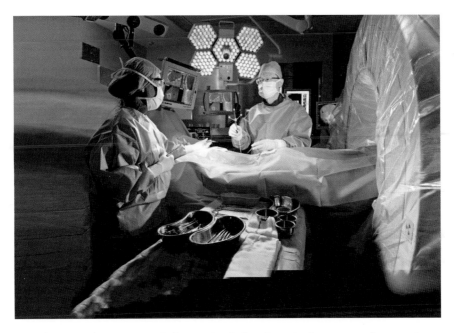

Newer techniques of treatment including minimally invasive robotics surgery allow our doctors to use the latest technology to tackle very complicated clinical problems, elevating us to world-class standards.

The heavy patient load also means that SGH clinicians have the privilege of treating rare and common illnesses with unusual variations. Not only do such cases test our diagnostic and treatment skills, they challenge our clinicians and health-care professionals to search for improvements or new procedures and treatments.

Such opportunities for care and research draw professionals who are passionate and motivated about improving healthcare and lives.

At SGH, we believe that we are a unique community that is able to offer the citizens of Singapore the necessary environment and support to deliver the sort of excellence that keeps us perpetually at the front line of medical advances.

Pioneering Care

2014 • SGH received Joint Commission International (JCI) — Academic Medical Centre accreditation

2012 • SGH starts world's first trial to determine optimal time to deliver electrical shocks to cardiac arrest patients
• SGH is first in South East Asia to be able to remove hard-to-reach cancers of the throat, tongue and tonsils using the *daVinci*™ robot-assisted surgical system for minimally invasive procedures

- SGH and National University Hospital jointly performed the first simultaneous pancreas and kidney transplant in Singapore
- A team of doctors from SGH, National Cancer Centre, Duke–NUS and Genome Institute of Singapore identified a mutated gene in Asians that makes some cancer drug less effective and found solution for it

2010
- SGH implemented the world's first fully integrated bed management system with RFID technology that provides real-time information on hospital bed occupancy and patient location tracking
- First dual-kidney transplant from an older donor is performed

2009
- SGH and National Heart Centre jointly performed Asia's first combined heart and liver transplant for a patient with familial amyloid polyneuropathy

2005
- SGH is the largest teaching hospital in Asia to achieve JCI accreditation

2002
- A combined team from SGH and National Dental Centre performed world's first modified jaw advancement technique for the treatment of obstructive sleep apnoea in Asians

2001
- SGH successfully separated a pair of craniopagus conjoined twins from Nepal in a historical 97-hour long surgery
- SGH and National University Hospital jointly performed world's first cord blood transplant for a patient with Thalassaemia Major

2000
- First lung transplant in Singapore was carried out by a multidisciplinary team from SGH, National Heart Centre and National Cancer Centre
- SGH team performed the world's first procedure of forearm attachment to shoulder blade

1998
- First stem cell transplant using unrelated cord blood is performed

1995
- The world's first peripheral blood stem cell transplant from a matched unrelated donor to a Thalassaemia Major patient is carried out

1993
- First hospital in Asia to use virtual reality surgery to successfully remove brain tumours and arteriovenous malformations

1992
- A surgical procedure in vaginal reconstruction devised by plastic surgeon Dr Julian Wee and paediatric surgeon Dr V T Joseph is termed "The Singapore Flap" and is adopted by doctors at the Mayo Clinic

1990
- Singapore's first heart transplant is performed
- First successful pregnancy in Asia achieved through surgical sperm retrieval
- Asia's first percutaneous endoscopic cholecystectomy, the removal of gall bladder using an endoscope, is performed

1989 • SGH performed Southeast Asia's first cochlear implant surgery which gives hearing to the profoundly deaf

1982 • First total knee replacement operation is performed

1981 • The new Singapore General Hospital is opened by Prime Minister Lee Kuan Yew

1977 • First two living-related renal transplants are performed

1970 • Singapore's first renal transplant is performed

1965 • First open heart surgery is performed

1821 • The first General Hospital opens

11.2 Changi General Hospital

Lee Chien Earn*

Changi General Hospital (CGH) is Singapore's first purpose-built regional general hospital serving the population in eastern Singapore, in line with the government's master plan for healthcare.

CGH was formed by merging two hospitals — Toa Payoh Hospital, and the old Changi Hospital (Fig. 11.2.1), inheriting the rich heritage of both its predecessors.

Old Changi Hospital was situated on Barrack Hill along Netheravon Road, and began operations in the mid-1930s as a small British military hospital known as the Royal Air Force Hospital.

Toa Payoh Hospital (Fig. 11.2.2) was known as Thomson Road Hospital from 1959–1975. It was formally opened on 20 May 1959 with only 2 doctors, 7 nursing staff and 1 commissioned ward! From these very humble beginnings, it steadily built its reputation as a medical institution providing quality care with a wide range of medical services, including neonatology, gastroenterology and urology. It also provided excellent postgraduate training for doctors. In September 1965, the School of Nursing for Pupil Assistant Nurses opened on its campus. The hospital continued to grow rapidly with the development of the surrounding HDB new towns and by the 1980s, its administrators were already looking to build a bigger and better hospital. Many possible locations were considered, including the land adjacent to the hospital.

After much deliberation, a new site in the fledgling Simei new town in eastern Singapore was agreed upon. Planned and commissioned by members of the Toa Payoh Hospital (and joined later by a team from Changi Hospital), "New Changi Hospital" began operations — within budget and on schedule — on 18 December 1996. However, by its official opening on 28 March 1998 (Fig. 11.2.3), the hospital was renamed "Changi General Hospital." The Guest-of-Honour at its official

---

*Chief Executive Officer, Changi General Hospital, Singapore.

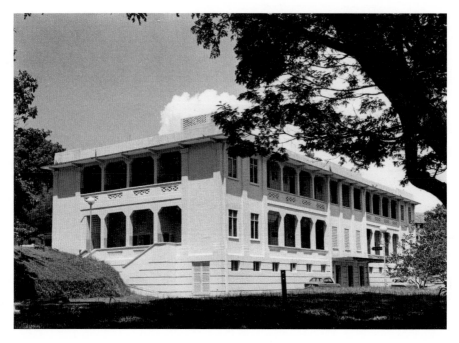

Fig. 11.2.1.   Changi Hospital.

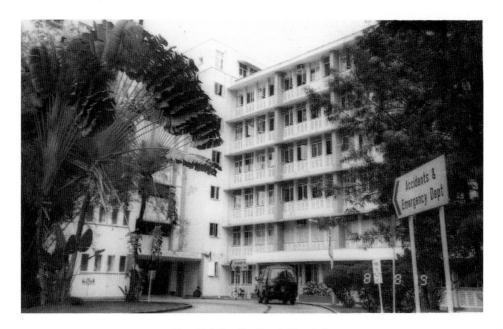

Fig. 11.2.2.   Toa Payoh Hospital.

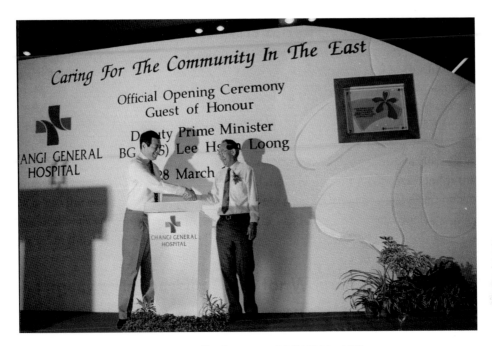

Fig. 11.2.3.   Official opening of CGH 28 Mar 1998.

opening — then Deputy Prime Minister, BG (NS) Lee Hsien Loong, explained that "The new name reflects [CGH's] role as a regional hospital offering a broad range of services, and the main provider of hospital services for the 750,000 Singaporeans living east of the Kallang Basin."

With this charter in place, CGH started to build its clinical services to provide a comprehensive range of specialities needed by the population in the region. Besides enhancing its clinical expertise, CGH also introduced new specialities such as dermatology, psychological medicine, geriatric medicine, respiratory medicine, renal medicine and sports medicine. CGH also systematically developed new specialist centres such as the Integrated Sleep Service, Breast Centre@Changi, the Endoscopy Centre and the Changi Sports Medicine Centre (CSMC). Since its inception in 2003, CSMC has become Singapore's largest multidisciplinary sports medicine centre providing leading sports medicine services and programmes.

In expanding its services, CGH has focussed on delivering clinical and service quality, and innovating in healthcare delivery wherever possible. For example, as early as 2001, CGH leveraged on the potential of the Internet by pioneering an online pharmacy to enable patients and the public to purchase homecare and re-tail medical supplies via the Web. CGH also went on to pioneer online healthcare assessment tools for corporations and individuals. CGH was the second hospital in Singapore to receive the Joint Commission International (JCI) Accreditation on 11 June 2005, and the first hospital in Singapore to have a JCI accreditation for its Heart Failure Programme and the Acute Myocardial Infarction Programme.

CGH has also sought to integrate its healthcare services with those of other institutions to meet the needs of the wider community. For example, with the Kandang Kerbau Women's and Children's Hospital (KKH) and the Singapore General Hospital (SGH), CGH introduced O&G outpatient services, to make it more accessible to women living in eastern Singapore. CGH also worked closely with the SingHealth polyclinics, a major primary care provider in eastern Singapore, to streamline referral processes and clinical protocols to better manage their patients' conditions.

In 2011, CGH embarked on a new chapter in its journey. CGH left the fold of SingHealth (which it had been a part of since 2000) and became a founding partner of the Eastern Health Alliance (EH Alliance), the new regional health system for the people of eastern Singapore. Together with the EH Alliance's other foundation partners — St. Andrew's Community Hospital, SingHealth Polyclinics, Peacehaven Nursing Home and the Health Promotion Board, the group has been working together to create and deliver innovative health programmes with each partner bringing to the table its unique and vital skills and

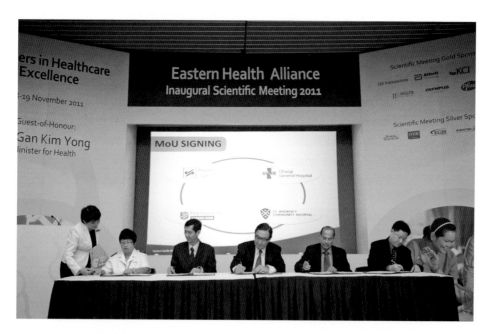

Fig. 11.2.4.   Signing of MOU by founding partners of EH Alliance.

expertise to deliver increasingly seamless quality care for the population in eastern Singapore (Fig. 11.2.4).

As the acute care partner within the EH Alliance, CGH is focused on four priorities — to save lives, restore optimal functionality, provide complex multidisciplinary outpatient care and to be a strong resource for EH Alliance. In partnership with the EH Alliance, CGH has helped develop and deliver many healthcare delivery innovations, such as the Health Management Unit that provides telecare support for discharged patients with chronic conditions; the Community Health Centres that support GPs with screening and ancillary services; the transitional care programme that helps bridge care gaps between hospital and home; GPFirst, a programme to reduce the number of less serious cases coming to the A&E; and the heart failure telehealth programme.

The population in the East has grown to 1.4 million and is rapidly ageing. CGH has grown in tandem to meet the needs of the community. In 2011, it embarked on the redevelopment of its campus in Simei to create new spaces, facilities and capabilities. This includes the building of The Integrated Building, a new 280-bed wing with St. Andrew's Community Hospital that began operations in December 2014 and was officially opened by President Tony Tan Keng Yam in July 2015, the ongoing construction of a new CGH Medical Centre that will by 2018 help transform CGH's specialist outpatient care model and capabilities, and the ongoing remodelling and expansion of wards, operating theatres, the Emergency Department, and overall public spaces within the CGH main building. This phase of development is expected to be completed by 2020 (Fig. 11.2.5).

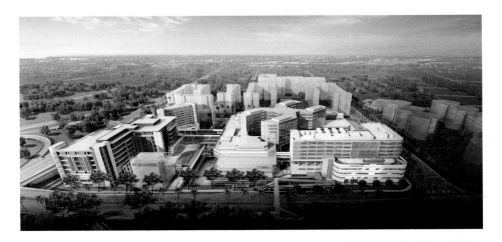

Fig. 11.2.5.   Simei campus 2020.

In summary, since its official opening in 1998, CGH has grown by leaps and bounds. For example, specialist outpatient attendances grew from less than 150,000 in 1997 to more than 350,000 in 2013. To better care for its patients, the hospital's medical specialities has increased from 14 medical specialities at inception to 29 presently. The number of patients has also increased exponentially in tandem with an ageing, growing population in the region. For example specialist outpatient attendances grew from less than 150,000 in 1997 to more than 350,000 in 2013. To care for its patients, CGH's staff strength has also increased more than two-fold in the last seven years to more than 5000 in 2014.

CGH is driving a new model of care that seeks to optimise recovery and rehabilitation of patients, and enable the delivery of care from hospital to home.

CGH, the first regional general hospital in Singapore, has throughout its history strived to be a leader in innovating the delivery of healthcare to its patient. CGH's vision is to continue to be a caring hospital trusted by patients and staff, renowned for clinical excellence and innovation, as it seeks to deliver on its mission to deliver the best patient care with passion and empathy.

11.3 Tan Tock Seng Hospital

Philip Choo[*]

The history of Tan Tock Seng Hospital (TTSH) spans nearly two centuries, from a humble makeshift shack in 1844, caring for the destitute and poor, to today's 7500-strong established multi-disciplinary hospital, caring for the masses.

The Birth and Growth

Set up 171 years ago to tend to the "diseased of all nations," TTSH was known as the "Chinese Pauper's Hospital." In 1860, the Hospital moved to Balestier Plains, where it continued to care for the poor and was nicknamed "Rumah Miskin" or "the House of the Poor." The Hospital relocated in 1909, this time to Moulmein Road, where it had a bigger space to accommodate some 1000 patients.

After the Japanese Occupation in 1945, there was a surge in the demand for medical treatment as Singapore grew rapidly in the wake of the post-war baby boom. TTSH needed to expand its capacity in terms of facilities, services, and manpower. The government took full control of TTSH in 1961 and started adding new wards and buildings.

In the 1990s, TTSH was restructured and it became the regional and referral centre for Respiratory, Geriatric, and Rehabilitation Medicine for Neurosciences, Rheumatology, and Immunology. The Communicable Disease Centre was also placed under the Hospital's direct administration in 1985.

Adopting Technology

On 1 April 2000, a new, modern TTSH was opened by then-Deputy Prime Minister, Mr Lee Hsien Loong.

[*] Professor, Group Chief Executive Office, National Healthcare Group, Singapore.

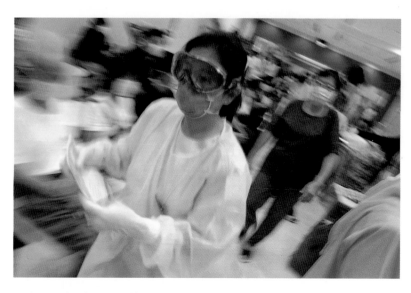

SARS — TTSH was the designated hospital to treat SARS patients in 2003. As a nation, we fought the battle together and won the Silent War.

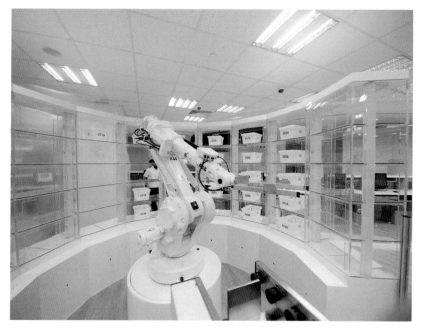

OPAT — TTSH's Outpatient Pharmacy Automation System, launched in 2014, features automation, robotic, and RFID technologies, to ensure a highly efficient and accurate medication packing and dispensing process for patients.

This new hospital was specially designed for the provision of comprehensive inpatient and outpatient services. Its specialist clinics, wards, and emergency department could manage high patient volumes. Even today, TTSH remains one of the busiest hospitals in Singapore and continues to operate from this present infrastructure.

Within the last 14 years, TTSH has greatly harnessed new technology and techniques to provide better care. It was the first in South East Asia to successfully perform macular translocation cases and fit-bone surgeries; it was also the first to introduce the Nailfold Video Capillaroscopy system for patients with rheumatic diseases; and robotic orthosis to provide better rehabilitation outcomes for patients with gait issues. It also set up a non-invasive ventilation unit and specialist clinics for conditions like heart failure and musculoskeletal disorders. TTSH became a member of the National Healthcare Group in 2000.

When SARs hit Singapore in 2003, TTSH became the designated hospital to treat infected patients and focused only on containing, treating, and protecting against the disease. There were many lessons from the short, but significant episode. TTSH remains vigilant to this day and is constantly strengthening its ability to contain, treat, and protect against infectious diseases. It is currently developing Singapore's National Centre for Infectious Diseases which will vastly increase Singapore's ability to handle outbreaks.

Enabling the Community

The health needs of Singaporeans have been altering dramatically over the years as a result of both economic progress and social-demographic changes. At the same time, chronic degenerative diseases such as cancer and heart disease have replaced infectious diseases as the major causes of death. Adding to the complexity of chronic diseases and their complications is the interaction between these diseases and their respective treatments.

For a more sustainable healthcare system, with an affordable and accessible quality of healthcare, care has to revolve around the patient and not the individual institutions.

There has been a concerted effort to widen TTSH's community of care and develop programmes to address care challenges at different levels.

Within the hospital walls, besides TTSH staff watching out for patients, volunteers are recruited to support patients in their times of need or to help keep elderly patients company in the wards. When patients are discharged, TTSH provides continued support through volunteers and has a mobile medical team to offer clinical stability and rehabilitation. There is also a home therapy programme to integrate the bedbound and elderly back into the community.

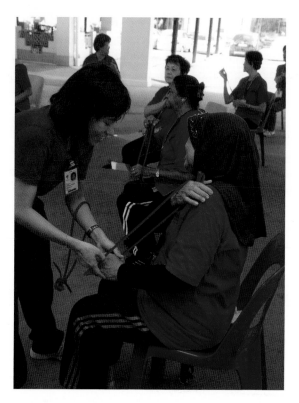

Community Outreach — More outreach programmes, volunteer groups, and patient support groups are set up at TTSH to better care for people in the community. "I am heartened that Tan Tock Seng Hospital continues in its mission to be 'The People's Hospital' today." — President Tony Tan at TTSH's 170th Founder's Day Celebrations Dinner in 2014.

In 2012, TTSH launched the Virtual Hospital initiative which brings care both medical and social directly into the homes of patients. This is possible only with the collaboration of several committed community partners.

TTSH has also ventured into raising the overall knowledge and capability of step-down care partners. In 2009, TTSH initiated Project Care to help raise the level of care in nursing homes. To date, it has collaborated with seven nursing homes. The Hospital also works with day care centres to improve their therapy programmes and facilitate systematic upgrading of their staff's skills.

Upstream, TTSH is also working with primary care partners to right site the care of patients, for instance those with dementia.

Beyond patients, TTSH is working with grassroots partners like community development councils to organise talks, activities, and screening to reach out, educate, and train more people to increase a community's ability to take care of itself.

The Future

Safer care often requires greater availability and participation by healthcare professionals as integrated team members. By working together, healthcare professionals and institutions are better positioned to recognise opportunities for improvement and are able to develop more effective systems of care.

Two key projects are being developed to enable better care for the population. The first is HealthCity Novena, a major integrated healthcare development in Novena that will set the ground for partner institutions to more ably respond to changing and complex healthcare needs. The second is the National Healthcare Group's Regional Health System which aims to transform the delivery of care in central Singapore such that patients at different stages of health can navigate the health system for accessible, affordable quality of care.

Moving forward, TTSH will continue to focus on nurturing better people to give better care. It will work more closely with like-minded partners to spearhead more positive transformations in care and care delivery. The goal is to make cost-effective care faster, better, safer and more readily available to the people of Singapore.

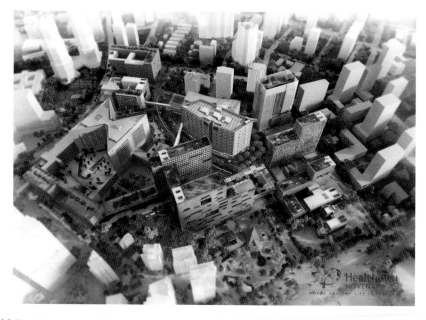

HealthCity Novena — TTSH plays a key role in the development of HealthCity Novena, a centre which integrates community healthcare, medical education, and research in a vibrant and sustainable communal environment to co-create better solutions for citizen's health.

11.4 Alexandra Health System

Caroline Lim*,a

Not so Humble Beginnings

The roots of Alexandra Health System (AHS) can be traced back to the British Military Hospital, opened in 1938 as the principal hospital for the British military personnel in the Far East. When the British withdrew from Singapore, the hospital was handed over to the Singapore Government in 1971 for a token sum of S$1, and renamed as Alexandra Hospital (AH). AH then was a well-built and well-maintained hospital with comprehensive medical services and handling 15% of all of Singapore's hospital admissions (Fig 11.4.1. The Alexandra Hospital). As one of only five hospitals in Singapore to have a neonatal intensive care unit, the Obstetrics & Gynaecology Department (O&G) of the hospital also provided relief to the Kandang Kerbau Hospital (KK Hospital). In addition, as the closest hospital to the burgeoning industrial activity in Jurong, AH handled most industrial accidents.

However, the glory of AH was not to last. With the restructuring of Singapore's public healthcare system in the mid-1980s, AH found itself outflanked by the new and improved Singapore General Hospital (SGH) and National University Hospital (NUH). Its O&G and Paediatric departments were closed and transferred to KK Hospital. By 2000, AH's market share had dropped to less than one-third of what it was in 1980s and it suffered from low staff morale and poor public perception. The future of Singapore's healthcare was advancing full steam ahead, and AH was being left behind.

From Caterpillar to Butterfly

AH was finally restructured on 1 October 2000 and became part of the National Healthcare Group, with Mr. Liak Teng Lit appointed as its Chief Executive Officer.

*Director, Alexandra Health Institute and Corporate Communications, Alexandra Health System, Singapore.
a The author is grateful to Dr. Wong Sweet Fun, Chief Transformation Officer of AHS and Ms. Claire Ooi for their contributions to this article.

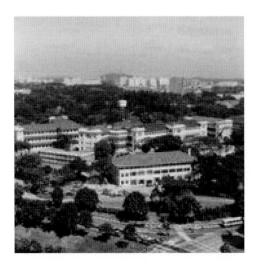

Fig. 11.4.1.   The Alexandra Hospital.

Together with his management team, they would attempt the daunting task of not just transforming the quality of clinical expertise, but also its efficient and effective delivery, while creating a more conducive environment for healing.

A revolutionary approach was needed — to be respected by its patients, the hospital would have to respect its patients as people, concentrating on their total well-being, treating them holistically while treating their specific diseases. A new concept of healthcare delivery emerged, which continues to be in practice today. "Fast medicine" is a matter of life and death, targeted at saving the patient's life first and foremost, at all costs. To this end, timely response was redesigned with the Department of Emergency Medicine placing senior doctors at the forefront, the triage counter, making them the first point of contact for patients, significantly reducing delay and waiting time. "Cruise medicine" goes beyond the firefighting of fast medicine to a more holistic approach to disease management. For example, a multidisciplinary team set up in the centre for diabetic care paid attention to patients' diet and lifestyle choices, as well as provided support for patients to manage their conditions independently. "Slow medicine," distinct from the high cost aggressive medical treatment given to all patients, instead focuses on comfort, patient preference and choice, especially with regards to palliative care. The AH Geriatric Centre was redesigned to offer not just acute hospital-based services, but also community-based outreach initiatives such as the Health for Older Persons Programme (HOP), aimed at preparing people for the challenges of ageing.

Changing the way healthcare was delivered would have far reaching implications on the structure of operations, facilities, and the whole culture of AH. Putting Mr. Liak's firebrand mantra of "learn from everyone, follow no one, look for patterns

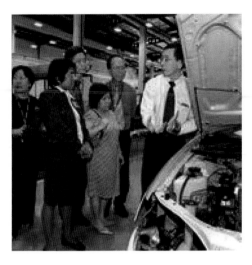

Fig. 11.4.2. AH management team on a study trip to Toyota to learn the best practices of the Toyota Production System.

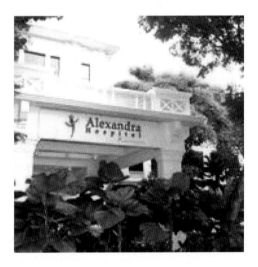

Fig. 11.4.3. The healing oasis.

and work like hell" into practice, the management team visited diverse successful organisations like The Ritz-Carlton, Citibank and even the prominent Japanese car-maker, Toyota, determined to find best practices that could be transformed in the healthcare context (Fig. 11.4.2). These visits spawned the "kaizens" and "kaikakus" that support the delivery of "better, faster, cheaper and safer" healthcare today.

The environment is a key factor in physical and mental wellbeing, and the AH management team strove to create a healing environment for its patients (Fig. 11.4.3). Taking inspiration from Singapore's reputation as a garden city, AH morphed from a dilapidated old hospital into a blooming hospital-in-a-garden, and its collection of free ranging butterflies was unrivalled.

The hard work and dedication of the AH management team paid off. Within a year of restructuring, AH attained ISO9001:2000 and ISO14001 accreditations. In 2001, AH achieved the People Developer Standard, Singapore Quality Class. For six consecutive years from 2006, AH was ranked number one among other restructured hospitals in the MOH's annual patient satisfaction survey, a far cry from the 1999 survey that indicated that 39% of the public would not have recommended AH to others.

Efforts in the environment also did not go unnoticed. In 2005, AH won the first prize in the inaugural "Community in Bloom" competition by the National Parks. AH further received the President's Award for the Environment in 2008. During the Singapore Garden Festival in the same year, AH won the Best Community Garden Award and Platinum Award of the Community in Bloom.

Taking Charge in the North

In 2004, when it was announced that Khoo Teck Puat Hospital (KTPH) (Fig. 11.4.4) would be placed under the management of AHS, Minister Khaw Boon Wan, the then Minister for Health, challenged the team to build "a hassle-free hospital" with "patients unambiguously at the centre of the focus, with technology fully exploited for the benefit and convenience of patients," and well-linked to other hospitals for seamless transfer.

From a single hospital, the Alexandra Health System (AHS) now has expanded into a public healthcare cluster that takes care of the needs of 700,000 residents in

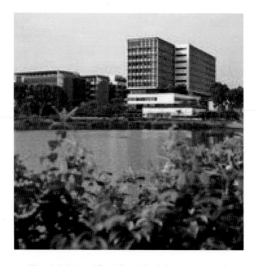

Fig. 11.4.4. The Khoo Teck Puat Hospital.

the northern part of Singapore. The AHS cluster, formed in 2008, retained the name "Alexandra" in dedication to the pioneering management team who contributed to the success of AH. AH itself was handed over to the JurongHealth.

AHS currently manages the 590-bed KTPH. In addition to KTPH, which is an acute hospital, the 428-bed Yishun Community Hospital will cater to the rehabilitation and sub-acute needs of patients when it opens in December 2015. Furthermore, the Admiralty Medical Centre, due to open in 2017, will be a one-stop medical centre with an emphasis on outpatient clinic consultation, day surgery, rehabilitation and diagnostic services as well as community health outreach activities. The Sembawang Primary Care Centre, a part of Sembawang Sports & Community Hub will be an integrated community hub with sports, medical and communal facilities and the Woodlands Integrated Health Campus which will comprise an acute hospital, a community hospital and a nursing home, will open progressively from 2020.

Shaping the Future of Healthcare, the Alexandra Health Way

Not content with making a positive difference to just patients, AHS has set its sights on establishing a health ecosystem in northern Singapore by engaging the community and residents to take care of their own health. The Alexandra Health Way opens up the possibility of a hospital without walls, and is personalised down to the individual, centred on preventive and rehabilitative care. For well and healthy residents, they are championed to become a sphere of good influence, and role models for their families and peers. For those at risk of developing chronic illnesses, the Population Health Screening programme spurs them to take proactive and pre-emptive action. And for those with existing chronic and medical conditions, the Community Nursing initiative and Transitional Care Service embeds nurses directly into the community to treat people in their own homes enabling residents to live independently and meaningfully after discharge, safe in the knowledge that help is at hand when they need it. For patients who are frail and nearing the end of their lives, Advance Care Planning facilitate ageing in place, and bring them and their families some relief, comfort and closure. In this way, healthcare becomes lifelong, anticipatory, and holistic.

AHS's mission has been to provide quality, affordable and hassle-free healthcare with science, love and wisdom. To this end, AHS promises to touch lives, pioneer care and make a positive difference in the health of our community.

11.5 National University Hospital

Joe Sim*

The Early Days and Close Links with the University

The National University Hospital (NUH) opened on 24 June 1985, with 280 beds and 180 staff. It was purpose-built as the principal medical teaching institution of Singapore and as a centre for medical excellence. More significantly, as Singapore's first restructured hospital, it was to take the lead in piloting innovative, more effective and responsive healthcare models. The experience at the NUH would later provide valuable insights and lessons for the restructuring of hospitals in Singapore. Mr. Khaw Boon Wan, Minister for National Development, was NUH's first Executive Director (Chief Executive Officer).

Though it opened only in 1985, the hospital's heritage goes much further beyond that; the origins of its clinical departments can be traced back to the beginning of NUS. When NUS was established in 1905 as The Straits Settlement and Federated Malay States Government Medical School, it was staffed by some of the most respected names in medicine. The departments relocated to NUH when it was established and these doctors would go on to form the majority of the medical team at the hospital.

Our Trailblazers and their Contributions to Medicine

Many well-known pioneers in healthcare played key roles in NUH's formative years, establishing or heading departments, where they led teams which achieved breakthroughs in medicine and in the training of doctors.

Among these pioneers was the late Emeritus Professor S.S. Ratnam, perhaps best remembered for his role in delivering Asia's first test tube baby through *in-vitro*

*Adjunct Associate Professor, Deputy Chief Executive (Clinical Enterprise), National University Health System; Chief Executive Officer, National University Hospital, Singapore.

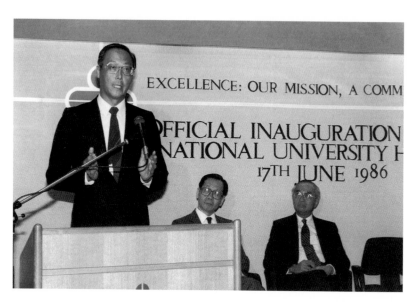

Official opening of the NUH by Mr. Goh Chok Tong, then First Deputy Prime Minister & Minister for Defence, on 17 June 1986. Among the distinguished guests who graced the event were Prof. Lim Pin and then Minister for Health and Finance, Dr. Richard Hu.

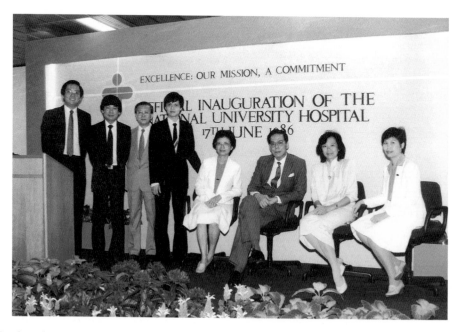

Our board members, then-Executive Director Mr. Khaw Boon Wan (standing, second from left) and Chairman Mr. Kwa Soon Bee (seated, in grey suit) at the official opening of the NUH in 1986.

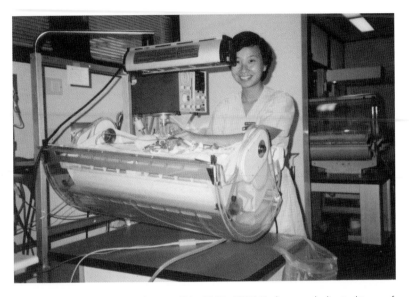

Keeping a baby warm in an open incubator at Ward 24 in 1987. Today, our dedicated team of neonatologists and nurses provide a full range of specialist care, including pre-delivery counselling for parents with high-risk pregnancy and care of the newborn.

fertilisation. Many of his former students are now established practitioners in the field of O&G, including Professor P.C. Wong, who is highly regarded in the fields of infertility and assisted reproduction.

Another well-known pioneer was the late Emeritus Professor Wong Hock Boon, who founded the Department of Paediatrics at NUS in 1962 and went on to head the department until his retirement in 1988. Known as the Father of Paediatrics in Singapore, he left a legacy of dedication and passion for teaching, research, and excellent clinical care for sick children in Singapore and in the region.

In cardiology, we have Emeritus Professor Chia Boon Lock, who headed NUH's Division of Cardiology, Department of Medicine and later, as Chief of the Cardiac Department from the 1980s to the late 1990s. Known as the Father of Cardiology, Professor Chia was one of the first two cardiologists to introduce echocardiography, as well as the first to introduce ambulatory blood pressure monitoring in Singapore.

Many of the pioneers are still with NUH today, among them University Professor Lim Pin, Emeritus Professor K. Shanmugaratnam, a highly regarded pioneer in the field of pathology; Emeritus Professor Robert Pho, fondly known as the Father of Hand and Reconstructive Microsurgery in Singapore, and Emeritus Professor Edward Tock, who headed the team responsible for the planning and construction of the NUH.

On the administrative leadership front, we have a league of outstanding and accomplished alumnus; among them National Development Minister Khaw Boon Wan, who was our first Executive Director (Chief Executive Officer); as well as

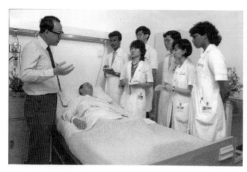
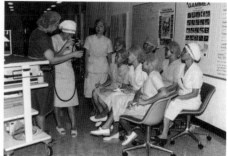

Nurturing the next generation of healthcare professionals has been and remains an important mission for NUH, being the principal teaching hospital of the NUS Yong Loo Lin School of Medicine.

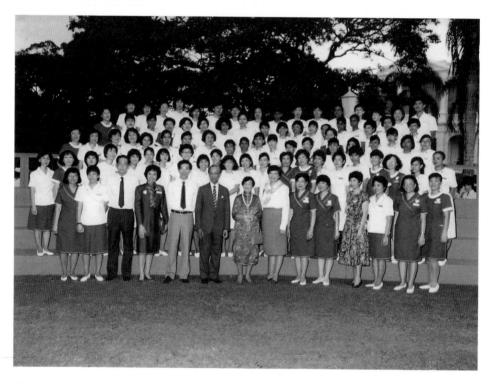

NUH nurses at the Istana in 1990. Every year, nurses in Singapore are invited to tea with the President and First Lady as part of the Nurses' Day Celebrations.

three Directors of Medical Services in Professor Tan Chorh Chuan, who is currently President of the NUS; Professor Kandiah Satkunanantham, veteran orthopaedic surgeon and A/Professor Benjamin Ong. Many of our colleagues have gone on to assume senior clinical and administrative leadership positions in both public and private healthcare institutions in Singapore.

Contributing to Healthcare in Singapore and Beyond

In the last thirty years, NUH has stayed true to its mission to provide quality patient care, spearheading many quality initiatives, and remain at the forefront of medicine.

In 2004, NUH became the first hospital in Singapore to receive the Joint Commission International (JCI) accreditation, an international stamp for excellent clinical practices in patient care and safety. Since then, the hospital has been re-certified three times, including being the first to achieve the new JCI Academic Medical Centre standards in 2013.

In 2006, NUH was the first hospital in Singapore to publish clinical outcomes data on its website, benchmarking against international outcomes, and providing greater transparency. This has since become a standard for restructured hospitals in Singapore.

NUH was among the first few hospitals in Singapore to welcome its pioneer Advanced Practice Nurses (APNs) in 2006. Today, it has one of the largest groups of certified APNs in the country. Nurses at NUH have embraced innovations to improve patient care and safety. We were the first to adopt the Trendcare Patient Acuity System in 2006 to better allocate nursing resources for different patient groups.

The team at NUH has also helped place Singapore on the world map with breakthroughs such as:

- 1989 — The world's first baby conceived via MIST (Micro-Insemination Sperm Transfer).

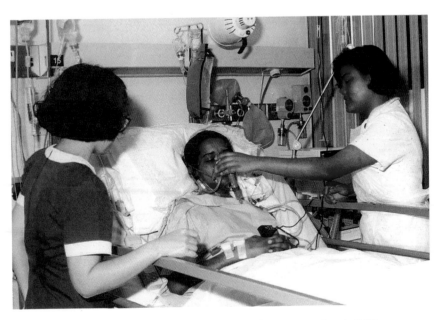

The team behind Singapore's first successful liver transplant in 1990.

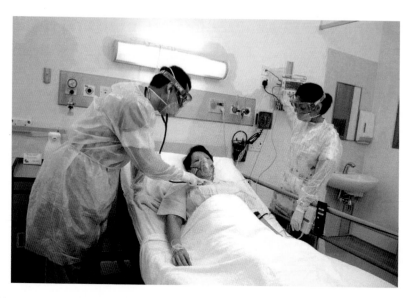

In 2003, everyone at NUH — doctors, nurses, frontline and support staff — played their roles and remained vigilant as they joined the rest of Singapore in their combat against SARS.

- 1990 — NUH's Department of Ophthalmology developed the world's first known software programme for colour vision testing.
- 1990 — Singapore's first successful liver transplant. This was followed by the country's first successful living-related liver transplant in 1996. Today, our transplant outcomes remain top-rated and NUH is the only public hospital in Singapore to offer paediatric and adult kidney and liver transplant programmes.
- 1997 — Cardiothoracic surgeons at NUH are the first in Singapore (and Asia) to perform open heart surgery on a "beating heart." The "door-to-balloon" time of 67 minutes for patients with a heart attack at the National University Heart Centre, Singapore is better than the international benchmark of 90 minutes.
- 2001 — With another hospital, NUH performed world's first successful cord blood transplant on a Thalassaemia Major patient.
- 2007 — The first-in-man early cancer clinical trial of a "new-generation" drug which slows tumour growth, commenced at the NUH, offering cancer patients new hope and putting Singapore on the world map.
- 2007 — A team at NUH discovered that genetics is the key to why different ethnic groups of patients require different doses of Warfarin, an anti-clotting drug, to achieve the same effect. This finding led the US Food and Drug Administration (FDA) to make it mandatory to state on Warfarin labels that genetic make-up can influence how one responds to the drug.

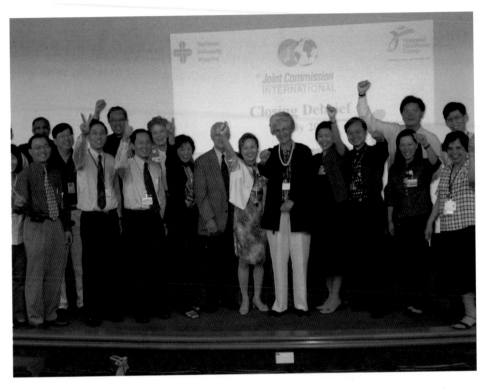

We did it! In 2004, NUH became the first hospital in Singapore to receive the Joint Commission International (JCI) Accreditation, an international stamp for excellent clinical practices in patient care and safety.

- 2007 — Singapore's first Translational Clinical Research (TCR) Grant went to a team led by A/Professor Yeoh Khay Guan, Senior Consultant in Gastroenterology & Hepatology; the $25 million grant would enable the investigators to research the genetic links, a screening tool and novel treatments for gastric cancer. The team was awarded a renewed grant of a second $25 million in 2013 for the second phase of work.
- 2009 — The transplant team at NUH successfully overcame medical barriers in living donor transplantation with a kidney transplantation involving blood group Incompatibility and Cross Match Positive.
- 2011 — The opening of the Centre for Reproductive Education and Specialist Training (CREST) marks Asia Pacific's first dedicated fertility training centre.
- 2012 — Singapore's first simultaneous pancreas and kidney transplant was successfully performed at the NUH, as part of an innovation and technology initiative funded by the Health Services Development Programme of the MOH.
- 2012 — NUH team developed a new personalised cancer treatment protocol for children with acute lymphoblastic leukaemia, offering safer treatment with less complications.

- 2013 — NUH received the JCI Academic Medical Centre Accreditation in May, making it the first local hospital to achieve new standards with its third re-accreditation.
- 2014 — Doctors successfully performed the first faecal microbiota transplantation in Singapore, giving hope to people with chronic gut infections.

Celebrating the Best Talents

As testimony of the high calibre of its people, the NUH team has featured prominently at the annual National Medical Excellence Awards (NMEA), the only one presented by the Ministry of Health to recognise contributions from health professionals for innovations in healthcare, patient safety, clinical quality and biomedical research, as well as outstanding clinical education and training. Since the awards were inaugurated in 2008, more than half of the individual and team award winners are from NUH.

On the nursing front, we have four recipients of the prestigious President's Award for Nurses, the highest accolade for the profession in Singapore.

In 2008 Professor Tan Chorh Chuan was awarded the National Science and Technology Medal for his distinguished contributions to the development of Singapore's scientific capability, particularly in the biomedical sciences sector.

In 2012, Professor Lawrence Ho from the Department of Medicine received the President's Technology Award for his role as co-inventor of the world's first flexible robotic endoscopy system, the Master and Slave Transluminal Endoscopic Robot (MASTER). The system was successfully used to perform endoscopic submucosal dissection in human patients.

Professor John Wong, Chief Executive of the National University Health System (NUHS) of which the NUH is a member, received the President's science and Technology Medal in 2014 for his distinguished and sustained contributions to Singapore's healthcare and biomedical sciences research. Professor Wong, one of the pioneers in Singapore's push for the biomedical sciences, was instrumental in shapping policies, recruiting top scientists and working with Singapore's economic agencies to attract pharmaceutical companies to Singapore.

Nurturing Future Generations of Healthcare Professionals

In 2010, NUH welcomed the pioneer batch of medical and nursing residents in Singapore.

To-date, we have 32 training programmes and over 500 residents, accounting for a quarter of total postgraduate training numbers in Singapore.

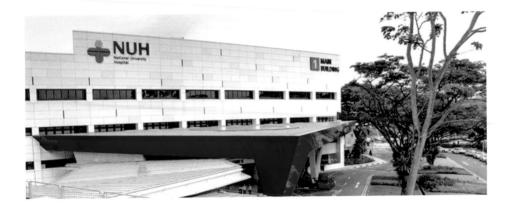

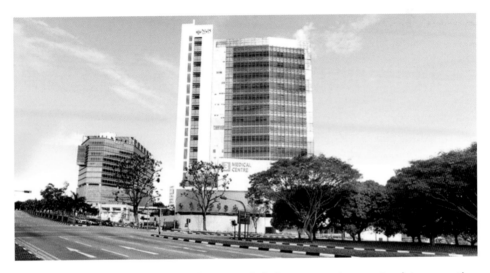

NUH today... with its latest medical centre which has a capacity to attend to more than 250,000 patient visits a year.

A first in Singapore, NUH's Nursing Residency programme offers an evidence-based curriculum developed for an academic medicine environment. It supports our new graduate nurses in their transition to become competent professionals.

Shaping Medicine for the Future

The well-being and interests of our patients remain our focus as we stay committed to providing Singaporeans with good quality and affordable medical care that come from the heart.

We will hold fast to our mission to train the next generation of healthcare professionals and to fulfil our role as part of an academic health system through translational research which paves the way for new cures and treatment, offering our patients, hope, and a new lease of life.

11.6 KK Women's and Children's Hospital

Kenneth Kwek*

Dedicated to the advancement of women's and children's health, KK Women's and Children's Hospital (KKH) has evolved, since its founding in 1858, into a leader in obstetrics, gynaecology, paediatrics and neonatology. Today, the 830-bed referral centre provides tertiary care for high-risk conditions in women and children. It is also a major teaching hospital for the nation's medical schools, leading in education for obstetrics and gynaecology, and paediatrics in Singapore, as well as continuing to train generations of midwives, nurses, and allied health professionals.

A household name in Singapore, KKH is the birthplace of more than a million Singaporeans. From 1945 to the 1960s, the hospital catered to the needs of the post-war population boom in Singapore, delivering record numbers of babies — over 100 every day. In 1966, the hospital made international news when the Guinness Book of World Records declared it to be the world's largest maternity hospital at the time, with up to 39,835 births a year at its peak. The hospital held this world record from the mid-1960s until the early 1970s.

Amidst ever-evolving healthcare needs, KKH continues on its mission of driving clinical advancements, medical education, and research to improve care and better the future of every woman and child.

---

*Chief Executive Officer, KK Women's and Children's Hospital, Singapore.

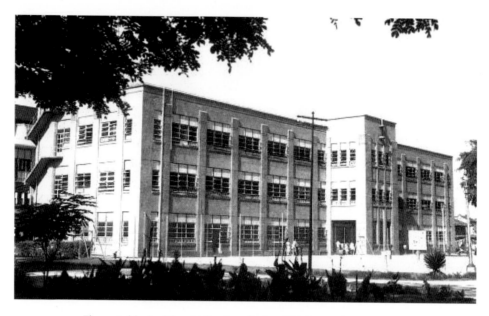

The main block of the old Kandang Kerbau (KK) Hospital in the 1940s.

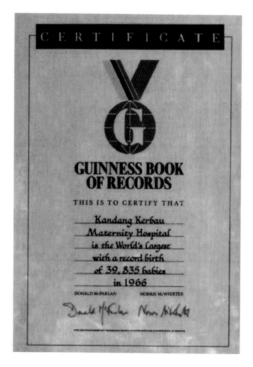

A Guinness Book of Records certificate declaring the then KK Hospital to be the world's largest maternity hospital in 1966.

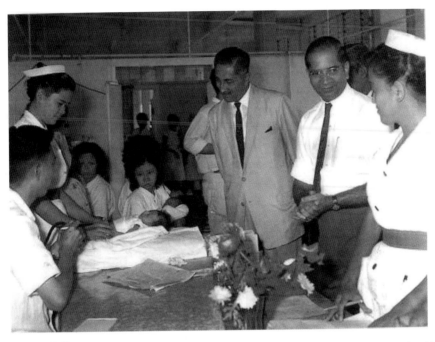

Singapore's Yang di-Pertuan Negara (and later first President), Yusof Ishak, tours KK hospital in 1962.

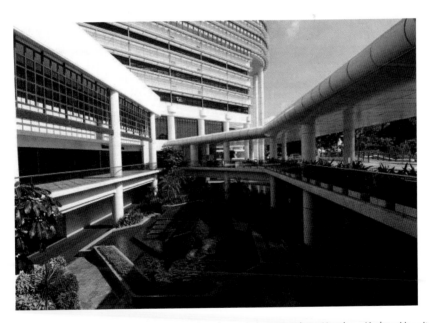

The current KK Women's and Children's Hospital — formerly known only as Kandang Kerbau Hospital — was built in 1997.

Clinical Care

As a leading tertiary care centre for women's and children's health, KK Women's and Children's Hospital (KKH) is the main referral centre for newborn babies suffering from complex and high-risk medical conditions. The hospital admits and manages about 400 to 450 such newborns a year. Multidisciplinary teamwork contributes to the hospital's low maternal, perinatal[1] and neonatal[2] mortality rates, which rank among the lowest in the world.

In its commitment to providing patients the highest standards of healthcare, KKH maintains the largest neonatal intensive care unit in South East Asia, and Singapore's only extra-corporeal membrane oxygenation (ECMO) mobile service. KKH is also the first and only vaccine sentinel site in Singapore to optimise the safety of childhood and women's obstetric vaccines. Additionally, the hospital helms the Singapore National Asthma Program, which aims to address the high burden of the respiratory condition in the local population.

"As a leader in children's health and a teaching hospital for over 100 years, we work closely with many healthcare institutions around the world to advance holistic

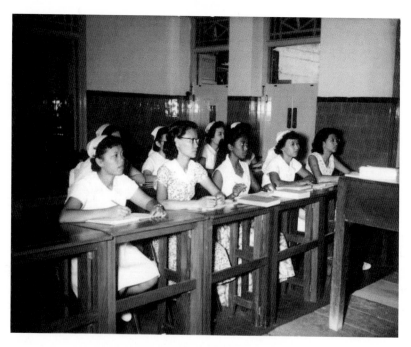

Nursing staff undergoing training in the 1960s.

---

[1] KKH perinatal mortality rate of 3.35 per 1000 live births as at 2013, excluding babies weighing less than 1000 grams at birth.

[2] KKH neonatal mortality rate of 1.99 per 1000 resident live births as at 2014.

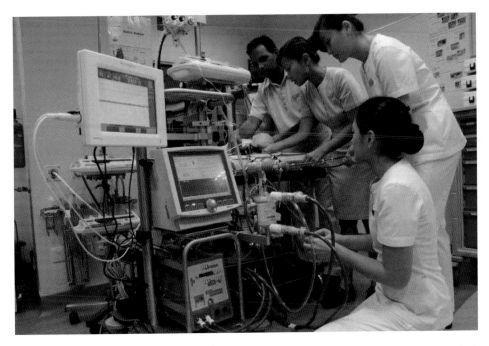

Current — ECMO specialist nurses conduct a training demonstration using the ECMO machine, which provides life-sustaining heart and lung support for critically ill infants and children.

and compassionate care for newborn infants and children in Singapore and beyond," says Adjunct Professor Victor Samuel Rajadurai, Head and Senior Consultant, Department of Neonatology at KKH. "The continual pursuit of excellence in clinical care improves infant survival rates, enhances the quality of life these children experience and gives hope to families."

Medical Research

In continual pursuit of better ways to care for patients, KKH developed the world's first fully-automated system to enhance blood pressure management for women undergoing caesarean section under spinal anaesthesia. In partnership with Singapore's Agency for Science, Technology and Research (A*STAR), KKH created an automated video surveillance system to watch over children with epilepsy as they sleep. The hospital was also a key collaborator in the international Magpie Trial, which proved the effectiveness of magnesium in reducing the risk of eclampsia, and its use as a prophylaxis.

"Research is the science behind medical care, allowing us to explore new frontiers of medicine to advance better diagnoses, treatments, cures and management

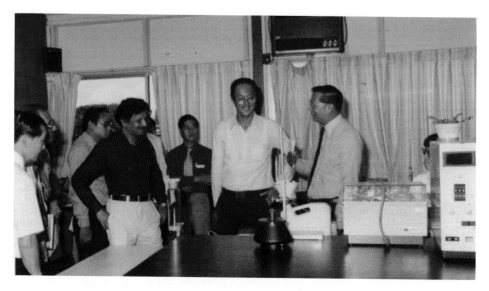

Then-Minister for Health, Mr. Goh Chok Tong (and later Prime Minister of Singapore), tours the hospital's research laboratory in 1981.

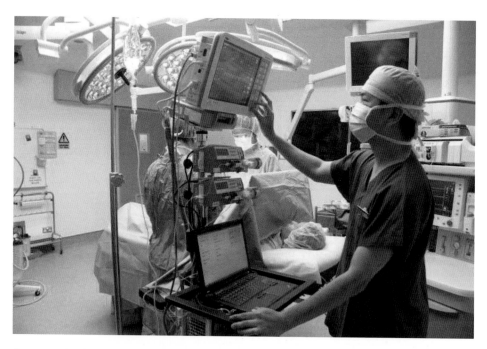

Current — Dr. Sng Ban Leong, Senior Consultant and Deputy Head, Department of Women's Anaesthesia, KKH, demonstrates the use of the world's first fully-automated system to enhance blood pressure management for women during caesarean section under spinal anaesthesia.

options," says Associate Professor Jerry Chan, Director, KK Research Centre, who is also Senior Consultant, Department of Reproductive Medicine at KKH.

Dr Chan continues, "Empirical evidence and robust research improve healthcare practices and drive optimal clinical care. These scientific discoveries, principles and values form part of the life-saving legacy that we bequeath to future generations."

Education

Continuing a longstanding legacy in education and instruction, KKH is a major teaching hospital for Duke-NUS Graduate Medical School, Yong Loo Lin School of Medicine, and Lee Kong Chian School of Medicine. The hospital runs the largest specialist training programmes for Paediatrics and for Obstetrics & Gynaecology in Singapore, both which are accredited by the Accreditation Council for Graduate Medical Education International (ACGME-I). To advance healthcare in Singapore and around the world, KKH also provides medical training and expertise to assist the sustained improvement of congenital cardiac, perinatal, paediatric, neonatal, and allied health care in countries such as Cambodia, China, India, Myanmar, and Vietnam.

To empower nurses and junior doctors to advance clinical education, research, and advanced care for patients, the hospital introduced the first paediatric Advanced Practice Nurse (APN) role in Singapore in 2013 for paediatric ambulatory and respiratory care, as well as Education Chief Resident and Administrative Chief

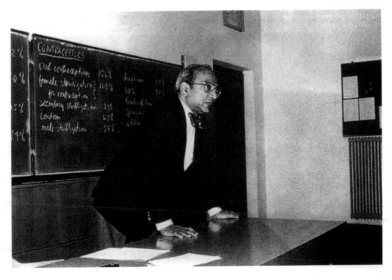

The late Professor S.S. Ratnam delivering a lecture on contraception. Prof Ratnam established the *in vitro* fertilisation programme at KK Hospital in 1982.

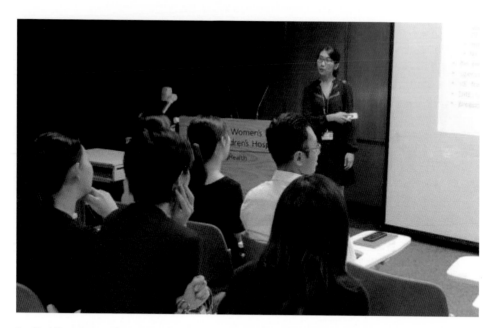

Dr. Ho Weng Yan, Administrative Chief Resident, delivering a lecture to fellow residents during a teaching session for the Obstetrics and Gynaecology National Training Programme (O&G NTP). The Chief Resident roles empower residents to share valuable input for the O&G NTP and provide guidance and training to junior doctors.

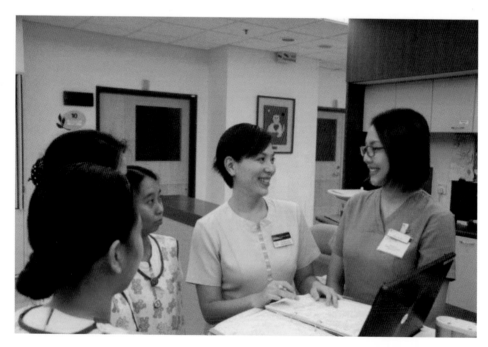

Advanced Practice Nurse (APN) Joyce Lim Soo Ting (centre) educating junior nurses in diabetes care. This role empowers nurses to play a greater role in advanced care for patients, and to engage in clinical education and research.

Resident roles. These allow medical staff to receive specialised training and mentorship while simultaneously providing guidance to others.

"To drive effective and sustainable care for patients now and in the future, a multiplier effect is necessary through the integrated education and training of healthcare providers, community partners, patients and caregivers," says Professor Chay Oh Moh, Campus Director, Education Office, who is also Senior Consultant, Respiratory Medicine Service, Department of Paediatrics at KKH.

"Our mandate is to equip the next generation to succeed and surpass us in knowledge, clinical skills, collaboration and most importantly, compassion for the sick and the wounded. Together with countless other doctors, nurses, allied health professionals and researchers, we continue to teach, train and mentor all who play a part in the health of our nation."

A Legacy of Pioneering Care for Women and Children

2014 — KKH leads the way as the first hospital in Singapore to establish a dedicated resuscitation code for cardiac arrest in pregnant women, termed "CODE RED."

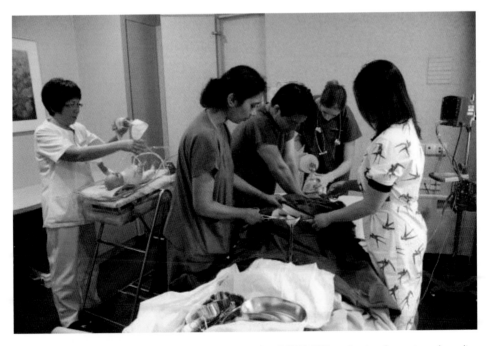

A multidisciplinary team during simulation training for CODE RED activation for maternal cardiac arrest.

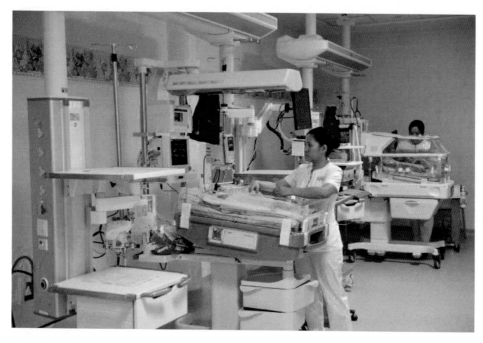

The enhanced neonatal intensive care unit at KKH, with greater capacity and new features, to further augment care for newborn babies suffering from serious medical conditions.

2013 — KKH establishes South East Asia's largest neonatal intensive care unit which has a survival rate of 93%.

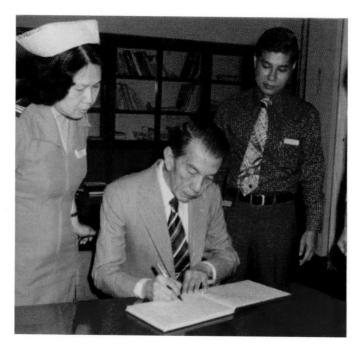

President Benjamin Henry Sheares with Matron Long Kwai Heng and Medical Director Dr. Ng Kwok Choy at the KKH Library in 1978.

2007 — KKH performs South East Asia's first open-heart microsurgery on premature infants weighing just over one kilogram.

2003 — KKH establishes a paediatric and obstetrics satellite facility at Tan Tock Seng Hospital for patients suspected to have Severe Acute Respiratory Syndrome (SARS).

2002 — The KK Gynaecological Cancer Centre is the sole Asian collaborator in the HPV Vaccine Trial — FUTURE II Study — a worldwide trial on a vaccine to protect women against the human papilloma virus (HPV), which causes cervical cancer.

1999 — KKH develops a single investigative method using high resolution ultrasound to diagnose biliary atresia in infants.

1983 — Singapore's first test tube baby is delivered by the late Professor S.S. Ratnam at KKH.

1965 — The late Professor Wong Hock Boon and Dr. W.R. Brown, a Research Associate of the Hooper Foundation, complete their research on kernicterus in Singapore. As a result, all newborns in Singapore are henceforth screened for Glucose-6 Phosphate Dehydrogenase (G6PD) deficiency.

1950 — Dr. Benjamin Henry Sheares (and later second President of the Republic of Singapore) pioneers a new technique to construct a vagina for women born without it, and achieves successful pregnancies.

11.7 Institute of Mental Health

Chua Hong Choon* and Daniel Fung†

Mental healthcare in Singapore has come a long way. The evolution of the Institute of Mental Health (IMH), the country's only tertiary psychiatric care hospital, mirrors the progressive shift in attitudes towards mental health, and the approach to mental healthcare system and services.

The hospital has gone through several incarnations in the last eight decades, evolving from a stigmatised mental asylum associated with confinement and social exclusion during its early years as Woodbridge Hospital, to a modern, restructured hospital within the National Healthcare Group, focused on mental wellness, recovery and rehabilitation.

To appreciate this journey of transformation and growth that IMH has undergone over the years, it is necessary to look back at the different eras of mental healthcare in Singapore.

The Early Years of Mental Healthcare

In 1928, a new hospital named The Mental Hospital was built in Yio Chu Kang to replace a 300-bedded psychiatric facility at Sepoy Lines.

This was a time when mental illness was thought to be incurable and the best course of action was to house the mentally ill in a safe place. Like most psychiatric facilities of that period, the hospital, fringed by the jungle and rubber plantations, was isolated from the local community. The hospital's sprawling architecture and forbidding fences reinforced its function as a custodial facility for the mentally ill, who were considered to be unpredictable and dangerous, and thus were often institutionalised for the rest of their lives.

*Adjunct Associate Professor; CEO, Institute of Mental Health; Deputy Group CEO (Clinical) National Healthcare Group, Singapore.
†Adjunct Associate Professor; Chairman Medical Board; Institute of Mental Health, Singapore.

As few medical professionals were trained in psychiatry, and treatment modalities were still in an infancy stage, there was a shortage of medical staff at the Mental Hospital. Patients were cared for by a handful of expatriate nurses with the help of health attendants. The health attendants were not trained in nursing, but nonetheless played a key role in managing the day-to-day needs of the patients. In fact, it was often said that health attendants ran the hospital in the early days. A precursor to rehabilitation for patients then was farm work, which was introduced in the later part of 1928 and remained an important activity for many years that followed.

The Foundations of Change

The post-war years saw developments in both the Mental Hospital and in psychiatric care as a whole in Singapore. One was the renaming of the hospital

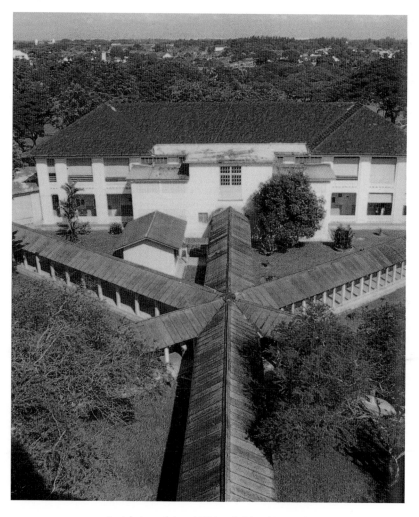

Aerial view of the old Woodbridge Hospital.

to Woodbridge Hospital in 1951 in an attempt to steer away from strongly entrenched stigma associated with mental illness. The other was that mental illness could now be treated with medications. Woodbridge Hospital gradually grew to become a 3000-bed hospital, which provided both acute mental health services as well as long-term care for persons with chronic mental disorders.

Beginnings of Multi-disciplinary Care

In 1954, the Psychiatric School of Nursing was established to provide specialised training for the care of the increasing number of psychiatric patients in the hospital. The concept of psychiatric nursing also started shifting in the 1960s towards an empowering and therapeutic care model with an emphasis on communication, behavioural therapy and recognising patients as individuals worthy of respect. The School continued its post-basic psychiatry training until its transition to Nanyang Polytechnic in mid-1994.

Alongside nursing, other areas of psychiatric care were also developed during this period. In 1955, the hospital established the Psychiatric Social Work and Occupational Therapy departments to alleviate apathy and help ease patients' transition back to a normal work environment. The medical social workers were initially concerned with providing food and shelter for patients who were discharged, but by the 1960s, their focus shifted to providing rehabilitation activities and trying to obtain work for patients.

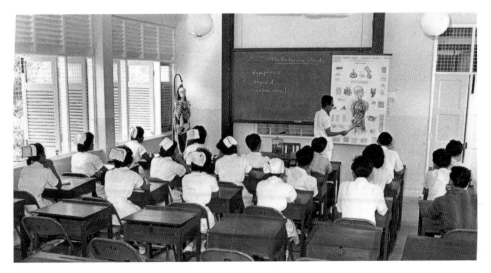

The Psychiatric School of Nursing began in 1954 to provide specialised training for the care of psychiatric patients in the hospital.

The hospital's Psychology Services began in 1956 with the aim of complementing psychiatrists' duties with IQ and personality assessments as well as helping patients manage personal difficulties and social maladjustments outside the institution. Through the years, the services provided by the department grew and various forms of psychological therapies were introduced.

The establishment of these departments sowed the seeds of the multi-disciplinary team concept practised in psychiatric care today with psychiatrists, nurses, clinical psychologists, medical social workers and occupational therapists working together to provide holistic care for patients.

Expansion of Outpatient Services

Going beyond the hospital, psychiatric outpatient clinics were started at the Bukit Timah, Paya Lebar and Kallang Dispensaries in 1957 to reach out to the community. In 1967, additional psychiatric outpatient clinics were opened at the Maxwell and the Queenstown Dispensaries. This helped the hospital to stay in touch with the psychiatric needs of the community and to develop appropriate programmes.

To cater to the needs of children and adolescents with psychological and emotional disorders, a Child Psychiatry Clinic was opened in April 1970. The clinic was staffed by a psychiatrist, a psychologist, a social worker and a nurse; and was started as a part-time service. By 1972, it was operating full-time to meet the growing need for better care for the young. In 1982, an 18-bed Child and Adolescent Inpatient Unit was opened at Woodbridge Hospital for the management of older children and adolescents with disturbed emotions and behaviours.

The Training of Psychiatrists

The 1980s saw great strides in psychiatric education in Singapore. Up to the 1950s, medical specialists were a rare breed in Singapore and almost all of them were expatriates. With an increasing need for doctors who were trained in psychiatry, the Singapore government embarked on a scheme to send local doctors overseas for training. Between 1967 and 1982, 20 medical officers were sent overseas for training in psychiatry. However, this measure was inadequate to cope with the growing demand for psychiatric services. In 1983, Woodbridge Hospital, in conjunction with the National University of Singapore Graduate School of Medical Studies, began local training of psychiatrists. The first locally-trained specialist with the Master of Medicine in Psychiatry graduated in 1985.

These developments were significant steps in the right direction. They heralded a sea change in the approach to mental health services in Singapore which has resulted in dramatic advances in the care delivery system, collaboration among healthcare and community partners, and the relationship between the healthcare service provider, patients and caregivers in the last 20 years.

Transforming the Care Delivery System

In 1993, Woodbridge Hospital moved to its present premises in Buangkok Green Medical Park and the name Institute of Mental Health (IMH) was included to reflect its added roles in research and education.

The main provider of tertiary psychiatric services in Singapore's healthcare system, IMH today provides a comprehensive range of clinical, rehabilitative and counselling services to meet the varied needs of children and adolescents, adults and the elderly. The hospital has a 24-hour Emergency Services clinic that provides urgent intervention for those experiencing acute mental health problems. It also runs Community Wellness Clinics in Geylang and Queenstown and a Child Guidance Clinic at the Health Promotion Board to make its psychiatric services more accessible to patients. IMH is also a recognised centre of excellence for research and education in psychiatric care. It became the first mental health institution in Asia to achieve the Joint Commission International Accreditation in 2005.

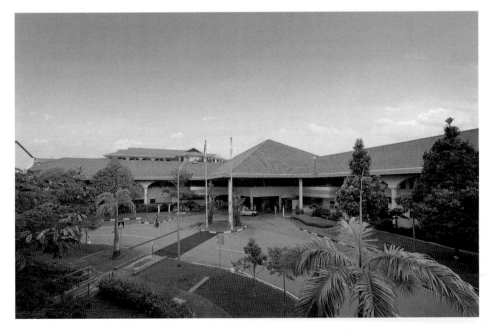

IMH is the only tertiary psychiatric care institution in Singapore.

Beyond the Walls of the Institution

Relocating the delivery of psychiatric care from the secluded premises in Yio Chu Kang to the heart of a then-developing residential neighbourhood in Hougang was a strategic move. It signalled a clear departure from the previous custodial care model to one of rehabilitation, recovery and integration, which would involve life beyond the walls of an institution.

The aim was for people with mental illness to live and work in the community even as they continued to seek treatment. The Community Psychiatric Nursing (CPN) service at Woodbridge Hospital, established in 1988, saw nurses regularly visiting discharged patients in their homes to provide continuing care and to ensure that they were coping well. Their services included administration of depot injections, assessing patient's mental state, observing side effects and effectiveness of medications and counselling. The CPN nurses also educated caregivers on the potential hazards of the patient's condition and preventive measures while providing psychological support.

IMH also set up Behavioural Medicine clinics around the island, as well as specialised services such as rehabilitation psychiatry to better prepare patients to return to the community while receiving follow-up treatment.

In 2004, IMH launched two programmes, the Assertive Care Treatment (ACT) and Mobile Crisis Team (MCT), to build on this service of bringing care into patients' living environment. ACT, comprising a multi-disciplinary team of doctors, nurses, administrators and allied health staff, monitored patients' condition, recovery progress and treatment to reduce the need for hospital re-admissions. MCT focused on reducing the impact of mental health emergencies through crisis resolution via its helpline service and home visit team.

The National Mental Health Blueprint

With increasing appreciation of mental health as a fundamental component of a person's well-being, the Ministry of Health's Director of Medical Services appointed a committee of policy-makers and mental health professionals in 2005 to formulate the first ever National Mental Health Blueprint (NMHB) for the years 2007 to 2012.

Launched in 2007, the blueprint looked at the entire spectrum of mental health and disease. The aim was to promote mental health as well as prevent the development of mental health problems, where possible, and reduce the impact of mental illness. To achieve this, the blueprint focused on four strategic thrusts:

mental health promotion; integrated mental healthcare; developing manpower; and research and evaluation.

The blueprint reinforced the move from a largely acute illness-centred, hospital-based healthcare delivery system towards a community-based model of psychiatric care, which would not only improve accessibility to services, but would also reduce the stigma associated with mental illness.

The NMHB introduced a range of programmes that tapped on community resources, as those on the ground, such as school personnel, general practitioners (GPs) and family service centres, were usually the first to observe early warning signs of mental illness. It also pushed for the right-siting of care, where services are provided at the appropriate setting, which may not always be in the hospital. This is especially so for milder cases of mental illness, where intervention in the community is better for the patient as it reduces stigma and keeps hospital beds for the severe cases.

Targeted Mental Health Programmes

IMH spearheaded several key programmes under the NMHB to address the needs of different demographic groups in Singapore.

Under the NMHB, IMH's ACT and MCT were combined in 2007 to become the **Community Mental Health Team (CMHT)**. CMHT set out to provide holistic healthcare in the community for those aged 18–65 with mental illness, and

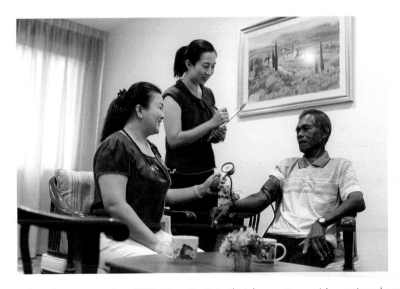

Multi-disciplinary teams from IMH visit patients in their homes to provide continued care.

it continues to do so today. The multi-disciplinary CMHT visits patients in their homes to provide regular assessment, treatment and rehabilitation, to promote their independence and integration in the community.

Studies have shown that patients who received close monitoring upon their discharge from IMH are less likely to be re-admitted to the hospital for treatment; and if they are re-admitted, the duration of their stay is significantly shortened. With CMHT, there has been a reduction in the burden of chronic mental illness on patients and their caregivers. Between 2007 and 2012, the number of hospitalisation episodes and length of hospitalisation stay decreased significantly.

The **Response, Early Intervention and Assessment in Community Mental Health (REACH)** programme is targeted at school-going children aged 6 to 19. It aims to improve mental health of children in the community, and to identify any emotional, behavioural and developmental disorders early.

When it was first introduced in 2007, the REACH programme focused on providing training and support as well as a helpline for school counsellors, but has since extended its services. The mobile multi-disciplinary mental health team works closely with school counsellors, community agencies and GPs to provide mental health assessment and intervention at the point of need such as schools, student care services and at home. It also helps Voluntary Welfare Organisations (VWO) that work with at-risk youths, out-of-school youths or those from dysfunctional families.

The **Early Psychosis Intervention Programme (EPIP)** is a landmark programme offering holistic, comprehensive and accessible service for those with early psychosis. It was initiated by the auspices of MOH in 2001 in response to findings that the condition of those diagnosed with psychosis often deteriorate significantly after the onset of symptoms. However, early intervention has shown to reduce the rate of deterioration. The programme was absorbed under the NMHB in 2007 and it aims to reduce the duration of untreated psychosis and improve quality of life of those with first-episode psychosis. It takes in those aged 16–40 who have been newly diagnosed with psychosis and provides individualised case management, psychological assessment, crisis intervention and support groups for both patients and their caregivers.

In order for early detection and treatment of mental illness to be effective, it is imperative that there is increased awareness of mental illness and wellbeing in the community. To this end, the **Community Health Assessment Team (CHAT)** was launched in 2009 to reach out to youths aged 16 to 30. With an online presence and a hub in Orchard Road, CHAT was designed to provide a safe, relaxed and convenient environment for young people to learn about mental illness and to seek assessment or advice. CHAT also networks and trains community partners who work with youths.

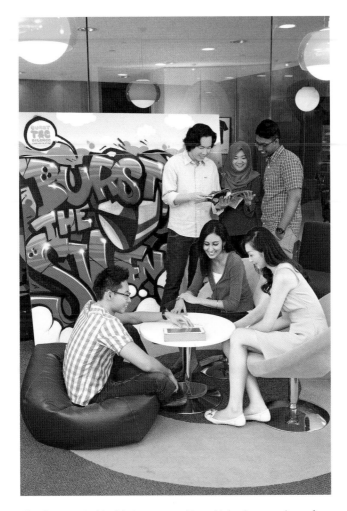

The Community Health Assessment Team Hub gives youth a safe environment to learn about mental illness.

A New Era of Collaborations

Alongside the evolution of the mental healthcare delivery system, there was a corresponding shift in how IMH worked. Previously, the responsibility for the care of people with mental illness rested mainly with specialised services in the public and private sector. However, a community-based care system requires a holistic and multi-agency approach to help patients receive continuous care and supervision. It requires re-thinking mental health as not just a health issue, but one that is also influenced by social factors. This reexamination saw IMH engaging and partnering with primary care and community services to provide support for those with mental illness, to improve access to mental healthcare services and to reduce stigma.

Working with GPs

Until recently, there was minimal involvement of GPs in mental healthcare. Yet, many patients with mild to moderate mental illness who are stable can be managed in the community with GPs providing continued care. In addition, mental disorders and physical health problems are not only associated with each other, but can often influence each other as well. As GPs are often the first point of contact for those who are unwell, they can play a significant role in detecting and subsequently providing primary care services to those with mental illness.

To this end, IMH launched the Mental Health (MH)–General Practitioner (GP) Partnership Programme to train GPs to better manage those with mild to moderate mental illness. The programme initially began in 2003 to right-site care of stabilised psychiatric patients from IMH to the GPs. In 2007, under the NMHB, it took on the role of providing liaison specialist services in order for patients to be referred to GPs as well as identifying, training and developing GPs with competencies to treat mental illness in the community.

With the training and an open channel of communication and partnership between GPs and psychiatrists, GPs are now better equipped to diagnose patients when they present with mental illness, and take necessary action. The programme

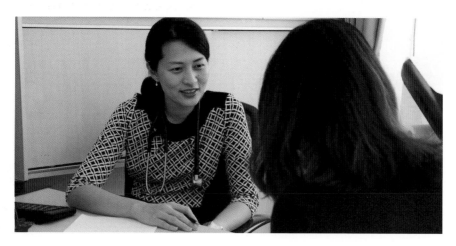

The Mental Health–GP Partnership Programme trains GPs to better manage those with mild to moderate mental illness.

also greatly benefits patients as they are able to receive treatment conveniently in their neighbourhood. Through this, there may also be less stigma for a patient to see a GP for follow-up treatments and thus may encourage greater compliance to follow-up.

Forging Community Partnerships

With the NMHB paving the way for the Community Mental Health Masterplan (CMHM) in 2012, focus shifted to stepping up efforts to build capabilities among community agencies and partners to provide accessible mental health services. Under the CMHM, IMH plays a key role in capability-building for Singapore's central region. It runs a national mental health helpline to support community partners in their work as well as manages programmes such as the Assessment Shared Care Team (ASCAT), where IMH provides support to NHG Polyclinic doctors and allied health staff through co-consultation and the Community Mental Health Intervention Team (COMIT), where IMH works with VWOs to provide psychosocial therapeutic intervention to support patients seen by GPs.

Case Management

Besides community partners, collaborating with the end user became critical. This required IMH to re-think how it engages its patients and connects them to the various social services and resources available to them. Patients often experience difficulties in performing day-to-day tasks due to their debilitating conditions; and this lack of personal autonomy may leave them feeling dejected and affect their recovery. Thus, it would be necessary to have someone help them navigate the hurdles that they face. Case managers emerged as a key link between the care team and the patient.

Case management was first introduced in IMH in 2000 for specialised pro-grammes. The service was extended to general wards in 2003 with four case managers. IMH's case management unit has now grown in both scope and number with 37 case managers, who keep in close touch with patients to ensure continuity of care and reduce defaults in treatment and follow-up.

IMH adapted a brokerage model to local needs with the objective of providing holistic, personalised care that prevents patients from falling through the cracks. At the core of this is a new way of coordinating care so each patient feels supported and assisted by his or her case manager, who takes on the role of counsellor, friend, advocate and broker.

Empowering Patients and Caregivers

Moving forward, IMH is working to empower patients and their caregivers to be more pro-active in managing their own care. Over the years, mental health patients lacked a voice and have laboured under the notion that they do not have the capacity to make decisions about their life or their treatment. This thinking needs to change — and it requires more knowledge-sharing between mental health professionals and those with mental illness and their caregivers. Well-informed patients are generally able to understand their condition better and tend to be more committed to take ownership of their treatment, and gain better control over their life.

To this end, IMH set up peer support groups, run by recovered patients, who lend a listening ear and share their experience and journey to recovery with others diagnosed with the same condition. In September 2014, IMH initiated an advocacy programme, called the Voices of Experience (VoE) with patients and caregivers appointed to be part of the committee. The programme is the first of its kind in the hospital. Besides advocacy to reduce stigma and promote social acceptance for persons with mental illness, it will also focus on providing peer support. Another key component of the programme is consultancy. VoE aims to serve as a platform for patients to get more involved in their care by providing feedback on service development and improvements as well as participating in the development of new facilities and programmes.

For caregivers, the Caregivers Alliance Limited (CAL), which was set up in 2011 specifically to meet the needs of caregivers of persons with mental illness, is a one-stop resource providing support, information, training and counselling services. CAL works closely with IMH and has a Caregivers Support Centre located in the main lobby of IMH to reach out to those accompanying their loved ones for treatment.

In addition, IMH has a small group of experienced caregivers who take on the role of peer support specialists under its Early Psychosis Intervention Programme. They come from various backgrounds and are matched with caregivers who are in a similar situation to lend a listening ear as well as share their own experience and caregiving strategies.

Other services, such as IMH's Job Club, which enables people with mental illness find employment, help patients find their feet in the community and build their self-confidence and self-worth — all of which are important in managing the condition, staying well and leading productive, fulfilling lives.

Changing the mindset of patients and caregivers to take control of their care is a challenging task and will take time. However, it is just as critical as an effective care delivery system and collaboration among community partners in IMH's on-going journey to advance mental healthcare in Singapore.

References

Institute of Mental Health. (2003) *Loving Hearts, Beautiful Minds: Woodbridge Hospital Celebrating 75 years.* ARMOUR Publishing Pte Ltd.

Ministry of Health. (2010) *Healthy Minds, Healthy Communities. National Mental Health Blueprint 2007–2012.*

Ng Beng Yeong. (2001) *Till the Break of Day, A History of Mental Health Services in Singapore 1841–1993.* Singapore University Press.

11.8 Parkway Pantai — An Integrated Healthcare Group

Tan See Leng*

A successful and thriving private healthcare system is the hallmark of a mature and developed country. In emerging economies, the development of core pillars such as infrastructure and property, logistics, financial services, telecommunications, and education often takes precedence over healthcare development. Private sector-funded healthcare provision is usually one of the last pillars to be developed.

In Singapore, private healthcare flourished as a result of the excellent ecosystem painstakingly built up by the government over the years.

From the time our longest-serving private hospital, Parkway East Hospital (PEH) — then known as Paglar Maternity and Nursing Home — opened more than 70 years ago, private healthcare has grown tremendously, particularly since the mid-1960s when Singapore first achieved its independence.

By the time Parkway ventured into the healthcare business in 1987, Singapore already boasted a robust medical infrastructure and world-class airport, which attracted even international patients who were seeking high-quality and affordable treatments.

This set the grounds for Parkway's growth. Within a decade, it became Singapore's largest private healthcare operator with Gleneagles Hospital, Mount Elizabeth Hospital, Parkway East Hospital, and the Shenton group of clinics under its fold.

Leveraging economies of scale, Parkway invested in each of its hospitals and expanded them into state-of-the-art facilities with multi-disciplinary capabilities delivering excellent clinical outcomes.

Today, Singapore's healthcare model is the envy of the world for its efficiency, cutting-edge medical facilities, well-planned healthcare structure, and excellent clinical quality. Public and private healthcare service providers compete in an open and transparent manner which is well regulated by the authorities.

The public sector, which encompasses academia, provides the necessary early training and honing of skill sets and expertise of doctors, allied healthcare professionals, nursing professionals, and research scientists. Additionally, the public

---

*Group CEO and Managing Director of Parkway Pantai, and Managing Director and CEO of IHH Healthcare.

sector also provides a stable and secure supply of medical logistics including quintessential blood and blood-related products. The government also ensures public health and hygiene standards, as well as health education and health promotion, are on par with the best in the world.

Public and private sector collaboration is key to ensuring that wastage of overlapping services is kept to a minimum and both the private and public sector providers can leverage and harness the competencies and capacities of the other.

It is this favourable climate and milieu of innovation and synergistic collaboration that has spawned the development of the private sector, allowing it to grow and flourish over the last half-century. The flexibility and free movement of healthcare workers have also contributed significantly to the continued development and maturity of the healthcare system as a whole. It has allowed the Parkway system of four tertiary hospitals, primary care network, imaging and laboratory services, and allied healthcare to flourish and contribute to the strategic growth of its parent company, IHH Healthcare Berhad, which is the world's second largest healthcare provider by market capitalisation of more than USD 12 billion.

In fact, Singapore medicine and the Singapore Inc have some of the best trademarks and brand equity in the world. Even in developed markets like the US and Europe, we are frequently held up as a model to emulate.

Brief Write-Up of Parkway Pantai HCIs in Singapore

(A) Hospitals

Mount Elizabeth Hospital (Orchard)

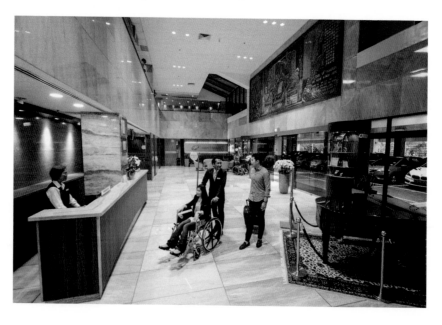

Mount Elizabeth Hospital (MEH) is a 345-bed tertiary care hospital located in the heart of Singapore's prime shopping district. Renowned for its depth of medical expertise, MEH provides a comprehensive range of medical and surgical services, with more than 450 qualified and experienced specialists under its roof. It is the first private hospital in Singapore to offer cardiac catheterisation, open-heart surgery, neurosurgery, and other advanced procedures. It continues to be a leading private hospital in Singapore in performing robotic surgeries and other complex, high intensity clinical cases. *For more information, please go to www.mountelizabeth.com.sg.*

Mount Elizabeth Novena Hospital

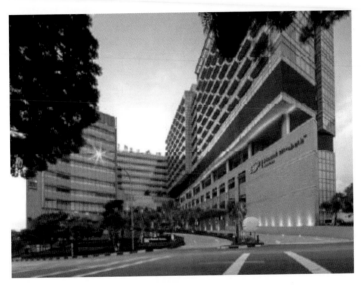

Mount Elizabeth Novena Hospital (MNH) is a fully single-bedded tertiary care hospital designed to accommodate up to 333 beds. The modern facility located in Singapore's premier medical hub in Novena has set new benchmarks for quality healthcare since opening in July 2012. As an extension of the Mount Elizabeth Hospital at Orchard Road, MNH provides patients access to Mount Elizabeth's medical expertise, reinforcing Singapore's reputation for delivering world-class medical services to both local and foreign patients. Adopting global best practices for quality patient care and clinical outcomes, MNH caters to the continuing demand for high quality and competitively priced healthcare services in Singapore and around the world. *For more information, please go to www.mountelizabeth.com.sg.*

Gleneagles Hospital

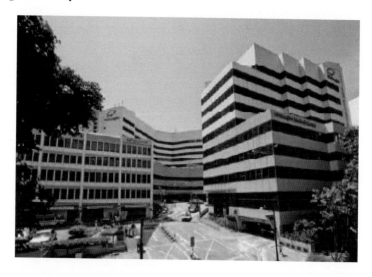

Gleneagles Hospital (GEH) is a 270-bed tertiary care hospital located in a prime residential district close to Orchard Road, Singapore's famed shopping street. The hospital provides a wide range of medical and surgical services including oncology, cardiology, general surgery, gastroenterology, liver transplant, orthopaedic surgery and sports medicine, along with obstetrics and gynaecology, which complements its multi-disciplinary approach to total management of patients. *For more information, please go to www.gleneagles.com.sg.*

Parkway East Hospital

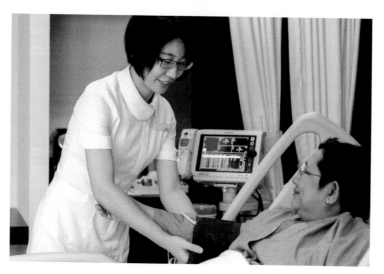

Parkway East Hospital (PEH) is a 113-bed tertiary care hospital located in eastern Singapore. It offers a comprehensive range of clinical disciplines and subspecialties including orthopaedics and general surgery, paediatrics, obstetrics and gynaecology, and cardiology. It is known for its personalised approach to the provision of healthcare. *For more information, please go to www.parkwayeast. com.sg.*

(B) Primary Care Network

Parkway Shenton

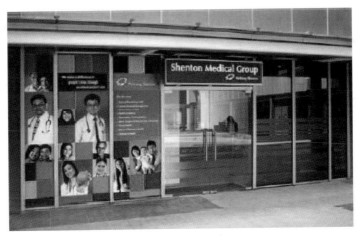

Parkway Shenton is a leading primary healthcare provider in Singapore, operating over 50 facilities island-wide including general practitioner clinics, in-house clinics for corporate clients, Executive Health Screeners, Accident and Emergency Departments or 24-hour clinics, and a Japanese clinic. Beyond that, Parkway Shenton also provides a total healthcare solution by combining its core competencies of professional medical care with healthcare insurance and third-party healthcare administration with claims services provided by its two sister companies. *For more information, please go to www.parkwayshenton.com.*

(C) Ancillary Services

ParkwayHealth Radiology

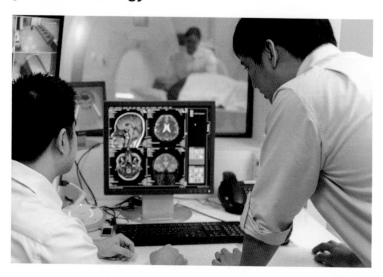

ParkwayHealth Radiology is a leading radiology and imaging provider in Singapore. Besides serving Parkway Pantai's four hospitals in Singapore, it also operates a network of nine radiology clinics that provide the medical community with high quality radiology and nuclear medicine services. Its comprehensive range of diagnostic and therapeutic offerings includes Magnetic Resonance Imaging, Computed Tomography (CT), Breast Imaging Services, and Ultrasound and Positron Emission Tomography (PET). *For more information, please go to www.parkwayhealthradiology.com.sg.*

ParkwayHealth Laboratory

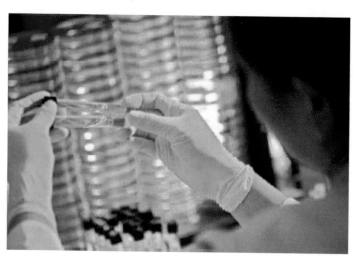

ParkwayHealth Laboratory provides high quality and cost-efficient services in the areas of clinical laboratory, histopathology, and genetics. It operates four well-equipped laboratories located within Parkway Pantai's four hospitals in Singapore, a satellite outpatient laboratory in Novena Medical Centre, and a reference laboratory at Ayer Rajah Crescent, to provide fast and accurate results for patients and medical practitioners. *For more information, please go to www.parkwayhealthlaboratory. com.sg.*

11.9 Mount Alvernia Hospital

Joyce See*

The Beginning

The story of Mount Alvernia Hospital (MAH) began with the arrival of the Sisters from the Franciscan Missionaries of the Divine Motherhood (FMDM) on 7 March 1949. They took over the tuberculosis wards at Tan Tock Seng Hospital, which eventually became known as Mandalay Road Hospital, and had also served "The Lepers Camp" — a community of lepers housed in Trafalgar Home in Woodbridge. Both centres were managed as self-contained units. Isolation was the treatment at that time.

In 1952, the Sisters were given an opportunity to start a private hospital to bring nursing care and services to Singapore's population. It was to be a well-planned and professionally managed hospital for everyone, especially for the poor and the disadvantaged.

In addition to pooling their savings and salaries, the FMDM Sisters started canvassing for donations all over the Singapore Island. There was also a promise from the Colonial government at that time to do a dollar-for-dollar matching grant based on the total collection. The Sisters set to plan and work towards building a 200-bed hospital (Fig. 11.9.1).

The construction of the hospital began in 1957 with the bulldozers moving in to clear the land. A.J. Braga who was then Minister of Health performed the ground breaking ceremony in 1959.

Though the Sisters' focus was on their mission of service, the consequences of political change could not be ignored. At the general election of 1959 with Singapore gaining self-government and competing priorities for limited funds, their matching grant was cancelled. The Sisters had to adjust their plans to cater for a

*Mount Alvernia Hospital, Singapore.

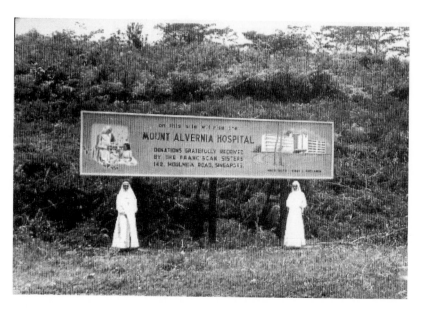

Fig. 11.9.1. The signboard erected at the foot of the "Thomson Hill Site"; advertising the future Mount Alvernia Hospital.

60-bed hospital instead of 200 but would be fully equipped to provide medical, surgical and maternity care.

On 4 March 1961, Mount Alvernia Hospital was declared officially opened. Staffing was done entirely by the Sisters who were professionally trained as nurses, midwives, physiotherapists, radiographers, laboratory technicians and other support services. The Sisters who ran the hospital received all their professional healthcare qualifications, religious training, and work attachment at a hospital in the United Kingdom.

At the time of opening, the hospital was equipped with two operating theatres, an anaesthetics room, a recovery room, two labour wards, a nursery and a milk kitchen. A physiotherapy department was also in place, as well as one outpatient department and a dispensary. An X-ray department was set up immediately. Ward duty for the nursing Sisters lasted from 7 am to 9 pm. Before and after official normal ward duties, the Sisters doubled up as housekeepers, chefs and meal servers as well.

Hospital Development

In 1963, the first extension to MAH was completed. This provided improved out-patient facilities, a new delivery suite, a third labour ward, a specialised nursery for premature infants and two more operating theatres. In the same year, the first Resident Medical Officer (RMO) joined the team and a second RMO was added two years later.

In 1964, one of the Sisters returned to Singapore after her training in England and Ireland to set up a department of pathology and a blood bank — making MAH the first hospital to have its own blood bank. MAH's blood bank was 90% self-sufficient and patients' relatives were encouraged to donate. With the seaport bustling with activities at that time, the Sisters also regularly went out to the anchored ships to drive blood donation from visiting seamen.

During the early years after independence, government-expanded medical services in primary healthcare focused on improving hygiene as inpatient care was not high on the government's priority list at that time. Hence, MAH saw the need to further develop to increase inpatient capacity and support services.

On July 1965, Prime Minister Lee Kuan Yew officially opened a new 5-storey wing, which brought the total number of beds to 127 (Fig. 11.9.2).

In 1969, MAH added another extension to provide care to chronically-ill patients. Within this building, another 22 beds were added.

PM Lee returned to the hospital again in 1971 to open another wing adding another 72 beds to the capacity. With this addition, the hospital now has 221 beds (Fig. 11.9.3).

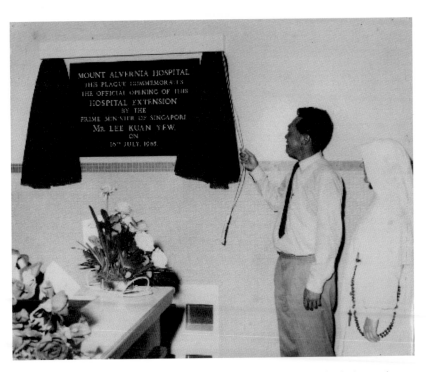

Fig. 11.9.2. The Nation's first Prime Minister, Mr. Lee Kuan Yew, officially declaring the new wing open.

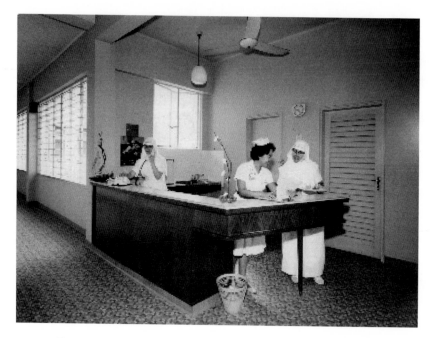

Fig. 11.9.3. Nurses' station in St. Francis medical and surgical ward.

The new wing included a much needed Intensive Care Unit and a Paediatric Ward. It also housed a new outpatient department with consulting rooms and a minor theatre. A radiography department and a pathology laboratory were expanded; while a hydrotherapy pool was also added to the physiotherapy department. For the convenience of patients and visitors, the hospital's public areas boasted a new coffee house and a pharmacy.

In the 1980s, a decision was taken to accommodate some specialist clinics on campus. Work began in 1989 to build a new medical centre. With on-campus doctors, increased in patient loads were expected. In 1991, a new wing was constructed to accommodate medical and consulting suites. This wing would also include a suite of six operating theatres, a delivery suite of 10 rooms, a 4-bedded first-stage room, a new physiotherapy and an occupational therapy unit.

MAH further stepped up support for specialist practices by expanding clinical services from the late 1990s onwards — services which included X ray, MRI, multi-slide CT-scan and digital mammography. Other developments included capabilities for laparoscope of Minimal Access Surgery. A Lithotripter Centre was also opened and a bone densitometer was added to the facilities of Diagnostic Imaging Department. Clinical support staff received training and skills upgrading with attachments at leading international institutions.

In addition to training its own staff, the hospital also ran courses for doctors. MAH scored a first as a private healthcare initiative by live broadcasting the procedure from the operating theatre for viewing in a separate training area. Foreign doctors were included in the training. The capability for laparoscopic surgery allowed MAH to include many more procedures in its Day Surgery services.

In 1986, MAH started accepting respite patients. This extension became known as Assisi Home. Two years later, it expanded into the area of Hospice Care. In 1992, a decision was taken to establish hospice care as a dedicated mission of the Assisi Hospice, housed in a separate building from the hospital.

MAH recognised that besides excellent care by physicians and nurses, a team of trained pastoral carers would be required to help to address the patients' emotional and spiritual needs, regardless of their religion, race, gender or ethnic background. The Clinical Pastoral Care Department was established by the FMDM sisters in May 1986 to provide a holistic healing environment for her patients.

In 1996, the new medical centre was finally opened and started admitting specialist doctors with full admission rights (Fig. 11.9.4).

Health screening centre was added to offer comprehensive and personalised services. The other one-stop service was the Day Surgery where the patient could register, checkout and collect medication in one place.

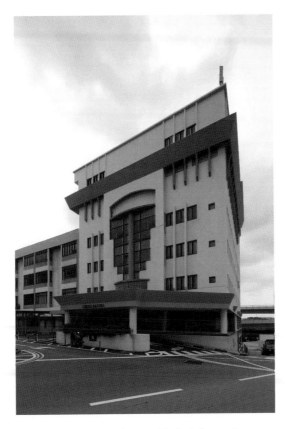

Fig. 11.9.4.   The new Medical Centre A.

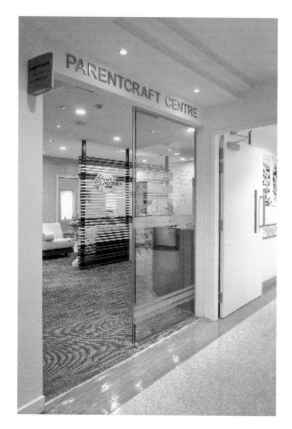

Fig. 11.9.5.   The Parentcraft Centre.

In 2004, allied health services were stepped up with the setting up of the Sports Medicine and Sports Surgery Centre functions in tandem with the rehabilitation centre. The following year, MAH added 24-hour outpatient clinic services to fill the gap when extended hours in Singapore public sector polyclinics were discontinued.

In October 2010, the Alvernia Parentcraft Centre was officially opened as a dedicated one-stop centre for ante-natal care, childbirth education and newborn baby care (Fig. 11.9.5). Equipped with cosy private consultation rooms and staffed by experienced lactation consultants and parentcraft counsellors, the Centre fulfilled the needs of both parents with newborns and those preparing for childbirth.

The following year saw more investment in several innovative IT initiatives such as electronic medical records, online medical test order by doctors, enhancement of pharmacy information system and customer relationship management system.

The new side extension facing Thomson Road was completed in 2012. It housed additional diagnostic imaging facilities, a bigger health screening centre, more

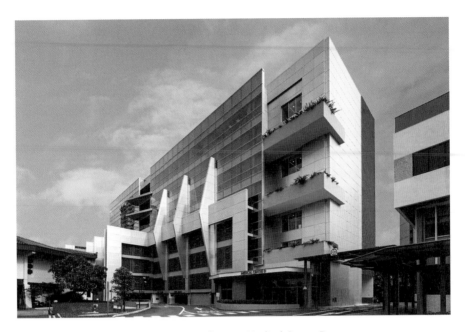

Fig. 11.9.6. The new Medical Centre D.

operating theatres and patient beds. It is served by a covered pedestrian walkway to provide easy access to Thomson Road.

The hospital Chapel had been an integral part of the infrastructure since MAH started in 1961. The Chapel went through a renovation and reopened in 2013.

The new Medical Centre D was finally completed and officially opened by Minister of Health, Mr. Gan Kim Yong on October 2014. This new 17,490 sq m new facility not only provides additional medical suites, but also the much-needed expanded car park space for the hospital. It is now home to over 60 specialist clinics covering 28 specialties (Fig. 11.9.6).

11.10 Raffles Medical Group

Lawrence Lim*

Raffles Medical Group (RMG) was founded in 1976 by two young doctors — Dr. Loo Choon Yong and Dr. Alfred Loh — who had the vision of starting their own private practice to give of their best to their patients. They laid the foundation for an institution based on a group practice model, pooling together talented doctors and leveraging their strengths to provide quality care for the patients.

Thirty nine years on, RMG has become a leading private integrated healthcare provider in Singapore. The multidisciplinary group practice has a staff of about 290 family physicians, specialists, and dental surgeons, serving more than 2 million patients, and over 6500 corporate clients, including government agencies and multinational corporations spanning various industries. The Group is publicly listed on the Singapore Stock Exchange since April 1997.

This is a far cry from the two-clinic practice when it started out in 1976 in the Central Business District in Singapore. From these humble beginnings, the Group expanded in the 1980s and 1990s in tandem with the growth of corporate businesses, branching out to the tourist belt, HDB heartlands, industrial estates, and the airport. Today, the Group comprises more than 80 Raffles Medical and Raffles Dental clinics in its primary care network (Fig. 11.10.1).

As it grew, the Group found itself needing to respond to demand for new services as well as integration of services. It took the direction of expanding along the healthcare value chain by adding secondary and tertiary specialty care by way of Raffles Surgicentre in 1993, which subsequently expanded and moved to Raffles Hospital when it was opened on 31 March 2001.

Raffles Hospital stands as the flagship of the Group, offering services in more than 35 specialties. Located at the heart of Singapore city, Raffles Hospital offers emergency care, multidisciplinary specialist clinics, dental services, Traditional

*Director, Corporate Development, Raffles Medical Group, Singapore.

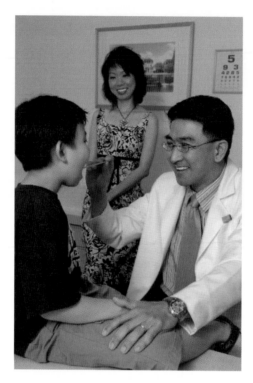

Fig. 11.10.1. Located where our patients work, live and play, our 80 multi-disciplinary clinics provide healthcare services to cater to the needs of the whole family.

Chinese Medicine, health screening, inpatient wards, delivery suites, operating theatres, intensive care units, and clinical support services. More than one third of the hospital's patients are foreign patients from more than 100 countries. Raffles Hospital has representative offices in Jakarta, Dhaka and Vietnam, and contracts and billing arrangements with more than 100 international healthcare insurance companies. The Hospital is ISO 9001:2008 certified and accredited by the Joint Commission International.

As a group, RMG actively participates in public-private sector collaborations that serve the interests of patients and the community. Raffles Medical and Raffles Dental clinics are accredited to serve patients under the Government-initiated Community Health Assist Scheme, Pioneer Generation package and Flexi-Medisave scheme. The hospital, in collaboration with the Ministry of Health (MOH), spearheaded a system which provides, starting from June 2015, for patients sent by Singapore Civil Defence Force ambulances to the hospital's Emergency Department to receive care at subsidised rates. This collaboration supports MOH's efforts in reducing waiting times at emergency

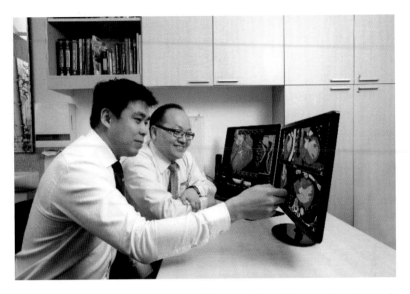

Fig. 11.10.2. As a group practice, doctors in Raffles Hospital provide team-based care, drawing on multi-disciplinary expertise within the Group for the benefit of our patients.

departments at public hospitals, and accords patients enhanced access to immediate medical care.

As a medical practice, RMG is unique in Singapore as the largest private healthcare group that is centred on a philosophy of institutional group practice, well established in renowned medical centres such as the Mayo Clinic. This model affords a structure of clinical governance with a staff of medical doctors and specialists working as a team and sharing a common commitment to the highest quality of medical service, teaching and research. As a group practice (Fig. 11.10.2), the physicians in RMG subscribe to clinical audit and peer review, adhere to a professional fee schedule, and adopt a team-based approach to integrated care. Patients with complicated or multiple diagnoses are able to benefit from coordinated and seamless care, and can draw on professional skills and capabilities across a number of clinical disciplines available under one umbrella.

The Group leverages on this team-based approach and integration of its medical services to customise health and wellness solutions for companies and individuals. Raffles Health Insurance, set up in 2005, operates as a healthcare insurance specialist offering healthcare financing solutions for organisations as well as individuals and their families. The Group's venture into consumer health under Raffles Health represents an extension of its commitment to the health and well-being of the individuals. Raffles Health develops and distributes the Raffles and Kidds brands of nutriceutical health products.

To strengthen its development as an institution, the Group set up the Raffles Healthcare Institute as its training arm, and the Clinical Trials Unit as a springboard for research. Raffles Healthcare Institute offers training for doctors, nurses, allied health personnel and healthcare managers. It partners with the universities, polytechnics and vocational institutes to provide clinical training for their undergraduates and postgraduates. The Group's Clinical Trials Unit serves as a one-stop resource centre to support clinicians to conduct high-quality clinical trials. It offers patients access to cutting edge treatments not yet available in the market, and clinicians a critical basis for innovation in disease treatment.

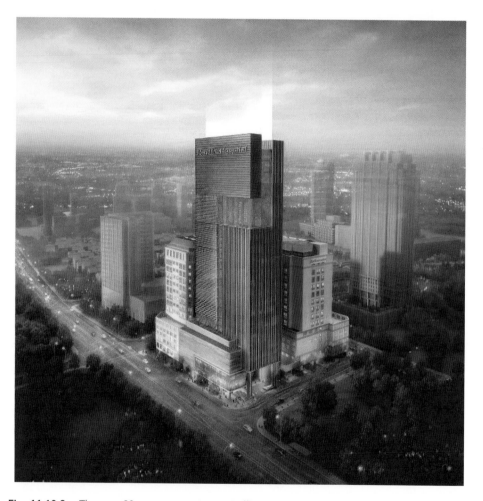

Fig. 11.10.3. The new 20-storey extension to Raffles Hospital, together with the existing hospital building, constitutes a compelling integrated medical campus well positioned to meet the growing needs of our patients.

In 2003, the Group set up the Medical Foundation as a channel for giving back to the community. The Group's charity arm was charged with the mission of helping the under-privileged, particularly those who required urgent medical treatment. It was renamed the Asian Medical Foundation in 2005 to reflect the regional scope of its work which included medical disaster relief in response to the Aceh tsunami in 2004 and the Nias earthquake in 2005.

As RMG looks forward to the future, it can expect in the next few years to develop into a private healthcare institution with an international outlook and presence. Beyond the Singapore shores, the Group operates medical centres and clinics in 12 other cities in Asia — Hong Kong, Beijing, Shanghai, Tianjin, Dalian, Nanjing, Shenzhen, Osaka, Hanoi, Ho Chi Minh City, Vinh Tuy and Pnom Denh. The Group has been the exclusive medical provider in the Singapore Changi Airport and Hong Kong's Chek Lap Kok International Airport since they started operations in 1990 and 1998, respectively.

In Singapore, Raffles Hospital's 20-storey (Fig. 11.10.3) new wing will add 220,000 sq ft of space to expand the hospital's specialty services. The Group's new-concept multi-disciplinary medical centres in Holland Village and Orchard Road will offer comprehensive services, including family medicine, dental, health screening, radiology, Traditional Chinese Medicine and specialist services.

Reflecting on the Group's growth plans, Dr. Loo Choon Yong, Executive Chairman, affirms: "Raffles Medical Group must exist for a greater cause than itself. We must grow and become stronger so that we can bring better healthcare to more communities and more people."

12 Ages and Stages: Five Decades of Community and Residential Services in Singapore*

Wong Loong Mun,[†] Nixon Tan,[‡] Toh Kong Chian[§] and Jason Cheah[¶]

In 1961, the Bukit Ho Swee fire displaced some 16,000 people. It happened two years after the 1959 fire at Kampong Tiong Bahru in which about 5000 lost their homes. Ironically, these fires were then considered a "blessing in disguise" whereby an enlightened government rehoused the "inert community" of squatters after a disaster and set the country on the right path towards progress and modernity."[1] These incidents "cleansed" the path and set the direction in how our young nation would proceed. These series of disasters tested the then newly convened Singapore Council of Social Services (SCSS), which was a statutory body and the predecessor of the National Council of Social Services (NCSS), formed to coordinate and promote the roles and contributions of Voluntary Welfare Organisations.[2]

*We are deeply appreciative of our friends and colleagues who shared generously with us. They are Theresa Yoong, K. Veloo, Eileen Magnus, Chew Sin Poon, Elizabeth Yee, Victor Seng, Yip Moh Han, Christine Loh, Doreen Lye, Ong Hui Min, Dennis Tan, Geraldine Tan, Swapna Dayanandan, K.V. Miyapan, Loh Yik Hin, Arthur Chern, Lawrence Ang, Teo Her Tee, Then Kim Yuan, Angel Lee, Pauline Tan and Geraldine Lim.

[†] Principal Consultant & Chief Care Transition Officer, Agency for Integrated Care.
[‡] Executive, Principal Consultant Office, Agency for Integrated Care.
[§] Executive, Community Mental Health Division, Agency for Integrated Care.
[¶] Chief Executive Officer, Agency for Integrated Care.

[1] Loh, KS (2013) Squatters into Citizens: The 1961 Bukit Ho Swee Fire and the Making of Modern Singapore. NIAS Press: Copenhagen.
[2] National Council of Social Services. (2008) For All We Care — 50 years of Social Services in Singapore 1958–2008. NCSS: Singapore.

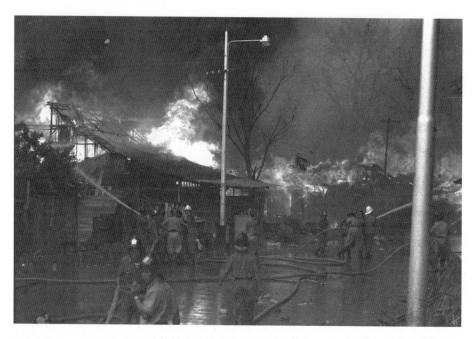

1961 — Firemen fighting to control the Bukit Ho Swee Fire. (Photo credit: Ministry of Information and the Arts Collection, Courtesy of National Archives of Singapore.)

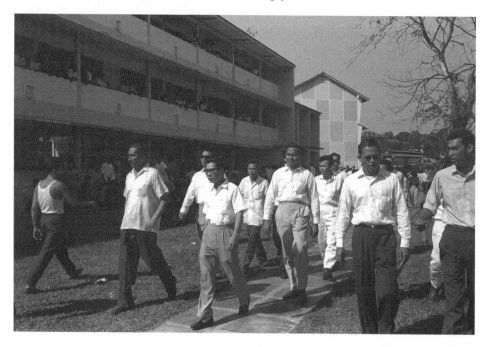

1961 — Yang Di-Pertuan Negara Yusof Ishak visiting the relief centre for victims of Bukit Ho Swee Fire. (Photo credit: Ministry of Information and the Arts Collection, Courtesy of National Archives of Singapore.)

Our journey about the residential and community care services starts from these successive fires soon after the People's Action Party (PAP) came to power in 1959. When we look back at the socio-political context of that time, the government faced great pressure to solve social problems resulting from such disasters and the social disorder at that time. After the British handover of power to the local administration, headed by the PAP, the foci of the government were to reduce the severe unemployment, expand primary healthcare services, make education accessible, tighten population control and implement large-scale housing.[3] The strategy then was to foster social integration through social investment and social welfare programmes while building the economic foundations in the country.[4,5]

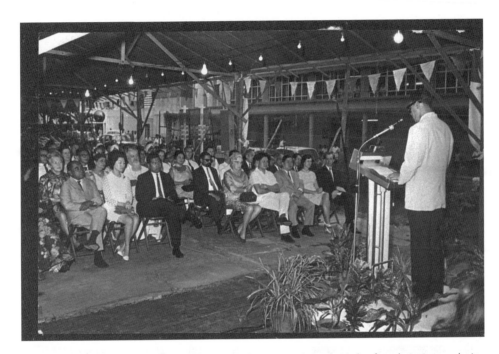

1968 — Minister for Social Affairs Othman Wok giving a speech at the foundation stone laying ceremony of the new Singapore Council of Social (SCSS) Service building. The SCSS is now known as the National Council of Social Service (NCSS). (Photo credit: Singapore Council of Social Service Collection, Courtesy of National Archives of Singapore.)

---

[3] Wijeysingha, V. (2005) The welfare regime in Singapore. In: A Walker & CK Wong (eds.). *East Asian Welfare Regimes in Transition. From Confucianism to Globalization* 187–211. Bristol, UK: Policy Press.
[4] Aspalter, C. (2006) The East Asian Welfare model. *International Journal of Social Welfare.* **15**: 290–301.
[5] Tremewan, C. (2005) Welfare and governance: Public Housing under Singapore's party-state. In: A Walker & CK Wong (eds.). *East Asian Welfare Regimes in Transition. From Confucianism to Globalisation*, pp. 77–105. Bristol, UK: The Policy Press.

Then, the efforts to provide social welfare were limited to those that came from private philanthropic efforts,[6] with the government only making occasional attempts into the social sector, e.g. to control epidemics. Colonial government was tied up with building infrastructure such as hospitals and in the management of diseases in congested areas.[7] It was only after the war in 1946 that the government established the Social Welfare Department to help the poor and needy segments. In 1947, a social welfare council was formed to acknowledge the importance of the voluntary welfare organisations.[8] During this period, the older person was not a social condition since the population was made mostly of younger people.

This chapter outlines the development of the residential and community care sector. In the early days of our nation, services were largely provided by religious groups, philanthropic individuals and families, mutual aid societies and clans, and that government was usually part of a larger patronage. It was relatively effective because our needs were simple then. As the nation grew, society became more complicated and individuals' needs complex. The government stepped in to define guiding principles on how we care for the old. It established successive committees to address the "problems of the old" and; in part also define the role of the Voluntary Welfare Organisation (VWO) vis-à-vis the residential and community care services[9] under the "Many Helping Hands Approach." Each committee defined the direction and development. The chapter ends with the last decade that highlights the growing pains of the sector.

Beginnings

Singapore's "welfare system" started during the colonial government where there were already informal ways of meeting needs before the establishment of social welfare services.[10] When Singapore was set up as a trading port, immigrants from China, India, Indonesia and surrounding countries migrated here to work. Then, there was hardly any support from the colonial government, immigrants depended

---

[6] Turnbull, CM. (2010) *A History of Singapore 1819–2005*. NUS Press: Singapore.

[7] Mudeliar, V, Nair, CRS, Norris, RP. (1979) Development of Hospital Care and Nursing in Singapore.

[8] Wee, A. (2004) Where we are coming from: The evolution of social services and social work in Singapore. In: KK Mehta & A Wee (eds.). *Social Work in Context: A Reader*, pp. 39–80. Singapore: Marshall Cavendish Academic.

[9] In our story about the sector, we make the assumption that the development of the services mirrors the development of the Voluntary Welfare Organisations (VWOSs). In Peggy Teo's (2004) review of the healthcare system for the older persons, she also collapses and blurs the distinction of VWOs and LTC services. While there are pockets of participation from the private sector, it is still very much a cottage industry in the long-term care sector. (Teo, P. (2004) Health care for older persons in Singapore. *Journal of Aging & Social Policy.* **16**(1): 43–67.)

[10] Wee, A. (2004) Where we are coming from: The evolution of social services and social work in Singapore. In: KK Mehta & A Wee (eds.). *Social Work in Context: A Reader*, pp. 39–80. Singapore: Marshall Cavendish Academic.

on one another and informal help from kinfolks, relatives and others from the same province of origin. The Chinese established a formal system of mutual aid known as clan associations. These clans were based on surname, dialects or province. The functions of the mutual aid societies included benefits to aged and disabled members, compensation for industrial accidents, payments to unemployed workers, nursing and maternity care, funeral expenses and provision of educational opportunities. Mutual aid societies provided a locally organised, self-help version of what we would call the welfare state.[11,12] These were the humble beginnings of some of our VWOs. As time passed, the communities prospered and large-scale associations begin to form based on language and/or province. They began to undertake projects such as schools and healthcare institutions. The Kheng Chiu (Hainanese) association formed a home for the elderly, while Kwong Wai Shui (Cantonese)[13] established a large hospital in the old Tan Tock Seng Hospital premises.[14]

Similarly, Man Fut Tong Nursing Home's founder, Venerable Ho Yuen Hoe left her family in Hong Kong in 1941. She started off as a maid and shared her quarters with Samsui women in Chinatown. After the war, she sold cooked food and worked as a hairdresser weaving plaits and buns for amahs and other Chinese women. In 1948, she joined a Buddhist group, became a vegetarian and led a life of austerity. This group functioned akin to a mutual aid society along the lines of gender, dialect and religion — the Man Fut Tong Mutual Aid Association. Through her entrepreneurship and smart investment, she procured lands and set up an old kampong-style two-storey zinc house that housed a temple and 40 single women. This home catered mainly for samsui women who had neither savings nor family. She created a mutual support environment where they took care of each other.[15] Through the years, the home grew to occupy the adjacent land, converted from

---

[11] Cheng, LK. (1990) Reflections on the changing roles of Chinese Clan Associations in Singapore. *Asian Culture*. **14**: 57–70.

[12] Kuah-Pearce, KE (2006) The cultural politics of clan associations in contemporary Singapore. In: KE Kuah-Pearce & E Hu-Dehart (eds.). *Voluntary Organizations in the Chinese Diaspora*, pp. 53–75. Hong Kong: Hong Kong University Press.

[13] Ou, R. (2010) *Kwong Wai Shiu Hospital Centennial Celebration*. Singapore: Toppan Security Printing.

[14] Kwong Wai Shui started as a result of the colonial government's call in 1910 for the Chinese community to establish their own medical facilities as growing number of locals were falling victim to infectious diseases. Wong Ah Fook and Leong Man Sau who were two leaders of the Cantonese community convened prominent personnel and raised more than $100,000. The facility was modeled after a well-known free hospital in Guangzhou. In 1911, under the Kwong Wai Shiu Free Hospital Ordinance, then Governor of Singapore, Sir John Anderson signed a memorandum of understanding with Kwong Ah Fook to transfer the land and the old premises of Tan Tock Seng Hospital to the hospital with a lease of 99 years and annual lease payment of $1.

[15] Man Fut Tong can be considered as a female Buddhist vegetarian house to provide lodging for unattached women. Many were immigrant Chinese women and some married women deserted by their husbands.

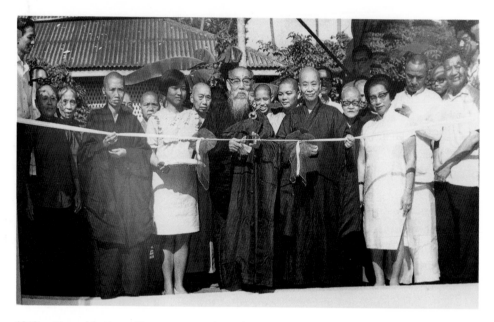

1949 — Venerable Ho and her youngest adopted daughter Venerable Lai Hui at the Opening Ceremony of the Man Fut Tong Old Peoples Home. (Photo credit: "Man Fut Tong — A Life for Others," p. 33. Courtesy of Man Fut Tong Nursing Home.)

a sheltered home to a nursing home and eventually, settled in its current location at Woodlands.[16]

Within the Indian community, migrants who worked in the construction and naval industries formed the Indian Association in 1923. This was a pan-Indian, rather than narrowly ethnic, language, religion, caste or region-based organisation. Mr. G. Bhanu and his Malayalee friends also set up a similar organisation — the Sree Narayana Mission — in 1946 in the context of post war hardships. The Mission started with the welfare of the immigrant community and cemented relationships across ethnicity, caste and dialects through festive celebrations, religious events, charity events and marriages. Their initial welfare initiatives consisted of the provision of financial assistance, working with youth and food relief programs. The Mission grew from relief efforts to establishing a residential home in Canberra Home. In 1979, it had 4 beds and by 1981, it grew to 53. By 1994, the home had 224 residents.[17]

Other faith based organisations, such as the Little Sisters of the Poor and St. Andrew's Mission Hospital,[18] were already established in the early beginnings of the nation. The St. Andrew's Medical Mission opened a dispensary in Bencoolen

---

[16] Rajan, U, Devi, GU (2006) *A Life for Others*. Singapore: Man Fut Tong Home.

[17] Ebrahim, N. (2013) *Generations of Giving: The Story of Sree Narayana (Singapore)*. Singapore.

[18] Reid, L, Thay, W. (2006) *A Light that Shines: The Story of St. Andrew's Mission Hospital*. Singapore: SAMH.

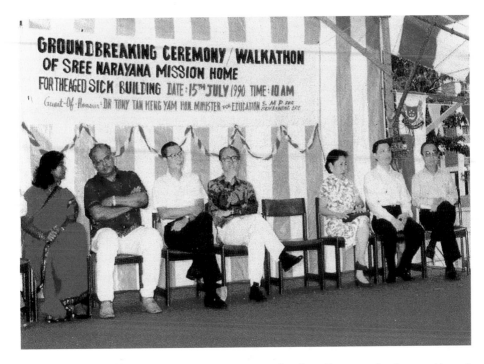

1990 — Dr. Tony Tan (4th from left) graced the Groundbreaking Ceremony for the new Home in Yishun in 1990. Dr. Onn (3rd from right) was involved in the fundraising for the home. (Photo credit: "Generations of Giving — The Story of Sree Narayana Mission (Singapore)," Courtesy of Sree Narayana Mission.)

Street in 1913 to provide free medical care for destitute women and children. Their service was very well received and in 1923, it opened the St. Andrew's Mission Hospital for Women and Children at Erskine Road. The hospital had 60 inpatient beds and an outpatient clinic. The Little Sisters of the Poor arrived in the 1930s and began their work of looking after the aged and destitute. The Little Sisters, which is a congregation of religious sisters known for their care of the sick and dying, setup a home in Derbyshire Road for 12 elderly folk in 1935[19] and eventually moved to the present home in 49 Upper Thomson Road in October 1939. The Sisters devoted themselves to the care of the sick and elderly under their charge, and worked tirelessly until 2000 when they transferred operations of the home to the Catholic Welfare Services.[20]

---

[19] The building of the Home was made possible by a $60,000 (1937 currency) donation by Mr. Aw Boon Haw and Mr. Aw Boon Par, who were Burmese Chinese entrepreneurs and philanthropists best known for introducing Tiger Balm. "Governor Lays Corner Stone for Home for Aged." The Singapore Free Press and Mercantile Advertiser, 8 June 1937, p. 9.

[20] Interview with Mr. Victor Seng, CEO of St. Theresa's Home on 19 September 2014.

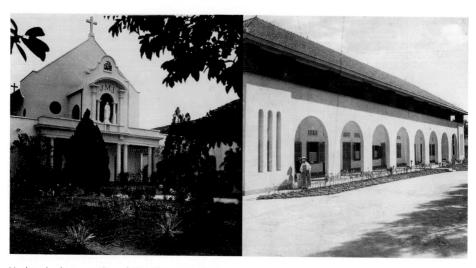

Undated photographs of St. Theresa's Home in its early days. (Photo credit: Mr. Victor Seng, administrator of St. Theresa's Home, Courtesy of Little Sisters of the Poor.)

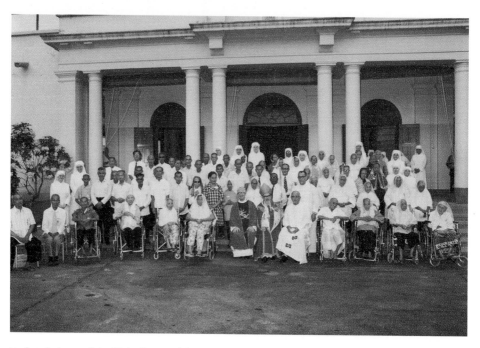

Undated photo of the Little Sisters of the Poor and key Catholic leaders (middle: Archbishop Michel Olçomendy) with residents of St. Theresa's Home. (Photo credit: Mr. Victor Seng, administrator of St. Theresa's Home, Courtesy of Little Sisters of the Poor.)

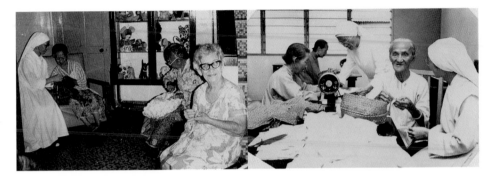

Undated photo of elderly staying at St. Theresa's Home enjoying an afternoon of knitting with the Sisters. (Photo credit: Mr. Victor Seng, administrator of St. Theresa's Home, Courtesy of Little Sisters of the Poor.)

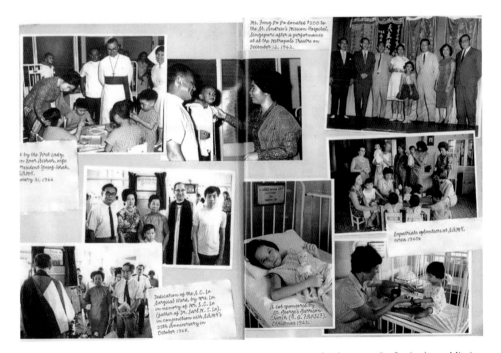

1960s — Photographs from 1960s of St. Andrew's Mission Hospital. (Photo credit: St. Andrews Mission Hospital "From Flicker to Flame." Courtesy of St. Andrews Mission Hospital & Singapore Anglican Community Services.)

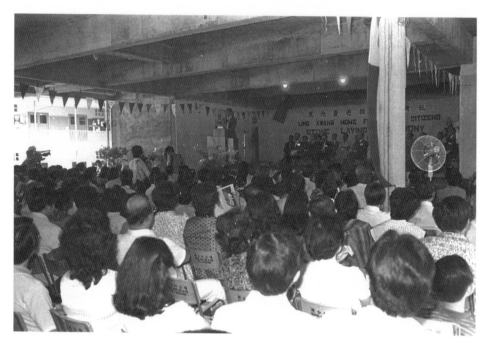

1983 — Then-Minister for Defence and Second Minister for Health Goh Chok Tong delivers a speech at Ling Kwang Home for the Aged at Serangoon Garden Way, during the stone laying ceremony. (Photo credit: Istana Collection, Courtesy of National Archives of Singapore.)

Other Christian organisations were driven by more proximate reasons. They were led by strong patriarchs with supportive family and congregation who ventured beyond church grounds to reach out to the indigent and old. For example, Ling Kwang Mission,[21] established by the late Reverend Dr. Quek Kiok Chiang under the auspices of Bible Presbyterian Welfare Services, started off as a welfare clinic in 1968. It offered free medical services to the poor and needy among the rural residents in the areas of Cheng San, Ang Mo Kio and Yio Chu Kang. In 1979, after the squatters occupying the plot of land behind the church were cleared, Reverend Quek built a nursing home for the elderly. The founder of Ju Eng Home, the late Mr. Ang Oon Hue, arrived in Singapore in 1930. Through hard work, he bought lands in the Jalan Kayu and surrounding estates. He set up the Chinese-educated Ju Eng Primary School in Jalan Kayu in the early 1940s but had to close in 1987 due to falling enrollment. So Mr. Ang donated the land to the government and set up a charitable home to serve the poor, frail and sick in that area.[22] Reverend Dr. Quek Kiok Chiang, who was a family friend, helped

---

[21] Email correspondence with Mr. Dennis Tan, CEO of Ling Kwang Home dated 16 September 2014.
[22] Oral history Interviews with Mr. Lawrence Ang Poh Siew. (2011) Interview 003396. Oral History Centre. National Archives of Singapore.

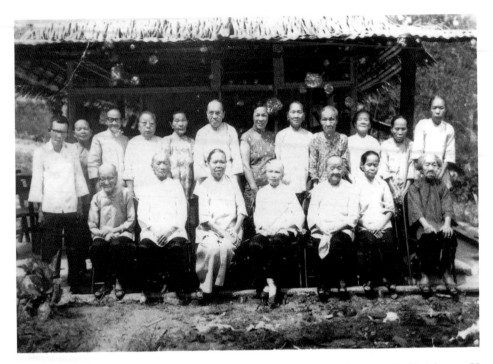

1974 — Residents of Singapore Christian Home in a group photograph. (Photo credit: "Celebrating 50 years of God's Goodness," p. 6, Courtesy of Singapore Christian Home for the Aged.)

set up the home. Both men also helped set up the Singapore Christian Home. The story of this nursing home started when three Christian friends — Madam Lau Kah Eng, Liew Choon Giok and Tan Kiat Jin — wanted a home to spend their last lap of their lives together. This was made possible after they met Madam Ang Soh Cheng who sold her home to them. Eventually, she joined them and gradually, more women some homeless required accommodation. They moved to Yishun and then, Sembawang where they were officially registered as Singapore Christian Home for the Aged in 1977.[23]

Faith-based groups must be understood in terms of their linkages with the larger social networks of which civil society is composed. These congregations created a caring community and worked across long-lasting personal friendships. These informal relationships played an important role in support and, helped each other through difficult times to achieve their goals to help the old and poor. Similarly, non-sectarian organisations — especially groups of volunteers united under a common cause — also contributed positively to the functioning of civil society and nation building.

---

[23] Singapore Christian Home for the Aged. (2011) Celebrating 50 years of God's Goodness.

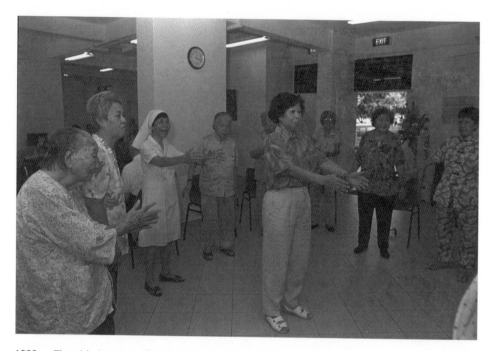

1993 — The elderly with staff at Apex Rehabilitation Centre located at Block 119, Bukit Merah View. Then-Minister of State for Health Dr. Aline Wong officiated at opening of the centre. (Photo credit: Ministry of Information and the Arts Collection, Courtesy of National Archives of Singapore.)

The Lions Clubs, for example, were established as small groups of dedicated professionals that met regularly to discuss about improving the well-being of the community. As early as 1972, local members across the diverse clubs made visits and gave daily essentials like biscuits, rice and soap to nursing homes. One such home that benefited from the largess of the Lions Club East was Singapore Christian Home. In 1977, former Deputy Prime Minister, Dr. Toh Chin Chye, encouraged the members to think ahead to deal with the fast and growing elderly population in the community. So eight clubs came together to convert a void deck at Block 403 Ang Mo Kio Avenue 10 into a four-room home for 18 elderly. This joint project materialised in 1980. Shortly, it moved to a 45-bedded home in Toa Payoh Rise in 1985 and in 1997, it became a 154-bedded nursing home in Bedok.[24] The story of Lions resonates with the Apex Club members who support the Apex Day Rehabilitation Centre and Apex Harmony Lodge. Similarly, after six years of visiting nursing home residents, the volunteers of the Sunshine Welfare Mission Home also decided to come together to set up a nursing home to care for the old, sick and poor.[25]

[24] Lee, D. (2009) *Our Lions Story: Singapore Lions Clubs — Celebrating 50 years of Community Service, 1958–2008*. Singapore: Lions Club of Singapore District 208.

[25] Information accessed from Sunshine Welfare Action Mission's website on 2 December 2014.

Then, there was a group of volunteers who responded to a news article about St. Joseph's Home that cared for the terminally ill. When the volunteers realised that the terminally ill with cancer were sent home to die, there was a need to reach out to help them. As they went around helping the dying at home, more needed their assistance and services grew. Hospice Care Association was thus formed in 1989.[26]

A few pioneers, such as the late Dr. Khoo Oon Teik, started out with more personal reasons. He bore witness to the suffering and death of his brother due to kidney failure; and was resolute that no one should suffer the same ordeal. In 1969, Dr. Khoo with his friends started the National Kidney Foundation in the attic of the Singapore General Hospital.[27] Mdm. Tsao Ng Yu Shun, who started the Tsao Foundation for the elderly at the age of 86, was also informed by her care work for her parents, in-laws and her favourite uncle — "I know what it is to grow old, and I deeply feel the desperation of those who face old age alone, who cannot get to a doctor when sick, and whose families cannot — for whatever reasons — adequately care for them. The pain of poor health is so much worse when you are frail and

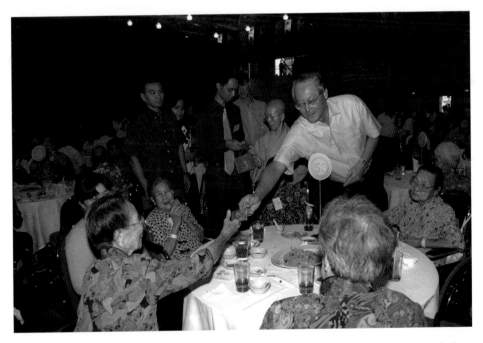

2002 — Prime Minister Goh Chok Tong distributing Angpow to elderly guests during Vesak Great Joy Party organised by Singapore Buddhist Welfare Services at Singapore Expo Hall 1. (Photo credit: Ministry of Information, Communications, and the Arts Collection, Courtesy of National Archives of Singapore.)

---

[26] Goh, C. (2003) Reflections and vision of SHC Chairman on hospice work. *Hospice Link.* **10**(3): 1,5.

[27] Information gathered from the National Kidney Foundation website (accessed on 2 December 2014).

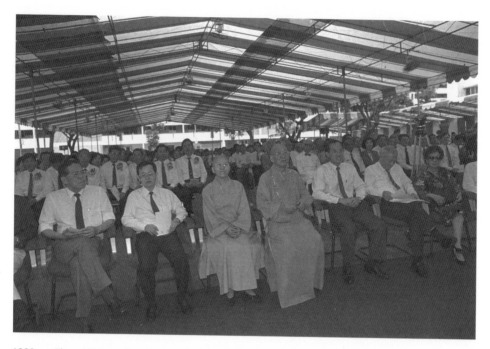

1992 — Then Minister for Information and the Arts and Second Minister for Foreign Affairs Brigadier-General (BG) George Yeo Opens Singapore Buddhist Welfare Services (SBWS) — National Kidney Foundation (NKF) Dialysis Centre at Block 114 Hougang Avenue 1 in 1992. SBWS President Venerable Kuan Yan and founder Venerable Yen Pei were seated with the Minister. (Photo credit: Ministry of Information and the Arts Collection, Courtesy of National Archives of Singapore.)

old."[28] There were other luminaries such as Dr. Ee Peng Liang,[29] Dr. Oon Chiew Seng, Venerable Yen Pei and Ms. Teresa Hsu[30] who set up St. Joseph's Home, Apex Harmony Lodge, Singapore Buddhist Welfare Services and Society for the Aged Sick respectively. Their legacies remained and remembered.

These faith and civil associations and individuals contributed to the effectiveness and stability of our nation[31] because they embodied the importance of social

---

[28] Tsao Foundation. 20th Anniversary (2013).

[29] Ee-Chooi, T. (1987) *Father of Charity and ... my Father.* Singapore: SNP Printing.

[30] Teoh, E. (2014) Welcome Address. Presentation made at the Official Opening of the Society for the Aged Sick's Tower Block.

[31] Majority of the sector were operated by faith-based charities and non-sectarian organisations. However, the commercial operators and government also ran some nursing homes. In the 1960s, there were large commercial homes such as the Dragon Lotus Homes, Yew Tee Home and Aljunied Home. But the conditions were deplorable. In 1971, SCSS set up an Ad Hoc Committee for the Aged Destitute and Chronic Sick to intervene in the conditions of the home. Later Villa Francis (Mandai Home) home was built to house all these needy elderly when it was opened in 1978. And a group of nuns from the Sisters of Franciscan Missionaries of the Divine Motherhood ran the home. But after 3 decades of running the home, the Sisters passed the responsibility to the Catholic Welfare Services. In terms of market share, the provision of nursing homes from the private sector has stayed relatively stable around 40%

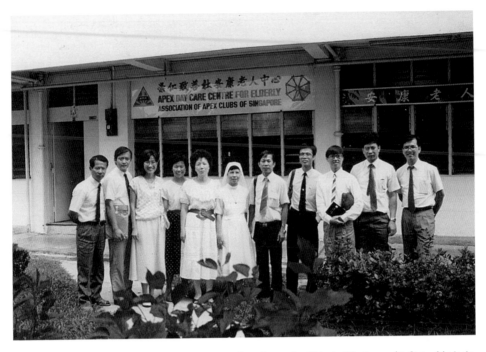

1990s — APEXian Club visitors to the APEX Day Care Centre for Elderly. (Photo credit: Sister Marjorie, Courtesy of APEX Day Rehabilitation Centre for Elderly.)

participation, cooperation and public-spiritedness. They provided assistance to the old and needy and also helped to bring people together and made possible for people to mobilise to achieve their values and satisfy their needs. More importantly, the community benefitted by the cooperation and cohesion of these individuals

---

with the rest from the VWOs. The government also ran large residential homes like the 700-bedded Woodlands Home that has a combination of the poor, destitute, sick and bedridden. However, the conditions were deplorable and eventually, dismantled where the destitute were sent to homes for the destitute and the sick were sent to nursing homes post 1989 (Veloo, KV. (2014) *Life & Times of a Social Worker: A Personal Memoir.* Singapore: SMU Press). Another pivotal point in the history is when Government set up Home Nursing Foundation in 1976. The role of the home nursing services was to serve the elderly who lived in the rural areas. And after 1984, they started to offer day rehab and day care within the polyclinic premises. In line with the government's approach to have charities run LTC services, HNF was devolved from government and restructured as a charity in 2001. A similar history awaited Apex Club and Ang Mo Kio Hospital. In 1980, SCSS also set up the first Day Care Centre for the elderly in Block 119 Bukit Merah to provide help for stroke survivors. It was also later handed over to the Apex Club to run (Apex Day Rehabilitation Centre: 30 years of Caring, 2010) in 1983. Similarly, in 1993, the government set up Ang Mo Kio Hospital (AMKH). This is a community hospital that offers inpatient rehabilitation and geriatric care for patients after their acute episode. Almost a decade later, AMKH was handed over to Thye Hwa Kwan Moral Society. It seems like we have come full circle with government's intention to run nursing homes.

while the individual also gains fellowship and help from the friends within these associations. These organisations may be driven by an idealistic altruism but it is also pragmatic readiness to cooperate with others similarly placed so as to surmount the conditions of a rapidly changing society in our young nation. At the core of these groups was practical reciprocity and collective solidarity in the face of insecurities peculiar to a growing nation.[32]

Pubescence — Growth & Development

After 1965, the planning for ageing services remained relatively small scale and efforts were focused on family planning to reduce our nation's high fertility. After the appointment of a committee to study the problems of the aged in 1982, ageing began to take precedence. The 1984 report[33] of the committee laid the foundation and policy recommendations towards ageing for the next two decades. It crystallised the eventual formulation of the national principles of eldercare — the family must play the primary role in caring for the elderly and placement in an institution can only be justified as a last resort. It emphatically states that the most cost-effective way to provide care can only be through voluntary welfare organisations, and they form an important part of an overall fabric to augment care and support provided by family members, relatives or friends. In 1988, the government commissioned the Advisory Council on the Aged[34] to undertake a comprehensive review of the status of ageing and the recommendations made were largely an extension of the 1984 Report. There was recognition that more community services are required to help the frail aged and their family. Some programmes such as befriender services, home help, home nursing and day care centres were in existent, but there was also a push for geriatrics, comprehensive home health and dementia services. It also elaborated that the government should convert the short term leases of buildings occupied by voluntary welfare organisations to 30-year term leases, provide purpose built facilities and bear the capital and recurrent costs of these VWOs on a cost sharing basis with the VWOs.[35]

---

[32] Wuthnow, R. (2004) *Saving America: Faith-Based Services and the Future of Civil Society*. Princeton, NJ: Princeton Press. Madsen, R. (2007) *Democracy's Dharma: Religious Renaissance and Political Development in Taiwan*. Berkeley, CA: University of California Press.

[33] Singapore. Problems of the Aged. Report of the Committee on the Problems of the Aged. Singapore: Ministry of Health, 1984. 54pp. Howe Yoon Chong, chairman.

[34] Singapore. Community-based Programmes for the Aged. Report of the Committee on Community-based Programmes for the Aged. Advisory Council on the Aged. September 1988.

[35] During this period, the government was very generous and offered much assistance to the VWOs to set up nursing homes. The government would bear 90% of the construction and development costs of the homes and will help with at least 50% of the operational costs of their residents (after means

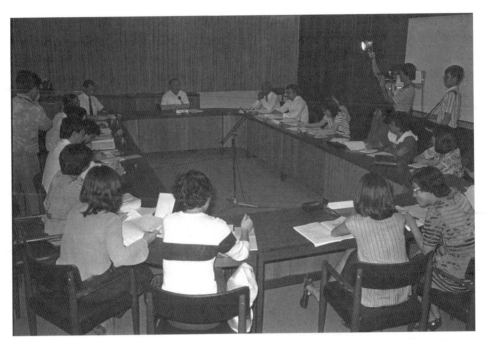

1983 — Minister for Health Mr. Howe Yoon Chong holds press conference on 'Senior Citizens' at Ministry of Health. (Photo credit: Ministry of Information and the Arts Collection, Courtesy of National Archives of Singapore.)

By the late 80s, there were four groups — private, government, temple and charity — of residential homes. In 1985, at the official opening of the Lions Nursing Home for the Elders, Mr. Dhanabalan (then the Minister for Foreign Affairs and Minister for Community Development) made the remark that the Homes for the Aged should limit admission of the ambulant aged because they require minimal medical care and are generally healthy enough to look after themselves. Homes for the Aged Sick should take the non-ambulant and bedridden patients. All the residential homes were subjected to the proverbial sorting hat — some were parked under the Home for Aged Act and the rest were placed under MOH's Private Hospital and Medical Clinics Act (and Specific Guidelines for Nursing Homes) in 1990. Henceforth, we have sheltered homes under Ministry of Community Development

testing). In part as Wong *et al.* (2014) has mentioned, the impetus for such generosity also came about from the demands of an ageing population and the overcrowding of our hospitals — where there is a shortage of facilities for the frail and sick patients. This only changed recently with the Built-Own-Lease model where the government owns the building and VWOs and private providers are invited to bid to be operators of the nursing home.

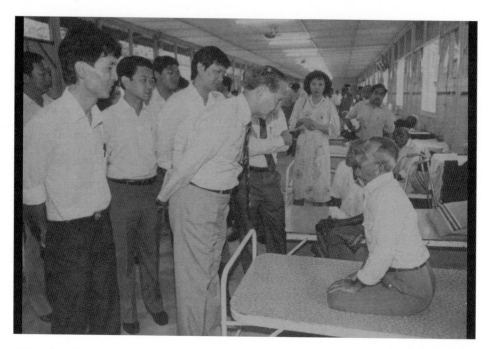

1987 — President Wee Kim Wee talking with a resident at the Woodlands Home for the Aged during his visit to the Home. (Photo credit: Istana Collection, Courtesy of National Archives of Singapore.)

(MCD) and nursing homes under Ministry of Health.[36] Government, in its more pragmatic ways, stepped in to put in place some requirements to safeguard the interests of the residents.[37]

With the government taking a more proactive role in ageing issues, there was a proliferation of community services after 1990s. This was in tandem with the recommendations put forth by the committees that encouraged ageing in place. For centre-based facilities, we had 9 in the 1990s and by the beginning of the new millennium, we had 34 and more than a decade later, we more than tripled in numbers. Likewise with home-based care, we had a meagre 2 and then, 10 in late 1990s and by 2005, we had doubled. Now, we have almost 70 providers. For residential inpatient settings, we grew from 50 in the 1990s to 95 in 2015[38] (please see a list of the current providers[39] in the Appendix).

---

[36] Sitoh, YY. (2003) Nursing Homes in Singapore. A quiet evolution. *Singapore Medical Journal.* **44**(2): 57–59.

[37] Wong, GHZ, Yap, PLK, Pang, WS. (2014). Changing Landscape of Nursing Homes in Singapore: Challenges in the 21st Century. *Annals Academy of Medicine.* **43**(1): 44–50. This is an informative article on the history of nursing homes in Singapore.

[38] These numbers include the voluntary welfare organisations and the commercial sector.

[39] List of current providers drawn from online eldercare resource repository Singapore Silver Pages, correct as at November 2015.

Hence, it was not a surprise that one of the main recommendations in the 1999 Inter-Ministerial Committee on Healthcare for the Elderly (IMHC)[40] was to focus on better coordination and integration of services. It encouraged different organisations — Ministry of Community Development (MCD), Ministry of Health (MOH), People's Association (PA), National Council of Social Services (NCSS) and Housing Development Board (HDB) — to develop multi-service centres where a comprehensive range of eldercare services could be co-located. This could provide the physical convenience for clients who require a range of services and also ensure a more efficient use of resources through the sharing of common facilities. Another similar recommendation was to encourage existing facilities for the elderly to provide certain types of community based services such as day care for dementia and home care services. Following these recommendations, MCD set up the Queenstown Multi-service Centre (QSMSC) in late 1990s. During its initial years, the tenants in QSMSC were Home Nursing Foundation, Dorcas

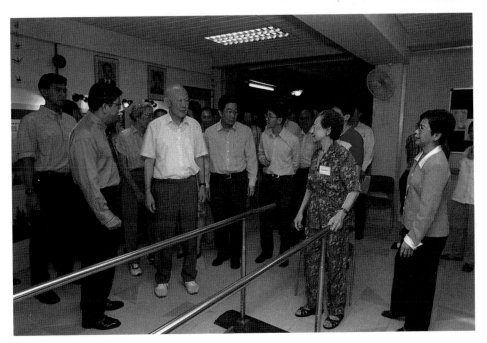

1998 — Senior Minister Lee Kuan Yew touring Queenstown Multi-Service Centre for the Elderly in Block 150A, Mei Chin Road after tree planting ceremony. (Photo credit: Ministry of Information and the Arts Collection, Courtesy of National Archives of Singapore.)

---

[40] Singapore. Inter-Ministerial Committee on Health Care for the Elderly. *Report of the Inter-Ministerial Committee on Health Care for the Elderly.* Singapore: Ministry of Health, 1999. 60pp. Yeo Cheow Tong, chairman.

Home Help Services, Queenstown Social Day Care and a satellite community development council. Meanwhile, MOH put in place the Framework for the Integrated Care for the Elderly that essentially used community hospitals and nursing homes to develop day rehabilitation centres and home care with support from the regional hospital.[41]

Another recommendation encouraged greater participation of private sector groups. While the VWOs are more focused in catering for the needs of destitute senior citizens, the private sector can help those who can afford to pay. The private sector was encouraged to provide eldercare services through the setting up of nursing homes. Within the next decade, six purpose built private nursing homes were set up — United Medicare in Toa Payoh, Orange Valley Homes in Clementi, Simei and Marsiling; and Pacific Nursing Home in Lengkok Bahru and Senja. The intention was to have more players that will create competition and enforce commercial discipline.

Against the backdrop of a national conversation about shared values in the 1990s, these successive policy reviews on issues related to older persons led to the crystallisation of a national policy on ageing in Singapore. The national policy on ageing reinforces the government's position that it does not take sole responsibility for the care of older persons. It advocates self-help and self-reliance of the older person. Family is the first line of care.[42,43] In order for the elderly to remain with their family and community, the residential and community care services via the VWOs support families in their care-giving roles. The community can play supportive and intermediate roles between the family and government. Meanwhile, the government can offer assistance through the funding of programmes and help ILTC providers to acquire land and HDB void decks. It can also regulate service provision and develop manpower capabilities. While the government's approach is clearly individualistic because it holds individuals personally responsible for their old age and expects them to be self-reliant, the flipside of "Many Helping Hands" can be seen as a communitarian approach to eldercare — As Mr. Ong Keng Yong said in his 2010 speech at the Centre for Social Development Conference, "The Many Helping Hands" approach was adopted and self-help activities through community organisations would make up for what the government was less

---

[41] Interestingly, in the latest Build-Own-Lease (BOL) tender for nursing homes, MOH has stipulated that the operator has to run a senior care centre and provide home care through the nursing home premises. The support from the hospitals to the community hospitals and nursing homes is not unlike the current arrangement of how some of the Regional Health Systems (RHS) are supporting the ILTC sector.

[42] Mehta, KK. (2008) A critical review of Singapore's policies aimed at supporting families caring for older members. *Journal of Aging & Social Policy.* **18**(3:4): 43–57.

[43] Mehta, KK, Vasoo, S. (2000) Community programmes and services for long term care of the elderly in Singapore: Challenges for policy makers. *Asian Journal of Political Science.* **8**(1): 125–201.

effective in delivering. The thinking was that caring for the needy and provision of services would best be done by dedicated, passionate people in the community and in non-government organisations rather than by civil servants.... government would provide the necessary support to make "many helping hands" work.[44–46]

Adolescence — Growing Pains

Since the adoption of the 1991 White Paper[47] on "Shared Values" where "Many Helping Hands" approach was first put into public awareness, the long-term care sector has grown; delicately balancing policy, funding, standards and frameworks. Over the last decade, the industry had to endure some growing pains.

Scandal and Standards

The legislation of residential homes in Singapore started in 1950s, when the City council passed the Nursing Homes and Maternity Homes Registration Ordinance, 1959.[48] In 1970, the newspaper carried a report on the *forgotten* old folks at Dragon Lotus Hill in Woodlands living in very poor conditions,[49] which prompted large-scale donations. The home was eventually closed down and residents moved to Woodlands Home for the Aged. In 1972, the abysmal conditions of living at Woodlands Home for the Aged were brought up in Parliament by Member of Parliament Mr. P. Govindaswamy,[50] *"the living conditions are bad. The old people are served with poorly cooked food. There are a lot of bugs in the beds."* Even then, the homes had minimal legislative purview. It was only after the 1989 Homes for the Aged Act and the Private Health Medical Clinic Act enacted in Parliament that mandated licensing matters in the Homes for the Aged and Nursing Homes. There were some improvements then, but standards were not elucidated explicitly.[51]

---

[44] Ong, KY. (2010) Singapore social policies: Vision, accomplishments and challenges. Speech at The Centre for Social Development (Asia) Conference. Shaw Foundation Alumni House, NUS.

[45] Rozario, PA, Rosetti, AL. (2012) "Many Helping Hands": A review and analysis of long term care policies, programs, and practices in Singapore. *Journal of Gerontological Social Work.* **55**(7): 641–658.

[46] Haskins, R. (2011) *Social Policy in Singapore: A Crucible of Individual Responsibility.* Ethos. Downloaded from the www.brookings.edu.

[47] Shared Values. (1991) Singapore. Singapore National Printers.

[48] A paradigm shift in regulating and running nursing homes in Singapore. *Journal of the American Medical Directors Association* **15** (2014): 440–444.

[49] "The forgotten ones...." *The Straits Times,* 22 March 1970, p. 7.

[50] *Singapore Parliamentary Reports, Budget Social Welfare,* 21 March 1972, Vol. 31 at col 951 (Mr. Perumal Govindaswamy, Member of Parliament for Anson).

[51] A paradigm shift in regulating and running nursing homes in Singapore. *Journal of the American Medical Directors Association* **15** (2014): 440–444.

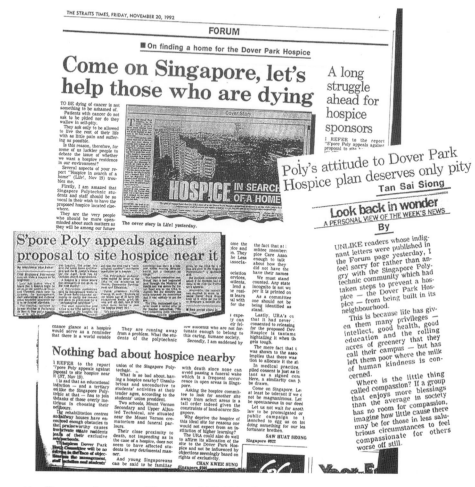

Headlines conglomerate of first case of NIMBY in Singapore — Dover Park Hospice site issues.

In June 2011, footage of Nightingale Nursing Home's staff mistreating a female resident was shown on local news bulletins and the incident immediately went viral prompting active and vivid discussions.[52] MOH released a statement divulging ongoing investigations on said Home and admitted to significant lapses of care standards and agreed that tight staff supervision should be in place when care was rendered to vulnerable patients. The Nursing Home was subsequently heavily fined for failing to render approved level of care.

The incident prompted the set-up of an industry-driven committee in 2012,[53] comprising nursing home operators and healthcare professionals to review the existing licensing standards and identify areas that can be enhanced. The committee then

---

[52] Tham Yuen-C. "Shocking scenes at nursing home." The Straits Times, 10 June 2011.

[53] Elizabeth Soh. "Industry weighs in on nursing home review." *The Straits Times*, 13 June 2011.

drafted an enhanced set of standards for the nursing home sector, due for introduction by 2015.[54] And soon to follow are standards for home and centre-based care.[55]

"Not-in-my-backyard" Syndrome — Negotiating Space Utilisation within the Finite

"I have held forth on the adversities — economic, social and emotional — that may befall many old people in modern societies where weakening family bonds and adulation of youth have made old age and therefore the aged outcasts of society — a category of untouchable to whom the young owe no obligation and who should be handed over to the tender mercies of the state to be looked until their death relieves us of this unnecessary obligation."[56]

"Not-in-my-backyard" or NIMBY was defined by Oxford Dictionary as one who objects to the siting of something perceived as unpleasant or hazardous in their own neighbourhood, especially while raising no such objections to similar developments elsewhere originated in the 1980s and gained traction in Singapore in the last decade due to several public incidents of siting of elderly facilities. Even before its popularisation in the recent decade, NIMBY was first invoked locally in 1992 when the management, staff association and student union of Singapore Polytechnic separately wrote to the authorities questioning the siting of Dover Park Hospice adjacent to the campus grounds.[57-59] The hospice eventually settled in its current site next to Tan Tock Seng Hospital in Novena, but public discourses of the days were generally negative.[60]

Fast-forward to 2011, where a relocation plan for Ren Ci Nursing Home to Bukit Batok was met with negative reactions from residents affected and displeased that their recreational space was removed.[61] NIMBY was brought up by the Prime Minister a month later in the Debate on President's Address and the spirit of compromise was invoked, where he stressed that the maturing democracy in Singapore required such

---

[54] *Singapore Parliamentary Reports, Head O — Ministry of Health,* 12 March 2013, Vol. 90 (Dr. Amy Khor Lean Suan, Minister of State for Health).

[55] Ibid.

[56] A speech by Mr. S. Rajaratnam, 2nd DPM (Foreign Affairs) at the 3rd Senior Citizen's week at the Victoria Theatre on November 15, 1981, at 2.30 pm.

[57] "Hospice in search of a home." *The Straits Times,* 19 November 1992, p. 2.

[58] Saw Huat Seong. "Come on Singapore, let's help those who are dying." *The Straits Times,* 20 November 1992, p. 37.

[59] Tan Sai Siong. "Poly's attitude to Dover Park Hospice plan deserves only pity." *The Straits Times,* 21 November 1992, p. 37.

[60] Ibid.

[61] Poon Chian Hui and Melissa Pang. "Ren Ci's move to Bukit Batok: Issues raised." *The Straits Times,* 21 September 2011, p. B2.

spirit for building of an inclusive society.[62] Subsequent in the next 24 months, NIMBY was significant on national news report from studio apartments in Toh Yi estate,[63] day care centres for elderly in Woodlands by Sree Narayana Mission[64,65] and at St. Hilda's Link in Kampong Arang. This was soon followed by the construction of Lions Home for the Elders in Bishan. In all of these cases, the original plan was delayed but not shelved. The government will build recreational and estate enhancements after the residents' feedback.[66,67] This information sharing was enhanced with grassroots organisations communicating plans and rationale to affected residents. This was a departure from the 'no comments' approach seen earlier in 1992 on Dover Park Hospice. In addition, NIMBY prompted a comment by Dr. Amy Khor in Parliament in 2012[68] that "… while the Government can plan to build the infrastructure, there needs to be a paradigm shift in the mindsets of people such that we are all attuned and aligned to the problems ahead… ." The agreement that "… a common under-stand(ing) of what we as a people face is …. meet the needs of the elderly, or for the common good of the population…" coincided with MP Ellen Lee's comment that "the needs of a greater majority have to be considered."[69] It is inevitable that the country has to realise that with an increasing ageing population, the network of facilities must surely then to be within reach in the community.[70]

Still Growing

The Community and Residential Care sector is in a process of renewal and evolution. As we bear witness to the passing of the founders and the ageing of our pioneers, we see the transition of the baton of leadership. And during this period of change, the government is injecting resources into this sector to catch up with the rapidly ageing population. In retrospect, we may have over-emphasised the importance

---

[62] *Singapore Parliamentary Reports, Debate on Presidents Address,* 20 October 2011, Vol. 88 p. 381 (Mr. Lee Hsien Loong, The Prime Minister).

[63] Janice Tai. "HDB stands firm on for elderly in Toh Yi." *The Straits Times,* 6 March 2012.

[64] Ibid.

[65] Tay Suan Cheang and Janice Tai. "Seniors' centre at void deck? No problem." *The Straits Times,* 4 February 2012.

[66] *Singapore Parliamentary Reports, Head T — Ministry of National Development,* 2 March 2012, Vol. 88 (Mr. Khaw Boon Wan, The Minister for National Development).

[67] Janice Tai. "HDB stands firm on for elderly in Toh Yi", *The Straits Times,* 6 March 2012.

[68] *Singapore Parliamentary Reports, Head O — Ministry of Health,* 12 March 2013, Vol. 90 (Dr. Amy Khor Lean Suan, Minister of State for Health).

[69] "Residents accept compromise plan." *The Straits Times,* 27 August 2012.

[70] Ang Chin Guan (letters). "An image makeover can change perception of nursing homes — From Nimby to Gimby …." *The Straits Times,* 1 October 2012.

of family values and self-help and under-estimated the need for supportive social structures in the community. While we should continue to emphasise on filial piety and family values, the evolving family structures, changing social climate and volatile economic situation requires a rethink in how we plan our system. The government is expanding the number of nursing home and bed numbers — 10 new nursing homes — and increasing to 10,000 home care spaces and 6000 day care spaces by 2016. There are massive infra-redevelopments to cater for the disabled, inventing new housing typologies and closing the persistent social-health chasm. Yet the sector is mired with challenges from recruitment of manpower and talent, getting the right balance of private and charity players and building fast enough to catch up with the ageing population. As government devotes more funds, they will demand that the monies be used in ways that are accountable to the public. It necessarily requires the application of standards of quality, efficiency and effectiveness. As expectations of standards rise and demands for greater professional and procedural norms are necessitated by government support, the sector will need to professionalise and apply levels of bureaucratic structure into their organisations. Yet this should not flatten the distinctiveness of this sector. The services run by VWOs are important as anchors for many of our relationships that tie civil society together. They are more enduring than many of ephemeral political projects that develop in local communities. They hold more possibilities for being there for the older person when illness or bereavement strikes. A cautionary note as government decides to run community hospitals and nursing homes, it bears reminding that the importance of faith and spirit of VWOs not be lost in these sites of slow medicine — nurturing, life affirming and healing.

Appendix

List of Current ILTC Providers — Home Care

1. 247 Home Nursing Services Pte Ltd
2. Abella Agency
3. Adventist Nursing & Rehabilitation Centre
4. Agape Methodist Hospice
5. Aged Psychiatry Community Assessment & Treatment Services
6. AgeWell Artsz
7. Allcare Nursing Services
8. Ang Mo Kio — Thye Hua Kwan Hospital
9. Angel Home Care

10. Assisi Hospice
11. Assist Care
12. Bethesda Care & Counselling Services Centre
13. Care for Elderly Foundation
14. Care Visions Singapore Pte Ltd
15. Caregiving Welfare Association
16. Cecilia Healthcare & Nursing Services
17. CODE 4 Home Care [A programme by the Care For The Elderly Foundation (Singapore)]
18. Comfort Keepers- Bedok
19. Comfort Keepers- Bukit Merah
20. Comfort Keepers -Toa Payoh Bishan
21. Community Rehabilitation and Support Services (Bukit Batok)
22. Community Rehabilitation and Support Services (Pasir Ris)
23. Community Rehabilitation and Support Services (Yishun)
24. Dorcas Home Care Services
25. Dover Park Hospice
26. eBeeCare
27. Econ Healthcare Group
28. ECON Homecare Services
29. Eden Rehabilitation Centre Pte Ltd
30. Ezyhealth Care @ Home Pte. Ltd.
31. Good Shepherd Loft
32. Handicaps Welfare Association (Whampoa)
33. HCA Hospice Care
34. Help-Serve (Homecare & Services)
35. Home Nursing Foundation
36. Hospice Home Care
37. KK Health Service Agent
38. Kwong Wai Shiu Hospital
39. Lotus Eldercare Pte Ltd
40. Loving Heart Multi Service Centre
41. Metta Hospice Care
42. MW Medical Pte Ltd
43. Nicole Consultancy Pte Ltd
44. NTUC Health Care@home
45. OmniMed Healthcare Holdings
46. One Care Zone
47. Onsite & Workplace Physio Pte Ltd

48. Pacific Rehabilitation
49. PhysioWay Pte Ltd
50. Physioworks Physiotherapy & Rehabilitation
51. Preciouz Kare Pte Ltd
52. QA Healthcare Pte Ltd
53. SATA CommHealth (Home Nursing)
54. SG Rehab
55. Singapore Cancer Society
56. SPD@Toa Payoh
57. St. Andrew's Community Hospital
58. St. Andrew's Nursing Home
59. St. Luke's Hospital
60. St. Hilda's Integrated Day Facility (SACH Home Care — Kg Arang)
61. Sunlove Home
62. Sunlove Rehab Centre
63. Sunshine Welfare Action Mission (SWAMI)
64. Tan Tock Seng Hospital Pte Ltd (Community Rehabilitation Program)
65. Tembusu Home Help Service
66. Tetsuyu Home Care Pte Ltd
67. THE LENTOR RESIDENCE
68. THK Home Help Service (East)
69. THK Home Help Service (West)
70. THK Seniors Activity Centre @ Ang Mo Kio 257
71. THK Wellness Hub
72. Thong Teck Home For Senior Citizens
73. Thye Hua Kwan Moral Charities Ltd
74. TOUCH Caregivers Support (TOUCH Community Services Limited)
75. TOUCH Home Care — AMK
76. TOUCH Home Care — Jurong
77. TOUCH Home Care — Toa Payoh
78. Tsao Foundation — Hua Mei Mobile Clinic
79. Tzu Chi Foundation
80. Yong-En Care Centre

List of Current ILTC Providers — Stay-In Facilities

1. St. Luke's Hospital
2. Ang Mo Kio — Thye Hua Kwan Hospital
3. Bright Vision Hospital

4. Ren Ci Hospital
5. St Andrew's Community Hospital
6. St Andrew's Mission Hospital
7. Assisi Hospice
8. Dover Park Hospice
9. St. Joseph's Home
10. Gleneagles Hospital
11. Mount Alvernia Hospital
12. Mount Elizabeth Hospital
13. Parkway East Hospital
14. Raffles Hospital
15. Thomson Medical Centre
16. West Point Hospital
17. Econ Medicare Centre (Braddell Road)
18. Econ Medicare Centre (Chai Chee)
19. Econ Medicare Centre (Choa Chu Kang)
20. Econ Medicare Centre (Recreation Road)
21. Econ Medicare Centre (Upper East Coast Road)
22. Econ Medicare Centre (Yio Chu Kang)
23. Econ Nursing Home (Buangkok)
24. Econ Nursing Home (SunnyVille)
25. Good Shepherd Loft
26. Green Avenue Pte Ltd
27. Greenview Nursing Home
28. Irene Nursing Home
29. LC Nursing Home
30. Lee Ah Mooi Old Age Home
31. Min Chong Comfort Home
32. Moonlight Home For The Aged & Handicapped
33. Nightingale Nursing Centre (Braddell Road)
34. Orange Valley Nursing Home (Bukit Merah)
35. Orange Valley Nursing Home (Changi)
36. Orange Valley Nursing Home (Clementi)
37. Orange Valley Nursing Home (Marsiling)
38. Orange Valley Nursing Home (Simei)
39. Our Lady Of Lourdes Nursing Home Pte Ltd
40. Pacific Healthcare Nursing Home Pte Ltd
41. Paean Nursing Home
42. Serene Nursing Home

43. Soo's Nursing Home
44. THE LENTOR RESIDENCE
45. United Medicare (Elizabeth Dr) Pte Ltd
46. United Medicare Pte Ltd
47. Windsor Convalescent Home
48. Sunlove Home
49. Tai Pei Social Service
50. Community Rehab Support Services (Singapore Anglican Community Services)
51. Singapore Association for Mental Health-Bukit Gombak Group Home
52. Econ Medicare Centre & Nursing Home
53. Ren Ci @Bukit Batok Street 52 (Nursing Home)
54. Tetsuyu Home Care Pte Ltd
55. Abdullah Shooker Jewish Welfare Home
56. Adventist Home For The Elders
57. AWWA Community Home for Senior Citizens
58. Bo Tien Home for the Aged
59. Evergreen Place — Home @ Hong San
60. Geylang East Home For The Aged
61. Henderson Senior Citizens' Home
62. Kheng Chiu Loke Tin Kee Home For The Aged
63. PERTAPIS Senior Citizens Fellowship Home
64. SBWS Happy Villa (Females)
65. SILRA Home
66. Singapore Baptist Convention Golden Age Home
67. St. Andrew's Cathedral Home For The Aged
68. St. John's Home for Elderly Persons
69. Zion Home For The Aged
70. ALL SAINTS HOME
71. All Saints Home — Tampines
72. Apex Harmony Lodge
73. Bethany Methodist Nursing Home
74. Bright Hill Evergreen Home
75. Grace Lodge
76. Jamiyah Nursing Home
77. JU ENG HOME FOR SENIOR CITIZENS
78. Kwong Wai Shiu Hospital
79. Ling Kwang Home for Senior Citizens
80. Lions Home for the Elders (Bedok)
81. Lions Home for the Elders (Toa Payoh)

82. Man Fut Tong Nursing Home
83. Moral Home For The Aged Sick
84. Ren Ci Nursing Home (Moulmein)
85. Singapore Christian Home
86. Society For The Aged Sick
87. Sree Narayana Mission (Singapore)
88. St Andrew's Nursing Home
89. St Theresa's Home
90. Sunshine Welfare Action Mission (SWAMI)
91. Tai Pei Old People's Home
92. The Salvation Army, Peacehaven Nursing Home
93. Thian Leng Old Folks' Home
94. Thong Teck Home For Senior Citizens
95. Villa Francis Home for the Aged

List of Current ILTC Providers — Day Care

1. Bo Tien Day Activity Centre for the Elderly
2. Care Corner Social Day Care for the Elderly
3. Caregiving Welfare Association
4. Econ Medicare Centre (Braddell Road)
5. Econ Medicare Centre (Chai Chee)
6. Econ Medicare Centre (Choa Chu Kang)
7. Econ Medicare Centre (Upper East Coast Road)
8. Econ Nursing Home (Buangkok)
9. Geylang East Day Activity Centre for Elderly
10. Goldencare Group Pte Ltd
11. Good Shepherd Loft
12. Jamiyah Senior Care Centre
13. Man Fut Tong Nursing Home
14. Marine Parade — Aspiration for Elderly Lodge
15. Marine Parade — Foo Hai Elderly Lodge
16. May Wong Social Day Care Centre for the Elderly
17. North East — Kampung Senang Activity Centre
18. Orange Valley Nursing Home (Bukit Merah)
19. Orange Valley Nursing Home (Clementi)
20. Orange Valley Nursing Home (Simei)
21. Our Lady Of Lourdes Nursing Home Pte Ltd
22. PCF Tampines East 3-in-1 Family Centre (Aged Care)

23. Queenstown Multi Service Centre
24. SASCO Hong Kah North Day Care Centre
25. SPD@Toa Payoh
26. St. Andrew's Senior Care Joy Connect
27. St. Luke's Eldercare (Ayer Rajah Centre)
28. St. Luke's Eldercare (Bukit Timah Centre)
29. St. Luke's Eldercare (Changkat Centre)
30. St. Luke's Eldercare (Clementi Centre)
31. St. Luke's Eldercare (Golden Years Centre)
32. St. Luke's Eldercare (Hougang Centre)
33. St. Luke's Eldercare (Jurong East Centre)
34. St. Luke's Eldercare (Serangoon Centre)
35. St. Luke's Eldercare (Tampines Centre)
36. St. Luke's Eldercare (Telok Blangah Centre)
37. St. Luke's Eldercare (Whampoa Centre)
38. St. Luke's Eldercare (Yishun Centre)
39. The CARE Library Private Limited
40. The Salvation Army — Peacehaven Bedok Multi-Service Centre
41. Wan Min Community Services
42. All Saints Home — Tampines
43. Apex Harmony Lodge
44. AWWA Dementia Day Care Centre
45. AWWA Family Service Centre
46. Montessori For Dementia Care
47. New Horizon Centre (Bukit Batok)
48. New Horizon Centre (Jurong Point)
49. New Horizon Centre (Tampines)
50. New Horizon Centre (Toa Payoh)
51. SASCO Day Activity Centre (Telok Blangah Rise)
52. SASCO Intergrated Eldercare Centre
53. Sree Narayana Mission Home — EEP (Woodlands)
54. St. Hilda's Community Services
55. Sunlove Home
56. Sunshine Welfare Action Mission (SWAMI)
57. Thong Teck Home For Senior Citizens
58. Yong-En Care Centre
59. Assisi Hospice
60. HCA Hospice Care
61. Community Rehab Support Services (Singapore Anglican Community Services)

62. Community Rehabilitation and Support Services (Bukit Batok)
63. Community Rehabilitation and Support Services (Pasir Ris)
64. Community Rehabilitation and Support Services (Yishun)
65. Institute Of Mental Health Day Centre — OcTAVE
66. Singapore Association for Mental Health-Oasis Day Centre
67. Ren Ci @Bukit Batok Street 52 (Nursing Home)

13 Our IT Journey: One Patient-One Record

Low Cheng Ooi* and Peter Tan†

The Evolution of Health IT

Singapore has been on the forefront of health IT implementation as a nation-state. It is a remarkable achievement, considering our small size and heavy patient load. This is especially remarkable since our public sector leads in IT implementation, across the spectrum from institutional systems to national systems.

The Early Years

The earliest record of a health IT system was from the Singapore General Hospital's Department of Pathology. In 1973, the Biochemistry Section was the first to get a mini-computer to handle the processing and management of the specimens for the lab. The system was Data General Nova with 16KB memory and two removable 5MB hard disk drives, including a paper tape reader, video terminals, and 180 cps printers. Even then, the system had an interface to instrument analysers. The user interface comprises the use of a stand-alone Teletype which punched paper tape in ASCII code, which were read by the paper tape reader into the computer, and paper reports as output. Fast forward 40 years, where we have home care teams accessing care records using touch tablets with 4G wireless connectivity — it is indeed a marvel at how far health IT has evolved!

However, true institution-wide IT implementations only started in the early 1980s, with the formation of the National Computer Board (NCB). The Civil Service Computerisation Programme (1980–1999) initially started with a focus on improving public administration through the effective use of IT. This involved automating

*Cheif Medical Information Officer, Ministry of Health, Singapore.
†Principal Architect, Integrated Health Information Systems, Singapore.

work functions and reducing paperwork for greater internal operational efficiencies. As the public hospitals were then-departments of MOH, computerisation was initiated under the programme, with the implementation of the Patient Care System (PCS). This was a mainframe system, initially deployed to registration clerks only, using TN3270 "dumb" terminals with their signature green text-only screens by 1983.

Subsequently, computer centres were set up to serve all five hospitals. Unlike today, computers meant mainframes, which were big and expensive to acquire and operate, hence this was probably the most cost-effective arrangement. The computer centre had data links to all five hospital sites, an achievement that is easy to trivialise in these days of ubiquitous connectivity. Implementation was contracted out in 1983, and it went live in 1985; and the computer centre in SGH campus is still operating today! The systems implemented were the Patient Master Index (PMI) and the Patient Billing System (PBS). Implementation started in AH first before progressing to the rest of the clusters, causing the pioneering team to face many challenges. Both the IT teams and users were new to the implementation of a computer system, and much time was spent on requirements study. The team studied the current workflows and diligently drew up many data flow diagrams. Given the technical constraints of early IT systems, even deciding which parts of the workflow should be computerised required careful consideration. The team was also bogged down with discussions into too many details such as screen design, a phenomenon that even Health IT teams today can empathise with. The project team was augmented by experienced implementers from overseas brought in by IBM. Even after such extensive preparation, in the initial days, the queue went from the registration counter to the road!

Restructuring and Administrative Systems

With the restructuring of the public hospitals in the late 1980s, the development of IT systems began to diverge. SGH formed its own IT department and one of her first projects was to modify the PCS into the Patient Management Patient Administration (PMPA) system to suit local requirements. One of the challenges it addresses was that we had different accounting practices, so there was a need to implement a proper system for everyone to follow. It was a challenge to change the hospital staff from their different ways of working, and the system had to be implemented five times for each of the different hospitals, with assistance from the SGH team. Each time, the team had to adapt the system to the different needs of each hospital. Despite the organisational challenges, the IT team tried their best to keep the codebase consistent across the PHIs, as the IT teams would come together to jointly develop and test code enhancements, before bringing back to their respective institutions for deployment. The cost sharing through transfer pricing became complicated to administer. Another key challenge was the incorporation of the requirements of Medisave when it was introduced in 1984. It would not be a stretch to say that the PMPA was a key enabler of Medisave implementation, as manual processing of claims could have been too impractical.

For outpatient patient administration, the SWI Paramedics system was implemented in TTSH, TPH, SGH, and KKH in 1990. It had much simpler outpatient registration and billing functionalities, but had by this time already included medication display, inventory, and purchase order functions.

In the late 1990s, driven by concern over the "Y2K bug," the public institutions all made plans to replace their existing computer systems. They independently came to the same conclusion to migrate out of mainframes to open systems. Through independent procurement processes, they all selected SAP, which was a mutual validation that the choice was a good one. Interestingly, no one broached the idea of sharing the new system, in spite of the common product selected. With hindsight, it would have been an opportunity to unify the administrative IT selected systems.

The public institutions were clustered into Singhealth and NHG in early 2000s, and the IT organisations had to be similarly reorganised, though with different philosophies. In Singhealth, a new Singhealth Infotech department was formed with responsibility for cluster-wide common systems and overall planning and governance, whilst leaving institutional IT teams intact to run operations and support unique institutional systems. On the other hand, NHG decided to centralise the IT staff into a single IT Division, resulting in a major human resource change management exercise lasting an entire year. These two different philosophies had an important bearing on the subsequent IT implementation journeys of the clusters. For instance, NHG embarked on the Naut1cus project, which successfully rationalised all the SAP implementations across her institutions into a single shared instance. This required painful harmonisation of processes, workflows, and data, which would not have been possible without strong resolve by the leadership. In contrast, the Outpatient Administration System (OAS) was implemented by Singhealth, which replaces SAP for specialist clinics and polyclinics, and allows for institutional variants whilst maintaining core commonalities, such as a single cluster patient master.

Clinical Systems

The evolution of clinical IT systems is a much longer, more varied one, which is natural since clinical practice is one of the most knowledge intensive professions, where each patient is different; and it is extremely challenging to codify and translate clinical workflows into instructions that can be executed by an essentially "dumb" computer. Typically, the journey starts with ancillary and specialty systems, as the problem space was sufficiently constrained to be "solvable" by current technology then.

For instance, in 1983, the SGH Department of Pathology upgraded the Nova computer to an Eclipse computer with application software from a US company, Meditech. The Meditech software was MUMPS based MIIS system, with 32MB of memory, and 2 × 300MB of disk capacity. We also progressed from the paper tape from the ten-year-old system to one where data entry was direct via a number of video terminals.

In 1991, there was a major upgrade and the computerisation was extended to the other sections like Haematology, Microbiology, and Histo Pathology. The technology has changed quite a fair bit over the years and this time, the server was 64MB Data General MV/8500 Eclipse computer with 8GB of disk storage space. Backup was on helical tape which was able to accommodate up to 14GB. Approximately, 100 video terminals were connected to the server via Ethernet at 10Mb/sec. Barcode printers were introduced to print labels that could be read by the instruments. The interface to the instruments were now bi-directional. The application software was upgraded to $T version which supported networking features. Apart from the operational labs, the system was also extended to cover pathology billing. This was also the beginning of integration of administrative and clinical systems, with interfaces to SAP for Admit/Discharge/Transfer (ADT) and Billing messages using the HL7 standard. The messages were transmitted through the Cloverleaf interface engine, which remains as the "heart" of health IT systems today.

The computerisation and digitalisation of imaging systems was another important development with huge productivity gains, as physical film is both cumbersome and expensive. This IT journey started in 1997 when the SGH campus implemented the first Radiology Information System (RIS) by Cerner, followed by a mini Picture Archival and Communications (PACS) by Siemens the next year. In 1998, NUH and NNI started their imaging journey with PACS by GE. In 2000, NCC implemented her PACS from Kodak and became the first centre to go filmless. By 2004, SGH campus went mostly filmless, including the operating theatres by 2005. Similarly in 2005, NHG Diagnostics implemented Kodak RISPACS solution and the NHG institutions progressively went filmless in subsequent years. This served as an important foundation for the implementation of off-shore Teleradiology services. Similarly, the hospitals in Singhealth recognised the need to share images within the cluster, which was implemented in 2007. That was also the year when Singhealth started experimenting with Teleradiology. By 2010, Singhealth consolidated the disparate RIS/PACS system into a new solution by Microsoft.

In 1993, TTSH embarked on the first Electronic Medical Record (EMR) project, to develop one specific for the Eye Clinic. The Eye Clinic was selected for two reasons, one of which was the assessment that the documentation requirements of the specialty would be constrained enough for software design to work and for development to be achievable. More importantly, the leadership of the clinic was open to participate in the trial, which was definitely a key factor for success. Thus a small team of five embarked on the project. The system incorporated many cutting edge design and technology elements for its day. Of note is its use of Pen for Windows, and the design objective to minimise the need for keyboard entry. Though the use of a point-and-click interface, the system allowed the doctor to capture notes of consultation visually, automatically translating into textual clinical notes. This was a remarkable achievement, considering this was 17 years before the launch of the iPad! In addition, the team also implemented a kiosk system for self-registration, experimenting with various plastic and metal kiosk designs.

A lot of lessons were learned through the project. Doctors were reluctant to abandon pen and paper to switch to documentation with IT system. This was partly due to a lack of IT literacy and acceptance at the time. It took time for users to learn how to use a mouse, and to also get over the concern that they could seriously damage the machine if a wrong instruction was issued, as desktop computers were expensive pieces of equipment costing thousands of dollars each. Additionally, the technology then was not as usable and reliable as today. Although the self-registration kiosks were intended to speed up registrations, they ended up taking longer than the manual counters, partly due to overloaded servers, compounded by the fact that patients at eye clinics often lack the visual acuity to see the instructions on the screen! It did not help that the TTSH campus server was situated on a hill and that power surges from lightning strikes led to frequent system failure. In spite of placing full-time staff beside the clinicians during rollout (a practice that is still done today for major IT changes), adoption could not quite take off. Hence the project was terminated in 1997. However, nothing was wasted. The servers and some of the software were repurposed. More importantly, the experience was invaluable in guiding future implementations. NUH similarly piloted a Procare system, which was eventually terminated due to poor usage.

The first forays into specialty systems started in the Accident and Emergency (A&E) departments in the mid-1990s. Perhaps a reflection of the fact that each hospital was structured as a separate company under HCS, each had implemented their own different A&E IT system. A&E are unique in the sense that they have to operate 7 × 24, have well-defined triage workflows, and are almost a mini-hospital after hours, with their own registration, bed management, and pharmacy requirements. Even after merging into dual clusters and till today, A&E systems are still different across the hospitals, though better integrated with other hospital IT systems.

We pick up the EMR trail again in the mid-1990s. SGH implemented the Carevision system in 1995, which was subsequently acquired by Eclipsys in 1999, and morphed into the Sunrise Clinical Manager. Due to later changes in company strategy, the software was licensed to iSoft from the UK, and was rebranded iSoft Clinical Manager (ICM), which became the cluster-wide EMR system in Singhealth.

On the "west" side, TTSH continued to implement various systems, such as the Electronic Discharge Summary System (EDSS), OT System, and a rudimentary form of ENT on the Lotus Notes platform. Once again, there were challenges faced with the technology, as Notes was a generic knowledge management platform. Around 1995, NUH embarked on the development of their first EMR system, which was the Electronic Prescription System (EPS). This later evolved to the Computerised Patient Support System (CPSS), which became NHG's cluster-wide EMR system.

Around 2004, both clusters initiated plans to make the next leap in EMR implementation: Computerised Clinician Order Entry (CCOE). Singhealth began planning to upgrade iCM to iSoft's next generation product Lorenzo. Meanwhile, NHG selected another commercial-of-the-shelf product after an RFP process. Unfortunately, it seemed that the Health IT industry had simultaneously hit a technical inflection point during this period, where most vendors were attempting to migrate from aging software foundations to more modern software development frameworks. Both vendors met with major technical challenges in their UK and US implementations respectively, and both clusters wisely took the painful decision to abandon their plans, and our health IT journey was stymied for about three years.

Both clusters took alternative paths around this "disaster" in the late 2000s. Fortunately for NHG, they were in the midst of building another IT system as a back-up for use during down-time of the planned new system. NHG quickly ramped up development of this system, codenamed Aurora, and incrementally developed their CCOE capability. This system has been incrementally enhanced over the years to become the CPSS2 system, which is the shared common EMR system across NHG and NUHS.

Singhealth elected to conduct an open procurement process in 2007. In the end, it chose it's previous vendor Eclipsys, albeit to an upgraded version of their SCM product. Similarly, this has now evolved into the shared common EMR across Singhealth and EHA. Subsequently, when KTPH was formed, the same EMR product was rapidly implemented there as well.

The CCOE journey has been a more challenging one. It was no longer just about providing clinicians with information at their finger tips; rather, it now actually required clinicians to move away from using pen and paper to issuing of orders via keyboard and mouse. The implementation journey in both clusters was a story of determined clinical leadership in the midst of pushback, coupled with hard work by IT teams on the ground, winning over users one site at a time. From draconian measures such as physically removing prescription pads to more subtle measures such as positioning the monitor to so as not to block clinician-patient interaction, the change management process was continually refined. However, the value in improved patient safety was realised, just from improved data quality alone; and more importantly, through safety checks and other clinical decision support. In addition, this was an important foundation for collecting clinical data, which previously could only be inferred from patient financial data.

Ministry and Stat Board Systems

While the institutions progressed along their IT journeys, the Ministry itself has also been exploiting IT in its own way. Up to the late 1990s, IT in AH, Woodbridge Hospital, and the polyclinics were still managed by the IT Branch in Ministry, and the implementation of SAP in the two hospitals during Y2K was executed by ITB.

One key system in the Ministry is the Central Claims Processing System (CCPS), which started in the early 1990s as a mainframe system developed by Singapore Network Services (SNS) to process Medisave claims. The infrastructure it resides on was also known as MediNet, part of a series of industry-specific Electronic Data Interchange (EDI) "Nets" following the success of TradeNet. In 2002, MOH migrated CCPS out to CCPS2, hosted in a Unix server and Medinet data centre owned by the government. In 2005, CCPS2 was migrated to Mediclaims running on Microsoft server and database platform, with Biztalk as the new integration service bus. Part of the impetus for the migration was to use a more modern software architecture that would be more inexpensive to operate, and more importantly, to change as the Ministry continued to innovate and fine-tune her Healthcare financing policies. The system has since proven relatively resilient, and has been extended to handle major policy changes over the years, such as the Private Medical Insurance integrated Medishield plans, Chronic Disease Management Programme (CDMP), and more recently the Community Health Assistance Scheme (CHAS). With each enhancement, the network grew, reaching the five private insurers and more than 1000 Medishield accredited institutions. Two other systems work in concert to effect the Ministry's health financing operations. The Casemix & Subvention (C&S) system receives submission based Disease-related Groups (DRG) for non-block piece-rate subvention. The Means Testing System (MTS) was also implemented in late 2000s, so that hospitals would have a means of consistently applying means-testing for patients.

The Ministry also started implementing clinical systems, such as the Perkin Almer system for pathology in the Dept of Scientific Services, and the National Immunisation Registry (NIR) for HPB in 1999, and subsequently, the National Disease Registry. In the late 1990s, the Ministry also implemented the School-based Health and Immunisation Programme (SHIP) System. In early 2000, the Student Health Assessment Programme (SHAPE) was developed by Ecquaria, which had a component to support the roving teams that performed health screening in schools. This was before the era of cheap wireless connectivity, so the system was designed so that each team of doctors and nurses would be trained to deploy notebooks and a simple local area network to capture student health screening data, returning every Saturday to sync with the mainframe. The IDEAS system was also implemented for the School Dental programme, complete with dental chart function. In fact, the school dental buses were amongst the early users of 3G data.

MOH HQ itself also implemented systems to enable its own operations. One particularly interesting system was to support regulations of Termination of Pregnancy/ Voluntary Sterilisation (TOP/VS) in early 2000s. It included a module deployed on a Personal Digital Assistant (PDA) running Windows CE — pre-cursors of the smartphones, without connectivity — that allowed field officers to tap through checklists and record findings during site inspection, and for reports to be subsequently generated back in office. Also, supporting the e-Government Action Plan, the Ministry launched the Health Professionals Portal, initially including e-transactions such as license renewal and mandatory reporting of infectious diseases (MD131 form).

IT contributed to the fight during the dark episode of SARS. A Contact Tracing System was quickly hacked up, using data feeds from MHA and MOE, which facilitated a literal army of NS men to manually call and update contact information, supporting the issuance of home quarantine orders. Subsequently, several systems were implemented to increase our emergency preparedness in the event of future disease outbreaks.

On the topic of tracking, the Forensic Integrated Operations Network Applications (FIONA) was a particularly interesting IT system implemented for HSA by NCS to support the work of the Forensic Medicine Division. Special clinical mobile notebooks (C5/F5 from Digimobile) were used in the autopsy suite for charting and notes. More interestingly, it had an integrated track and trace capability, using RFID tags on body parts to ensure that all movement is properly tracked and parts accounted for from receipt till claim or disposal. Some of the IT implementors tell stories of strange inexplicable occurrences during implementation. Were they truly phantasmic in nature, or simply the result of imagination triggered by the macabre setting, no one will ever know.

National Clinical IT Initiatives

National Clinical IT is the holy grail of many healthcare jurisdictions around the world and honestly speaking, Singapore can be considered a pioneer of this field. As early as 1991, an IT Sectoral Study Group for the Healthcare Sector already published a report on the subject, though actual implementation progress would happen in spurts over the decades.

In 1994, the National Patient Master Index (NPMI) was implemented in MediNet, storing patient demographics, allergies, and a set of six medical alerts. This can be considered as the first ancestor of the NEHR; with the storage of clinical data in the form of allergies and alerts, it became the first national clinical database. One little known fact is that in the original specifications there were plans to also store discharge summaries, though this was never implemented. Because the NPMI pre-dated EMRs, institutions accessed from and reported to it through their SAP patient administration systems, which meant that non-clinical registration staff had to ensure that allergies and alerts were printed out in labels and properly attached on paper medical files. This anomaly was not corrected till 2006, with the migration of NPMI to the Critical Medical Information Store (CMIS). Only after that could clinicians directly access and report drug allergies without relying on other staff. One side benefit was that we were able to also fork a data feed to HSA Pharmacovigilance Unit. This resulted in a happy problem; being used to information coming in drips via the fax machine, they were unable to cope with the sudden deluge of reports, and immediately requested their IT team to filter and throttle down the feed!

In 1997, plans were discussed for a National Health Information System. Unfortunately, the required investment was deemed too high, and so plans were shelved. The definition of a Minimum Data Set for clinical data and the enhancements to the MOH Data Dictionary were conceived then as a basic building block to the National Health Information System.

In 2000, an IT Masterplan for Healthcare Sector was developed, called "Health-Net.21." Under the auspices of this masterplan, a National Health Data Standards Committee was formed, with four subcommittees for Data Administration, Data Protection/Access, IT Security, and Data Exchange. It identified three initiatives:

- A national network to share electronic medical records (EMR);
- A health information portal to educate and empower patients and the public; and
- A health professionals' portal to support healthcare professionals in clinical decision making, research, training, and continuing education;

supported by a strong framework to ensure privacy/security, participation, and commitment by all members of the healthcare sector, national data standards, and adequate network infrastructure.

The most successful achievement of the committees was the MOH Data Dictionary, being the first National Health IT Standard to be established. The ministry continued to maintain the dictionary, with quarterly updates of code tables. The bulk of the updates were for the healthcare establishment code, which had to be updated regularly as institutions and GP clinics evolve. In fact, the hospitals came to rely on these code tables to encode data of the referring GP clinic during registration. Over the years, this has morphed into the National Health Data Dictionary developed by MOHH today.

In 2001, a Common Cross IT System meeting identified the following five areas with the potential for adopting common systems:

- Hospital Information System (HIS)
- Financial/Materials Management System
- HR Systems
- Electronic Medical Record (EMR/Intra-cluster)
- Supply Chain Management

However, translating into action proved an insurmountable challenge then.

In 2003, post-SARS, Minister Khaw Boon Wan identified Exploit IT Maximally as one of his eight priorities, and a small WG comprising MOH and IDA staff and cluster CIOs was formed in September 2003 to work on action plans. The WG identified the sharing of EMR across clusters as a potential quick-win, and four sub-groups were formed: Medico-Legal, Culture and Change Management, IT Architecture and Data Standards, and Publicity. It studied past initiatives and drew the following lessons:

- That it was important not to lose focus;
- To be realistic and not get too engaged in philosophical debates;
- Political will to drive change was important; and
- The key to success lay in 3 words: Implementation, Implementation, Implementation!

The Exploit IT WG focused on areas where the "market" was performing sub-optimally, and operated on the principle of applying the lightest touch possible. The three criteria used for prioritisation were patient outcomes, costs, and efficiency. The WG decided to begin with public sector institutions first, to establish the business case for private and people sector to join in the future. The WG was prepared to live with diversity, balanced with what makes economic sense.

The Medico-Legal subgroup tackled the biggest roadblock first, by reconfirming with AGC a position established by previous committees, which is that implied consent given by the patient through the act of seeking healthcare treatment was sufficient basis to enable EMR sharing. However, AGC advised the ministry to conduct a publicity effort, as common public knowledge is an important premise for implied consent. Hence, the Publicity Sub-Group printed brochures in four languages, and organised a media blitz for the EMRX launch, culminating in a press briefing on 30 March 2004.

Learning from the NHG's Cluster Patient Record Sharing system architecture, the Electronic Medical Record Exchange (EMRX) pilot was rapidly developed in a short three months on top of the MediNet. It was launched in 1 April 2004, starting only with hospital inpatient discharge summaries. EMRX's key objective is to allow all public hospitals and polyclinics in Singapore to share patient records online. These digitized records can be easily shared online across IT-enabled healthcare institutions. This improved patient care outcomes significantly as doctors can make more accurate diagnoses and prescriptions, hospitals would be able to provide better coordinated care and patients would be able to enjoy lower costs. Over the year, the team progressively rolled out the following documents on a quarterly basis: allergies, lab, and radiology reports, as well as medication.

As the pilot system was hardwired to work across just the two clusters, the ministry tendered for a more robust system that used an enterprise service bus architecture, so that it could be easily extended to more documents and institutions. In 2005, this new EMRX which ran on Microsoft Biztalk went live, with HPB's NIR immunisation data, and school health records being made available in 2006. The flexibility of the new system proved fortuitous when an outbreak of Vancomycin-Resistant Enterococci (VRE) occurred in July 2005, when MOH could implement in one month a quick and dirty solution on EMRX to alert hospitals of VRE-positive patients.

An interesting effect of driving quick implementation first was that it revealed the need for the non-IT aspects of national health IT work; for instance, disparity of data and workflows across clusters became more apparent through electronic sharing vs the paper world. Hence, the first Health Team IT Steering Committee was convened on 27 January 2006 as a platform for IT-related policy issues that cut across the healthcare ecosystem. The approach to establish key governance instruments were endorsed at this committee, such as the eHealth Interoperable Architecture and the Common Support Framework. The EMRX Clinical Committee and EMRX Audit WG were also established under this committee. Key programmes such as IDA's GP Clinic Management System programme were endorsed at this committee. The policy against storing of EMR on patient-carried devices was also endorsed at this committee.

An EMRX Clinical Committee was established to provide the clinical stewardship to enhance the EMRX. Key clinical practices advanced by the committee include:

- Sharing of unvetted HIDS;
- Feedback process to source institutions on erroneous EMR;
- Access by pharmacists and nurses; and
- Transfer of CMIS drug code maintenance from an ad-hoc Drug Code Team to HSA.

In 2007, initial forays were made beyond the public sector. EMRX access was extended to Community Hospitals. Subsequently, a pilot e-referral system between TTSH and Community Hospitals was implemented; this has since evolved into the integrated Referral Management System operated by AIC today. Clinical indicators collected for the chronic disease programme, were also made available on CMIS as a "quick-win" for EHR. Interestingly, it faced resistance from clinicians because the data was deemed to lack clinical value.

In 2008, MOH Holdings took over the reins of national health IT development. One of the key achievements was the formation of Integrated Health Information Services (IHIS). The impetus for this was the impending restructuring of Singhealth and NHG into smaller Regional Health Systems (RHS), as well as the formation of new RHS around new hospitals such as KPTH. It was simply not viable to distribute the limited IT staff with healthcare expertise across all the new entities, and there would be diseconomies of scale in duplicating infrastructure and functions. Also, it was felt that Singapore's healthcare system would benefit from a dedicated entity that could focus on developing healthcare IT capability.

EMRX had drawbacks; it is essentially a document-level exchange with no standardised or structured data. In order to realise the vision of "One Singaporean, One Health Record," the idea of National Electronic Health Records was birthed in 2008. In 2009, the National Electronic Health Record Architecture (NEHRA) Blueprint was completed, and the NEHR system finally went live in July 2010.

The Future

One of the challenges of penning this chapter has been to decide where to stop the story. At time of writing, there are many IT initiatives under way, from more sophisticated automation with pharmacy robots, supporting care teams beyond institutional walls, extending access beyond public sector care providers, empowering patients, improving care coordination across different providers in the ecosystem, and attempting to draw insights from the rich sources of data to improve care for each individual patient and for the system as a whole. The story of these myriad initiatives will have to wait for a future tome.

With the benefit of a retrospective birds-eye view, it would seem that our health IT journey progressed through several eras, as illustrated by the diagram below. Not counting the early years in the 1990s, health IT focused on providing View-only access to results from ancillary departments. This resulted in great improvement in clinician productivity, as they were freed from tracking down reports and handling physical film, so adoption was much easier. The 2000s was the era of Order Entry; which presented a larger change management challenge, as it started to impinge on the way clinicians practice. But both clusters were able to find committed clinicians who collaborated with the IT teams to implement site by site, improving with each implementation. The 2010s is now the era of Documents: not only has the data become more complex to include unstructured content such as clinical notes, the workflow has also become more complex, such as e-referral across institutions and care settings. Could it be that Health IT has a natural decade-long cycle in terms of major advancements? If so, the road ahead as Singapore Health IT progress towards 2020 should be an exciting one.

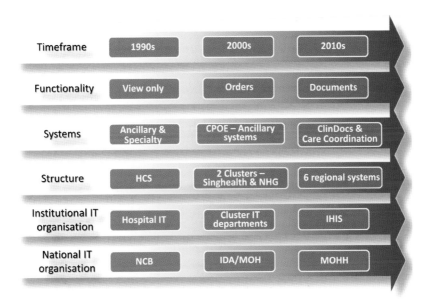

	1990s	2000s	2010s
Timeframe	1990s	2000s	2010s
Functionality	View only	Orders	Documents
Systems	Ancillary & Specialty	CPOE – Ancillary systems	ClinDocs & Care Coordination
Structure	HCS	2 Clusters – Singhealth & NHG	6 regional systems
Institutional IT organisation	Hospital IT	Cluster IT departments	IHIS
National IT organisation	NCB	IDA/MOH	MOHH

It is worth noting that all current and future successes will not have been possible without the rich history of pioneering efforts, including the so-called failures. Healthcare IT has always been a complex endeavour, and there are no guarantees of success. We are optimistic that future generations of health IT professionals will be inspired by these pioneering stories to continue innovating on top of our strong foundations.

Acknowledgements

The recollection of our Health IT's history and developments recorded in this chapter would not have been possible without the help of the following past and present Health IT pioneers and stakeholders, namely *Mrs. Chng Wong Yin, Dr. Chong Yoke*

Sin, Dr. Colin Quek, Ms. Florence Tew Lay Tin, Mr. Mark Ang Cheng Siew, Ms. Tan Swee Hua, and *A/Prof. Yip Wei Luen James.*

Our deepest appreciation to Ms. Poh Ming Ting and Ms. Victoria Tan Shi Ying for their tireless efforts in interviewing, collating and consolidating the information needed to piece this chapter together.

Thank you all for your contributions to this chapter.

14 Traditional Chinese Medicine

Ng Han Seong*

Singapore's healthcare system is largely based on modern medicine with Traditional Chinese Medicine (TCM) playing a complementary role. Treatment modality in TCM includes herbs, acupuncture, and *Tuina*. Despite the accessibility and advances in modern medicine, TCM is popular and well accepted by Singaporeans. A survey conducted by the Ministry of Health (MOH) in 2004 showed that 53% of the population had consulted a TCM practitioner (TCMP) in the previous one year. The figure was 45% in 1994. More recently, data collected from the National Health Survey 2010 in Singapore showed that 39.6% surveyed had visited a TCMP, 26.0% sought treatment for general well-being, 25.8% for acute minor injuries such as sprains, 20.6% for chronic aches and pain like headaches, back pain and rheumatism, and 17.5% for acute minor illness, for example, the cough and the flu.

TCM is considered part of the Chinese cultural heritage and tradition. Among all the Traditional Medicines (Chinese, Indian and Malay), TCM has the highest number of practitioners and patients. TCM practice in Singapore (with the exception of Acupuncture) is primarily confined to outpatient care. At present, there are about 2900 TCMPs[1] (please see Annex A) and 1000 TCM clinics in the community.

Early Days

During the early 19th century, Singapore was a young immigrant society, and our forefathers came from the Malay Peninsula, China, and the Indian sub-continent, bringing along with them their Traditional Medicines. Many of these early immigrants worked as coolies and labourers, and suffered from illnesses due to poor living conditions and a lack of proper medical care. Traditional Medicines, collectively

*Head (TCM) Primary and Community Care Division, Ministry of Health, Singapore. Registrar, TCM Practitioners Board, Singapore.
[1] As of December 2013, there were 2873 TCMPs registered with the TCM Practitioners Board.

called "Traditional Chinese Medicines" (TCM) for the purposes of this history, provided care and treatment for the early Chinese immigrants.

Spurred on by the need to help the sick and the poor, the local Chinese community established charitable organisations such as Tong Ji Hospital (1867) which subsequently evolved into the present Singapore Thong Chai Medical Institution (1983); and the Singapore Chung Hwa Medical Institution established in 1956, at Telok Ayer Street, with the primary aim of providing affordable treatment in the form of TCM to the local people and new immigrants. Today, there are more than 40 charitable TCM organisations providing accessible and affordable TCM treatment in Singapore.

Setting Standards and Regulation of TCM Practice and Chinese Medicines

After Singapore's independence in 1965, living conditions improved considerably and the people had greater access to modern healthcare services. Nonetheless, TCM continued to play a complementary role in our healthcare system.

In 1994, then-Minister for Health and Minister for Information and the Arts, BG (NS) George Yeo, appointed a Committee[2] on TCM, chaired by Dr. Aline Wong, then-Senior Minister of State for Health and Education, to review the practice of TCM in order to recommend measures to safeguard patient interest and safety, and to enhance the standard of training of TCM practitioners in Singapore. The Committee recommended a phased approach, starting with self-regulation of the TCMPs in the initial phase, followed by statutory regulation at the later stage. It also made recommendations to upgrade the standard of training of TCMPs and control of Chinese Medicinal Materials (CMM).

Visit to Singapore Thong Chai Medical Institution (Year TBC)

A TCM Unit was set up in MOH in 1995. As part of self-regulation, the following committees were formed to represent the local TCM community:

> Singapore TCM Organisations Coordinating Committee (STCMOCC) to represent the main TCM practitioners organisations; and

> Singapore TCM Organisations Committee (STOC) to represent the organisations dealing with the trade and retail of CMMs.

---

[2] Committee chaired by Dr. Aline Wong. Members include: Mr. Chia Chin Hua, Mr. Leong Mun Sum, Dr. Chia Tet Fatt, Prof. Tan Wan-Cheng, Dr. Kwa Soon Bee, Dr. Wong Kum Leng, Mr. Tan Tock San, Ms. Francis Low Pooi Fong, A/P Edmund Lee, Dr. Tan Kok Soo, Dr. Chen Ai Ju, and Mr. Tan Kiok K'ng.

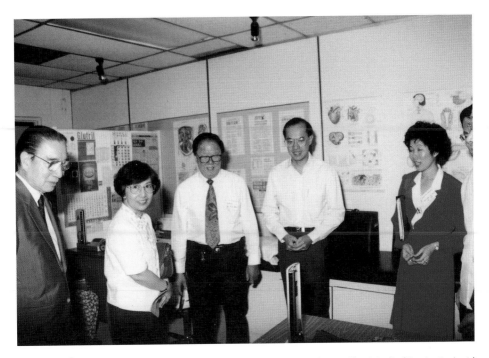

In the centre is the late Mr. Tan Tock San (Chairman of Singapore Thong Chai Medical Institution) with the Minister for Health and Minister for Information and the Arts, BG(NS) George Yeo on his left, and Senior Minister of State for Health, Dr. Aline Wong on his right.

Recognising that TCMPs' qualifications and skill levels were key in maintaining acceptable standards of TCM practice, the TCM Practitioners Act was passed in 14 November 2000 and the TCM Practitioners Board (TCMPB) came into operation the following year, 2001, for the purpose of regulating the profession. The registration of TCMPs started in 2001, starting with the acupuncturists, and followed by the TCM physicians in 2002.

Members of the First TCM Practitioners Board 2001–2003

In effect from 1 January 2004, all who wish to practise TCM are required to be registered with the Board and possess valid practising certificates. The Act requires TCMPs to be registered with the TCMPB. Besides registering TCMPs, the Board also accredits TCM schools and courses, and regulates the professional conduct and ethics of registered TCM Practitioners. The Board also published the Ethical Code and Ethical Guidelines in 2006.

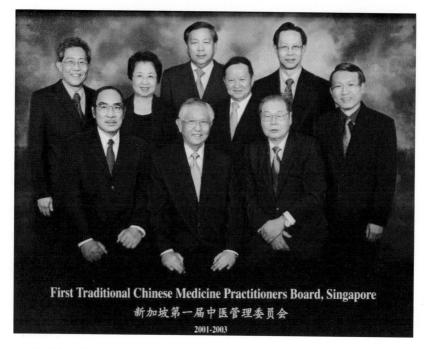

First Traditional Chinese Medicine Practitioners Board, Singapore
新加坡第一届中医管理委员会
2001-2003

L-R seated: Dr. Wong Kum Leng (Registrar), Mr. Ch'ng Jit Koon (Chairman), and Mr. Neo Say Hai.
L-R standing: Mr. Ong Boo Gong, Mrs. Chuo Peck Hiang (Executive Secretary), Mr. Teo Eng Kiat, Mr. Sia Bak Chiang, Prof. Hong Hai, and Prof. Lee Tat Leang.

During this time, the Health Sciences Authority (HSA) had also started the regulation of Chinese Proprietary Medicines (CPM) in the form of tablets, pills, and liquid preparations. CPMs are subjected to licensing requirements, listing, and labelling criteria, as well as the mandatory submission of tests reports on toxic heavy metal and microbial counts for every consignment at point of import. These products must thus comply with a set of safety and quality criteria before they are allowed for sale. To date, about 10,000 CPMs have been listed with HSA. CPMs are also subject to post-market surveillance checks, which include targeted sampling and testing.

Although there are no specific licensing requirement for raw CMMs, CMMs must not contain toxic or prohibited substances, be adulterated with Western drugs, contain excessive levels of toxic heavy metals, and must not make reference to their use for 19 diseases[3] stipulated in the Schedule of the Medicines Act.

With statutory registration of TCMPs and tighter regulatory controls on CPMs, Minister for Health, Mr. Gan Kim Yong, announced the lifting of a three-decade

---

[3] The 19 conditions are: Blindness, cancer, cataracts, drug addiction, deafness, diabetes, epilepsy or fits, hypertension, insanity, kidney diseases, leprosy, menstrual disorders, paralysis, tuberculosis, sexual function, infertility, impotency, frigidity, conception, and pregnancy.

ban on CPMs containing *Berberine*, in effect from 1 January 2013. HSA will continue to monitor the situation and consider extending the lift to CMMs containing *Berberine* as well.

Training of TCMPs

The following TCM training institutions are accredited by the TCMPB to train TCMPs:

> Singapore College of TCM (SCTCM) at 640 Lorong 4 Toa Payoh, Singapore 319522;

> Institute of Chinese Medical Studies (ICMS) at Sims Avenue Centre #04-04/05, 540 Sims Avenue, Singapore 387603; and

> Nanyang Technological University in a joint program with Beijing University of TCM at the School of Biological Sciences, located at 60 Nanyang Drive, Singapore 637551.

Both SCTCM and ICMS upgraded their TCM Diploma to Bachelor degree courses in 2006, with bachelor's degree courses by SCTCM and ICMS conducted in conjunction with Guangzhou University of Chinese Medicine and Beijing University of Chinese Medicine (BUCM), respectively. NTU also started a 5-year double degree program with BUCM, with NTU awarding a Bachelor of Science in Biomedical Sciences, and BUCM awarding the Bachelor of Medicine (Chinese Medicine).

In 2006, SCTCM started a two year part-time Graduate Diploma in Acupuncture course for registered medical and dental practitioners interested in providing needle acupuncture as a complementary form of treatment to mainstream medicine. These medical and dental practitioners must pass the Singapore Acupuncturists Registration Examination (SARE) and must also register with the TCMPB.

Apart from the above, TCM Bachelor degrees from TCM institutions in China are also recognised by the TCMPB, namely: Beijing University of Chinese Medicine, Chengdu University of Traditional Chinese Medicine, China Academy of Traditional Chinese Medicine, Guangzhou University of Chinese Medicine, Nanjing University of Chinese Medicine, Shanghai University of Traditional Chinese Medicine, Shandong University of Traditional Chinese Medicine, and Heilongjiang University of Traditional Chinese Medicine.

To date, about 19% of the 2900 TCM practitioners possess Bachelor degrees in TCM. This is an increase of about 14% compared to 5.2% with Bachelor degrees in 2006.

Training of CMM Dispensers

The following institution provides training for CMM dispensers:

1. TCM College (Singapore) at 371 Beach Road Keypoint #02-37. Singapore 199597.

In 2002, TCM College started a diploma course for CMM dispensers jointly organised with BUCM. From December 2005, those who graduated with intermediate and diploma modules can be listed voluntarily with the TCMPB.

Introduction of Acupuncture in Health Care Institutions

TCM in Singapore is mainly practised in private and charitable TCM clinics. Following the recommendations made by the Committee on Acupuncture and *Tuina* Practices (2004) chaired by Prof. Lee Tat Leang of NUH, acupuncture is allowed in hospitals and nursing homes since 2005. TCM clinics are permitted to co-locate within the premises of public healthcare institutions e.g. hospitals, as private entities to provide outpatient TCM treatment.

Upgrading Standards and Research

To strengthen and upgrade professional knowledge and practice standards amongst TCMPs, the voluntary Continuing TCM Education (CTE) programme was introduced by the TCMPB on 1 January 2013. TCMPs are encouraged to participate in the programme during this voluntary phase.

There was a need to seek more evidence in clinical practice of TCM with regards to safety and clinical efficacy. MOH had allocated a $3 million research grant in 2012 to encourage clinical TCM research. This calls for collaboration between doctors and researchers from modern medicine and practitioners from TCM institutions to carry out TCM clinical research, tailored to Singapore's context, especially in the area of chronic diseases.

Regional and International Cooperation on Traditional Medicines

A Memorandum of Understanding (MOU) and Plan of Cooperation (POC) on TCM were signed by PRC's Vice-Minister for Health Prof. Zhu Qingsheng and Senior Parliamentary Secretary Mr. Chan Soo Sen at the State Administration of TCM (SATCM) in Beijing on 22 July 1999.

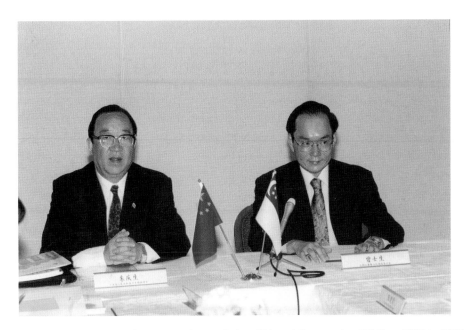

Signing the Memorandum of Understanding (MOU) and Plan of Cooperation (POC) on TCM by PRC's Vice-Minister for Health Prof. Zhu Qingsheng and SPS Mr. Chan Soo Sen at the State Administration of TCM (SATCM) in Beijing on 22 Jul 1999.

PRC's Vice-Minister for Health Prof. Zhu Qingsheng & Senior Parliamentary Secretary for Health, Mr. Chan Soo Sen.

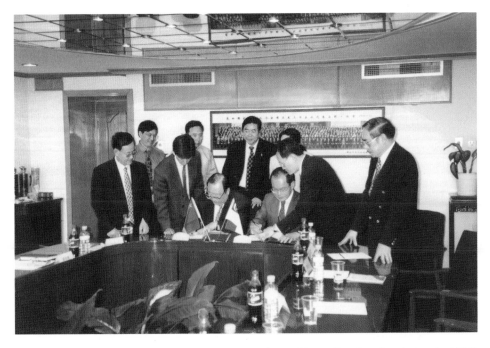

Prof. Zhu Qingsheng & Senior Parliamentary Secretary for Health Mr. Chan Soo Sen signing the MOU.

The MOU aims to formulate cooperation plans and facilitate the mutual exchange of information and expertise on teaching, practice, research, and regulation of TCM between both countries. Under the MOU and POC, PRC's experts have been invited to Singapore to assist in training of practitioners and to also conduct the Singapore TCM physicians Registration Examination (STRE). In return, health management training programs have been conducted annually since 2001 for PRC officials to learn about hospital management, medical care, and financial policies in Singapore.

In May 2013, Dr. Amy Khor, Minister of State for Health and Manpower, led a six-member delegation from MOH and the HSA, for the signing of the 5th POC in Beijing.

The MOH is also committed to participate in other regional and international meetings and workshops on Traditional Medicine organised by ASEAN and WHO. During such events, information on education, training, research collaboration, adverse reactions, and events associated with traditional medicines are shared among member states.

Chronology of Events (Summary)

Year	Event
1994	Then-Minister of Health and Minister for Information and the Arts, BG (NS) George Yeo, appointed a Committee on Traditional Chinese Medicine (TCM), chaired by Dr. Aline Wong, then-Senior Minister of State for Health and Education, to review the practice of TCM and to recommend measures to safeguard patient interest and safety, enhancing the standard of training of TCM practitioners in Singapore.
1995	The Ministry of Health accepted the recommendations in the report submitted by the Committee on TCM: • To adopt a phased approach to TCM regulation — self-regulation by the TCM community, followed by statutory regulation of TCM practice; • To upgrade the standard of TCM training; • To tighten control of Chinese Medicinal Materials (CMM). A Traditional Chinese Medicine (TCM) Unit was set up in MOH (which was subsequently renamed TCM Department) and to work closely with two local TCM associations, namely the Singapore TCM Organisations Coordinating Committee (STCMOCC) and the Singapore TCM Organisations Committee (STOC), to coordinate and implement the Committee's recommendations.
1997	As part of self-regulation, a list of 1807 TCM practitioners was published by STCMOCC.
1998	Chinese Proprietary Medicine (CPM) product regulation was gazetted under the Medicines Act.
1999	Signing of the Memorandum of Understanding (MOU) and Plan of Cooperation (POC) on TCM by PRC's Vice-Minister for Health Prof. Zhu Qingsheng and SPS Mr. Chan Soo Sen at the State Administration of TCM (SATCM) in Beijing on 22 July 1999. In effect from 1 September 1999, CPM product regulation was implemented to promote safety and quality of CPM products available in the Singapore market.
2000	TCM Practitioners Act was passed in Parliament on 14 November 2000.

(Continued)

(Continued)

Year	Event
2001	The TCM Department in MOH was renamed the Traditional & Complementary Medicine Branch (please see Annex B). Formation of Traditional Chinese Medicine Practitioners Board (TCMPB) on 7 February 2001. Main functions of TCMPB include: • Registration of both acupuncturists and TCM physicians; • Accreditation of TCM training institutions and TCM courses for the purpose of registration; and • To determine and regulate the conduct and ethics of registered TCM practitioners. Statutory registration of TCM practitioners began in phases starting with the acupuncturists.
2002	Statutory registration of TCM physicians started. TCM College (Singapore) started a diploma course jointly with Beijing University of Chinese Medicine, to train CMM dispensers.
2004	From 1 January 2004, practitioners who wish to practise TCM in Singapore are eligible for registration only if they possess the following: • TCM qualifications approved by the TCMPB; and • Pass the Singapore TCM Physicians Registration Examination (STRE).
2005	The Transmissible Spongiform Encephalopathy (TSE) Guidelines was issued to minimise the risk of contamination in Chinese Proprietary Medicines, Traditional Medicines and Health Supplements. Acupuncture services are now allowed as part of the service package for hospital and nursing home inpatients. Private TCM clinics are permitted to co-locate in hospitals and nursing homes to provide TCM services to outpatients. Nanyang Technological University started a double degree programme in Biomedical Sciences and TCM, jointly offered with Beijing University of Chinese Medicine. From December 2005, CMM dispensers who graduated from the Singapore TCM College's CMM dispensers training course (Intermediate and Diploma module) are voluntarily listed with the TCM Practitioners Board.
2006	The Ethical Code and Ethical Guidelines for TCM Practitioners were published by the TCMPB. The Singapore College of TCM started a Graduate Diploma in Acupuncture Course, conducted in English, to train registered medical and dental practitioners interested in learning acupuncture. Graduates of the course who pass the Singapore Acupuncturists Registration Examination (SARE) can be registered as acupuncturists by the TCMPB. The Singapore College of TCM and Institute of Chinese Medical Studies upgraded their TCM diploma programmes to bachelor degree courses, jointly with PRC TCM Universities (Guangzhou and Beijing respectively).
2007	Guidelines were revised to allow acupuncture services within western medical clinics.
2012	Minister for Health, Mr. Gan Kim Yong, formally announced the lifting of a three decade ban on *Berberine* effective from 1 January 2013, during the Foreign Experts TCM Symposium held at Thong Chai Medical Institution. As a safety precaution, HSA will lift the prohibition on CPM containing *Berberine* first, with a possible lifting of the prohibition on herbs containing *Berberine* by 2015. Minster Gan also announced that a new research grant would be set up for researchers interested in collaborating with TCM institutions to carry out TCM clinical research tailored to Singapore's context, at the 10th ASEAN Congress of Traditional Chinese Medicine cum 3rd Asia Advanced Forum on Acupuncture-Moxibustion organised by the Singapore Chinese Physicians' Association.
2013	The TCMPB introduced the voluntary Continuing TCM Education, or CTE, programme in an effort to strengthen professional knowledge and practice standards amongst TCM practitioners.

Annex A

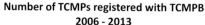

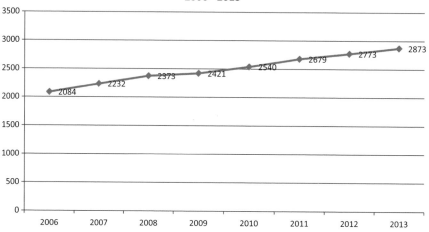

Annex B

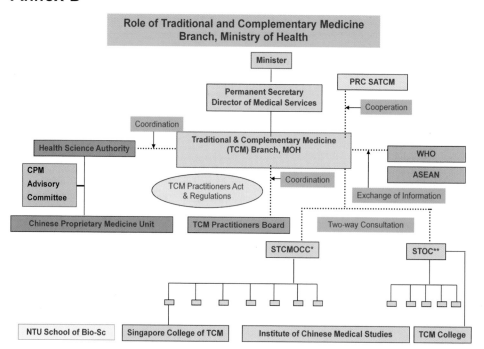

*Singapore TCM Organisations Coordinating Committee
**Singapore TCM Organisations Committee

Acknowledgements

Complementary Health Products Branch, Health Sciences Authority.
Traditional and Complementary Medicine Branch, Ministry of Health.

References

Ministry of Health Singapore (October 1995) *Traditional Chinese Medicine — A Report by the Committee on Traditional Medicine.*
National Health Survey 2010.
TCM Practitioners Board. *Annual Reports 2001–2012.*

15 Global Health — Singapore's Contributions

Yeo Wen Qing[*], Lyn James[†],
Derrick Heng[‡] and Chew Suok Kai[§]

Unless you know what you are looking for, you have no tools to find it
— Mike Leahy, Virologist. On SARS Outbreak

Introduction

In 2003, the Severe Acute Respiratory Syndrome (SARS) caused rampage across Asia and Canada, costing economies US$30 billion in merely four months.[1] In Singapore alone, the SARS outbreak killed 37 victims, and caused a major impact on any non-health sectors including education, tourism, transport, foreign affairs and the economy. In 2001, the anthrax scare infected 22 persons, killed five and cost more than US$1 billion to clean up.[2] In 2009, influenza H1N1 killed 284,000 people in the first year alone.[3] HIV/AIDS has been spreading silently for many years. Up until early 2014, Ebola, a disease thought to be confined to some remote villages in central Africa, has caused havoc across West Africa, and sending chills across the world.[4] For the Ebola outbreak, the crisis is as much a political catastrophe as it is a virological one. Just fresh from civil wars across Liberia and Sierra Leone, trust is lacking making rescue effort extremely excruciating.

On a quieter front, non-communicable diseases (NCDs) such as diabetes, high blood pressure, and heart diseases continue to kill silently. Tobacco and alcohol

[*] Deputy Director, International Cooperation, Singapore Ministry of Health.
[†] Director, Epidemiology & Disease Control Division, Singapore Ministry of Health.
[‡] Group Director, Public Health Group, Singapore Ministry of Health.
[§] Deputy Director of Medical Services, Singapore Ministry of Health.

intakes reach a high level with global tobacco and alcohol companies introducing new and innovative products such as e-cigarettes and alcohols pills, always a step ahead of the legislative curve. Cancer is the number one cause of death in Singapore as more and more people are plagued with mental illnesses and other chronic diseases. As we fight hard to keep non-communicable diseases at bay, at the same time, Singapore's population is growing older.[5] The issue of a rapidly ageing population is causing countries, developing and developed alike, to scramble for the best solution to tackle the unprecedented increase in their respective elderly populations. We are constantly sourcing for innovative ways to improve our health systems, formulating forward-looking policies to adapt to a rapidly changing environment, and to stay ahead of the curve.

This is the reality of healthcare around the world. To add to the challenge, health has become a global enterprise, intricately connected with one another. Diseases respect no borders; countries bear similar burdens of non-communicable diseases and other healthcare challenges.

Domestically, Singapore healthcare is undergoing a revolutionary transformation even as the world struggles to contain some of the worst outbreaks and epidemics. The question then is, how can we strike a balance in this ever-changing world, balancing our domestic demands versus our role in the global community? More specifically, what role can Singapore, an island state with a land-size of 716.1 km^2 and a population of 5.3 million, play globally?

What is Global Health?

What exactly is global health? A seemingly self-explanatory term, it is not yet widely understood. Experts have traced global health diplomacy to multiple origins. The earliest origins involve trade and exchange of gifts between nation states. As the understanding of the role of personal health in national economic development becomes better understood, negotiations over access to health services becomes an important part of bilateral relationships between countries.

Preserving access to basic health services even in times of war and natural disasters is a globally accepted norm. Even in the most intractable conflict situations, there is a reasonable expectation that access and "respect" for health services should be maintained. The observance of intermittent pause in hostilities during major conflicts to evacuate the dead, the dying, and the wounded creates additional respect for health services. Almost by rote, the restoration of basic health services is often one of the first orders of business in post-crisis situations.

Hence, it is not surprising that health programmes have become extremely important over the last fifty years in bilateral and multilateral development initiatives. Donor and host nations negotiate technical and financial support for health programmes.

The emergence of transnational health threats such as H1N1 influenza, SARS, and HIV/AIDS has helped concentrate global attention on health issues and has assisted in galvanising action at the highest levels of government and in the private sector.

In the last decade, the emergence and influence of high profile and media savvy public/private/civil society alliances on health has contributed to the increased attention on global health issues by policy makers around the world. Therefore it is no surprise that World Health Assembly and UNICEF events can sometimes become star-studded events where advocates are who's who in political and entertainment circles with the likes of Bill Gates, Angelina Jolie, and Michael J. Fox, championing their pet topics. One could say that the success of a health programme depends as much on medical advancement as its publicity and draw of their respective spokespersons or advocates.

In sum, global health diplomacy is an emerging field in global health and international diplomacy. As boundaries become blurred between global health and multilateral diplomacy, there is a growing call for health experts and development experts to become adept in international relations issues and for trained diplomats to become knowledgeable about global health issues.

A Flight Away — Importance of Global Health Diplomacy to Us

From Singapore's perspective, global health diplomacy revolves around bilateral and multilateral relationships. It provides an avenue for us to articulate our national health priorities and to contextualise these priorities within the framework of existing and future diplomatic and development initiatives.

To put into perspective the importance of global health diplomacy to Singapore, consider this: based on 2014 figures, on average, more than 140,000 people passed through Singapore's Changi Airport on a daily basis, with another 50,000 or so vehicles crossing the Causeway from Malaysia to Singapore everyday. We have also one of the busiest ports in the world and we practise an open-door, tourist- and business-friendly environment. With such openness comes a certain amount of vulnerability for diseases to enter Singapore unnoticed. There is always a possibility that some disease outbreak in a remote part of the world will find its way to Singapore's shores in no time. Simply put, any outbreak is just a flight or ride away.

Short of closing the borders or setting up strict surveillance at check-points each time an outbreak is declared in another part of the world, we need to adopt a more proactive approach. This entails strengthening our international cooperation outreach and building friendships with strategic partners and countries.

Such international cooperation in healthcare has been shown to be invaluable during global public health crises, such as the H1N1 influenza in 2009, and more recently the Middle Eastern Respiratory Syndrome-Coronavirus (MERS-CoV) and Ebola outbreaks. Bilateral and multilateral cooperations built over the years enable us to openly share information with our neighbours and supra-national organisations such as the WHO. It enables us to be well-positioned in terms of domestic readiness to handle pandemic outbreaks and prevent further cross-border spread of diseases.

When there is no pressing health crisis, international networks are equally important to us, as many countries are tackling common challenges like keeping their ageing populations healthy, and shaping financially sustainable, high-quality healthcare systems. Therefore, we see great value in forging stronger links with the international healthcare community to share and exchange experiences, technical know-how, and professional expertise.

Our international engagements have allowed us to refine our own system by learning from some of the world's best practices. It has also helped us in engaging global healthcare experts to work with us to further refine our policies and methods, and to keep ourselves at the forefront of healthcare policy thinking. We have been able to attract professionals and technical experts to work for Singapore, thus contributing to our human capital. Dr. David Heymann, a renowned expert in public health who had tackled the SARS outbreak and poliomyelitis eradication, was one of them. He has worked as a part-time consultant to Singapore after he retired as Assistant Director-General of the World Health Organisation.

Overall, Singapore worked closely with international organisations such as the World Health Organisation (WHO), the Association of South-East Asian Nations (ASEAN), and we actively participate in other forums such as the Asia Pacific Economic Cooperation (APEC) and the United Nations. Our international engagement efforts and growing networks facilitate the engagement of global healthcare experts in collaborations to further refine domestic policies and keep ourselves at the forefront of healthcare policy thinking.

Soft Diplomacy in Health

Since 2003, the Ministry of Health (MOH) and our healthcare institutions have participated actively in international fora. For examples, Singapore had seconded officers to WHO offices in Jakarta Country Office, the Western Pacific Regional Office in Manila, and its headquarters in Geneva. These officers were seconded for periods ranging from six months to three years. Officers were also deployed for short term emergency assignments such as during the H1N1 pandemic and in the aftermath of the Indian Ocean tsunamis in 2004 and the 2014 typhoon in the Philippines. More recently in early 2015, Singapore hosted the Ministerial Meeting on Universal Health Coverage.

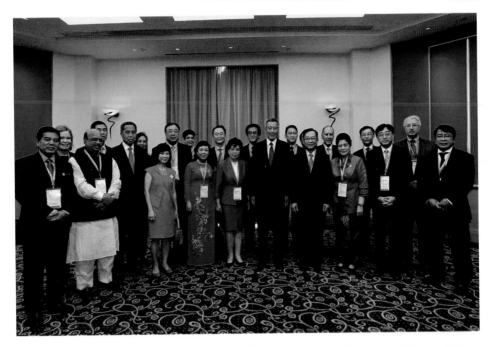

Figure 1. Ministerial meeting on Universal Health Coverage held in Singapore, February 2015.

The meeting was graced by Prime Minister Lee Hsien Loong and attended by Health Ministers and Senior Officials, include; WHO Director-General, Dr. Margaret Chan (Fig. 1).

The benefits of such direct exchanges are multi-fold for Singapore. Firstly, these exchanges allow MOH to develop direct linkages with senior officials of WHO, ASEAN, and individual member states. We also gain insights into the decision making process and build up personal friendships. Secondly, we allow our healthcare workers and administrators the invaluable experience and exposure of systems beyond our own domestic context. Lastly and most importantly, we can use these experiences to contribute and to exert influence in the development of global health despite being a small nation.

Increasingly, WHO is looking to Singapore to provide sound technical advice. Many of our doctors and senior administrators play an important role at Technical Advisor Groups (TAGs) as technical consultants or as Temporary Advisors to select expert groups. Our expertise is much sought after in areas such as communicable diseases, risk communications, and laboratory capacity building.

As a nation, we also play an active role in providing assistance to members of the global community. During the H1N1 Influenza Pandemic in 2009, Singapore responded to WHO's Director General's request and donated 50,000 doses of the pandemic influenza vaccine and 200,000 doses of the anti-viral drug, Tamiflu, to WHO to assist less developed countries during the difficult time.

Forging Stronger Relationships Bilaterally

In parallel with our outreach effort at multilateral platforms, bilateral relationships play an equal if not more important role in Singapore's health diplomacy. Our relationships with senior officials of key countries, in particular our ASEAN neighbours, have facilitated the regular exchange of information and data regarding the spread of the disease outbreaks in the region, which would otherwise not be readily available from public sources. Singapore also provided capacity-building training to health officials so that they would be better able to handle local outbreaks and to prevent the spread of communicable diseases to the region.

Beyond communicable diseases, Singapore initiated the ASEAN Health Policy Fellowship programme in 2011 to forge closer exchanges that go beyond a meeting or a short study trip. Under this programme, officers would be attached to a division within the MOH or Healthcare Institutions to get some hands-on experience. Attachments lasting from one to six weeks allows officers to know one another on a personal level. Such friendships go a long way in the careers of the fellows as well as receiving countries. Furthermore, MOH conducts regular engagement programmes or study trips to key countries to learn about their systems and touch base and network with senior officials.

Our Engagement at the
World Health Organisation (WHO)

Singapore became a member of WHO in 1966. In WHO, Member States are divided into six geographical regions — African (AFRO), American (PAHO), Eastern Mediterranean (EMRO), European (EURO), South-East Asian (SEARO), and Western Pacific (WPRO). Singapore comes under WPRO. The grouping of countries into regions was done by the United Nations during the post-Cold War era, to separate countries with potential and perceived political conflicts.

The significance of WHO lies in its mandate and legitimacy in global health governance. As a norm-setting body and the world's foremost authority in public health, the WHO provides guidance on international health issues and sets global health legislation, as well as coordinate member states' ability to tackle global issues of pressing concern.

Singapore has been active in the WHO circuit especially over the past ten years. We have established good personal relationships with key WHO personnel at the WHO headquarters in Geneva and we also enjoy close professional links with many WHO officials at the regional and country levels.

Singapore is also seen as being able to provide sound technical advice to the workings at WHO. As of 2014, WHO has designated 10 departments and agencies in Singapore as WHO Collaborating Centres (WHO CC) in specialised fields such as occupational health, health promotion, and transfusion medicine. These also include the MOH, Ministry of Manpower, Health Promotion Board, Health Sciences Authority, National Cancer Centre, National University of Singapore, Public Utilities Board, and the National Environment Agency.

Further, MOH officials have been invited to provide professional advice on steering committees and task forces, which provided valuable networking and engagement opportunities. These included the Asia Pacific Technical Advisory Group on the Asia Pacific Strategy for Emerging Diseases (APSED), Advisory Group of Independent Experts to review the smallpox research programme (AGIES), Pandemic Influenza Preparedness (PIP) Framework for the Sharing of Influenza Viruses, and Access to Vaccines and Other Benefits, International Health Regulation Emergency Committees, and the Global Outbreak And Response Network (GOARN).

In 2006, Singapore was elected to the WHO Executive Board (EB) for the first time. The late Dr. Balaji Sadasivan, then-Senior Minister of State (Health) was Singapore's representative on the Board. During Singapore's three-year term on the EB from 2006 to 2009, especially our term as Chair of the EB from 2007 to 2008, we gained valuable goodwill with other Member States (Fig. 2).

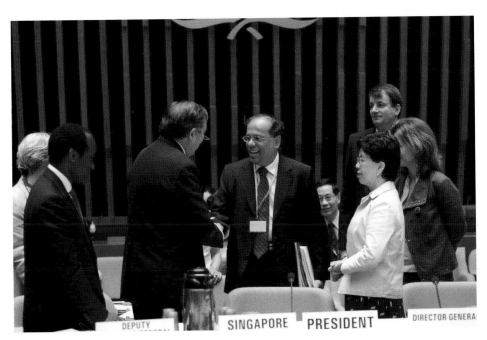

Figure 2.   The late Dr. Balaji Sadasivan assuming the role of President of the Executive Board in 2006.

Association of South East Asian Nations (ASEAN)

ASEAN was established in 1967 primarily with the aim of promoting economic, social, and cultural development in the region through joint collaboration and mutual assistance. At the ASEAN Heads of State Summit in 2000, the Initiative for ASEAN Integration was launched calling for greater economic and social integration, with the clarion call for an "ASEAN Community" to be formed by end of 2015. This led to the formation of the three pillars — namely economic, political, and socio-cultural, each with its Blueprint and Implementation Plan in preparation of an integrated ASEAN. Health Development falls under the Socio-Cultural pillar, under the supervision at Senior Officials level (SOMHD).

ASEAN SOMHD has since remained the main platform for regional health cooperation, where member states are obliged to participate at the annual meetings of different subsidiary bodies and are obliged to fulfil commitments made under the existing work plans. ASEAN offers stability in an established code of practise whereby content in meetings are guided by the ASEAN Secretariat (ASEC) with the Chair (usually the host country) having influence over the proceedings as well as the structure of these meetings. All issues will then be discussed and agreed upon at the Senior Official Level (SOM) before being raised for endorsement by the Ministers at the ASEAN Health Ministers Meeting (AHMM), and finally to the leaders at the ASEAN Summit. SOM is held annually whereas AHMM convenes once every two years. This is to allow for sufficient time lapse and the completion of work plans. The chairmanship at the SOMHD and AHMM level, rotated alphabetically, proceed in different orders.

In July 2010, Singapore hosted the 10th ASEAN Health Ministers Meeting in Singapore with the theme, "Healthy People, Healthy ASEAN," as well as the 4th ASEAN plus Three (China, Japan, and Korea) Health Ministers Meeting (Fig. 3) Singapore was the SOMHD chair for the period 2013 to 2014 after having taken over from the Philippines. During our chairmanship, we kick-started the discussion and process of our raison d'être for post-2015. This included starting the conversation on consolidating our collective efforts and sharpening the focus of ASEAN SOMHD.

Going forward, ASEAN remains as an important platform for us to engage our health counterparts. In particular, we should work with ASEAN Member States in the strengthening of health systems reforms, combatting of NCDs and use of tobacco, and continue our close cooperation in the surveillance and control of infectious diseases.

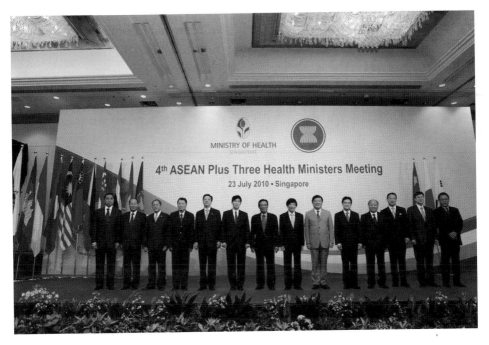

Figure 3   ASEAN plus Three Health Ministers Meeting in Singapore, July 2010.

Asia Pacific Economic Cooperation (APEC)

The Asia Pacific Economic Cooperation (APEC) was established in 1989 primarily for facilitating economic growth, cooperation, trade, and investment in the Asia-Pacific region. APEC comprises of 21 member economies. Unlike the World Trade Organisation (WTO) or other multilateral trade bodies, APEC has no treaty obligations required of its participants — decisions made within APEC are reached by consensus and commitments are undertaken on a voluntary basis. APEC Economies engage in economic and technical cooperation to attain sustainable growth and equitable development in the region, and to improve overall economic and social well-being. The Economies voluntarily take turns to host the meetings. Singapore last hosted APEC in 2009.

Though APEC is primarily a trade-related forum, the APEC Health Working Group (HWG) saw its genesis after the SARS outbreak in 2003 as the economies realised the impact of health, especially pandemic diseases, on trade. It started as a Health Taskforce in 2003 and became a permanent Working Group in 2007. The HWG meets bi-annually at the senior officials' level, and its main priorities include: (a) preparedness and response to public health threats (including avian and human pandemic influenza, vector-borne diseases, and HIV/AIDS); (b) building capacity of health promotion and prevention of lifestyle related diseases; and (c) strengthening health systems of the economies including health financing.

While health is not a core business of APEC, it is the only organisation that explicitly links health with economic growth and progress. Hence, two of APEC HWG's priorities are on: (i) communicable diseases, which if untamed, would cause considerable damage to the economy; and (ii) strengthening of health finance systems to ensure long term sustainability. Furthermore, the smaller nature of HWG (21 economies as compared to 194 member states in WHO) ensures nimbleness and flexibility in HWG's efforts.

APEC HWG provides Singapore the platform to engage several strategic partners that fall outside the ambit of ASEAN and WHO Regional Office, such as Russia, USA, and Canada. It also allows for us to profile our thought leadership, exchange views on global and regional issues, and directly engage other economies beyond our usual partners. Overall, Singapore enjoys a positive reputation with our APEC partners as we are viewed as having a strong and resilient healthcare system. Lately, we have been looked upon as having strong technical competency, having the capacity to front high-quality health projects, three of which had received funding and support from the APEC in the past two years.

Conclusion

In conclusion, international cooperation is an area that is likely to grow as transnational health threats grows and as the world becomes increasingly inter-dependent. It will continue to play an important role in our outreach and engagement efforts both bilaterally and multi-laterally. These engagements have allowed us to contribute to the international health agenda as an objective and constructive global player, and to help develop solutions to emerging health issues. Through our international relations, we learn from some of the world's best practices. In turn, we contribute to international health capability by sharing our own experience and expertise, as well as by providing technical assistance and training to other countries.

Being a small country makes us nimble and effective in pushing our policies, hence setting the benchmark for other countries. On the flip side, we can be easily forgotten or passed over in the world of giants and big players. Singapore needs to continuously find our niche and standing in the global world of health diplomacy, fitting in where we fit best and sharpening our focus and engagements. There is also the on-going challenge in striking equilibrium between our international engagements and domestic requirements without stretching our resources too far.

The final challenge is how to maintain the current non-partisan support of policy makers on global health issues over the long term. Global health diplomats must have a good grasp of domestic policies and interest vis-à-vis international direction and flow. Sometimes what we deem as viable in a local context may not be conceivable when expounded to an international audience. We need to be flexible and skilled in our interactions with fellow counterparts. Only then, can we further our influence beyond our shores, and always be viewed as a trustworthy nation in the complex world of health diplomacy.

References

1. MA Dixon, OA Dar, DL Heymann. (2014) "Emerging Infectious Diseases: Opportunities at the human animal-environment interface." *Veterinary Record. BMJ.* **174**(22): 546–551.
2. www.cdc.gov/niosh/nas/rdrp/appendices/chapter6/a6-45.pdf
3. "Why Global Health Security Matters." *Global Health,* United States Government. Website accessed at: http://www.globalhealth.gov/global-health-topics/global-health-security/ghsmatters.html.
4. Garret, Laurie, Renwick, Danielle. (2014) "Epic failures feeding Ebola crisis." *Council on Foreign Relations.* Accessible at: http://www.cfr.org/public-health-threats-and-pandemics/epic-failures-feeding-ebola-crisis/p33465
5. Prime Minister's Office, National Population & Talent Division. (2013) "A Sustainable Population for a Dynamic Singapore: Population White Paper."

16 Challenges in Healthcare

Lee Chien Earn* and K. Satku†

While we have done well in the last 50 years and have evolved to become one of the better health systems in the world, there are several issues ahead that threaten to disrupt the system's capability to serve Singaporeans well. Some issues, such as the management of chronic diseases, are surfacing now because of our success thus far, such as in managing communicable diseases. These issues are complex and are not easily solved. They are also not unique to Singapore and arise from an interplay of both international and local factors, including those outside of healthcare. We are already working on addressing most of these issues, some more definitively than others.

Investing Wisely

Singapore has been spending less on healthcare than other developed countries, but this expenditure will inevitably increase to meet future challenges. Singapore is able to increase its expenditure as evidenced by the increased spending on infrastructure and Pioneer Generation subsidies at a time when other governments are facing a budget crunch because of Singapore's prudent economic policies and management.

However, wealth can be easily squandered if it is not used wisely. Wrong decisions, especially those related to infrastructure and subsidy policies, can have long tails and increase the burden on future generations. However, making the right

---

*Chief Executive Officer, Changi General Hospital, Singapore.

†Chairman, Health Sciences Authority, Singapore. Professor, Department of Orthopaedic Surgery, National University Health System, Singapore. Professor of Health Policy, Saw Swee Hock School of Public Health, National University of Singapore. Former Director of Medical Services (2004–2013), Ministry of Health, Singapore.

decisions will become increasingly more difficult as systems become more complex. Reductionist, mechanical and linear methods of problem solving tend to flounder against the laws of unforeseen consequences and incomplete information. There is also the mismatch between the lifecycles of different elements in the healthcare system which may render investments obsolete. For example, technological changes occur at a much faster rate than the building of major infrastructure (e.g. hospitals) such that even as the hospital is being built, changes already need to be made to accommodate new technology. Another challenge facing decision makers is the need to take into account implementation issues, as a good decision implemented poorly may do more harm than good.

Some of the systems-level questions that need to be addressed include the role and governance of Regional Health Systems, the role of speciality centres vis-à-vis regional hospitals, the role of community hospitals (and whether they should be built adjacent to acute hospitals or as standalones in the community), and financing schemes that enable healthcare to be affordable, accessible and sustainable. In addition there are the myriad service-level decisions ranging from the mundane to the esoteric.

With increasing complexity, monolithic centralised command and control structures will impede the timeliness and appropriateness of decisions being made. For a resilient system, there must be strong decision making capabilities across the different layers of the healthcare systems. Even though Singapore is a small country, this can be challenging, with the growth in the number of healthcare institutions in both public and private sectors, where both new and existing institutions would want greater autonomy in introducing more services. How do we optimise flexibility and responsiveness while ensuring alignment for objective? How will the Ministry guide healthcare institutions as to which practices or services to pursue and which to scale down or discontinue? What are the levers to encourage "compliance"?

One of the key enablers is having the necessary intelligence to guide decision making. Data from the electronic records of the hospitals and healthcare systems is increasingly being collected and analysed for outcomes and cost-effectiveness. The mining of performance data could help to identify wasteful practices and guide policies and strategies for an efficient and effective provision of healthcare. The information explosion can however be a double edged sword as it further increases the challenge facing decision makers in separating the chaff from the wheat — discerning which data would be important to use and which would be just "noise" that is distracting or misleading.

The Ministry of Health is placing increasing emphasis on our health systems' performance assessment by building in-house capability (including health technology assessment) and funding the recently established Saw Swee Hock School of Public Health. These initiatives reflect the country's continuing investment and faith in public health to offer an independent academic analysis to help shape our policies and strategies. We will need to quickly boost our expertise in this area, marrying analytics with ground realities so that data is interpreted within the proper context, recognising our differing perspectives that may bias our conclusions.

Moving from Healthcare to Health

Countries around the world recognise that healthcare is not an end in itself, but a means to health. One of the key determinants of health is lifestyle choices. As such, Singaporeans need to see themselves as responsible active participants rather than passive recipients of services.

We also need to contain increased demand for healthcare services by reducing illness. Our strategies for reducing illness are premised on the assumption that if people lead healthier lives they will have less chronic illness, fewer episodes of hospitalisation and a shorter period of disability at the end of their years.

Changing health-related behaviour has however never been easy, especially when the consequences of choices made today manifest only sometime in the future. Presently, an additional obstacle is the immediate access to a plethora of information that is sometimes contradictory, alarmist or misleading. As a result, even those who want to make the right lifestyle choices may be confused as to the correct thing to do.

In this climate, the provision of reliable and accurate information as part of health promotion has never been more important. Health education is not only about providing information, but about instigating behaviour change. Health promotion needs also to go beyond persuading the individual to make better choices to enabling these decisions through the physical and social environment, the marketplace, supportive health services and regulations. This requires a multiagency approach beyond the Ministry of Health or even the public sector, to include the private and people sectors too.

The government's efforts in this respect include providing funding for health promotion, supporting behaviour change by providing services like smoking cessation clinics and screening programmes, making new regulations e.g. to curb smoking, and changing the environment to make healthier choices more available — for instance, helping hawkers to make their recipes healthier, having more stalls sell healthier food, identifying healthier alternatives sold in shops and supermarkets, making more provisions for exercise facilities in housing estates and so on.

The Ministry has recently articulated a Healthy Living Master Plan, to make healthy living the "default" choice. While ambitious, this master plan must succeed, albeit with adjustments, in securing health for all as lessons are learnt from the implementation experience. Within the plan are special considerations for promoting mental health care, an area of need that has been given adequate focus only in more recent years, but which is critical for health in the next several decades.

Another key area of focus is our diet. At the time of independence, Singapore was struggling to contain malnutrition in the form of under-nutrition. With economic success and the easy availability of food, we now encounter malnutrition in the form of high calorie foods coupled with indulgence. There should be no let-up in our health promotion efforts. We need to be innovative if the Healthy Living Master Plan is to make healthy lifestyle the default choice for us.

Providing Care that Matters to Patients

1. Containing Fragmentation of Care

We have the expertise to provide care for some of the most complicated conditions, but do so in a fragmented way. The care in the public hospitals has, in part, been driven by professional interest and increasingly sub-specialisation is seen as the norm — as part of the pursuit of excellence — and the general specialist is increasingly displaced. This leads to the fragmentation of care, with care provided by multiple specialists even within the same specialty. This results in increasing costs to the patient and the system. Sometimes, despite seeing various specialists, what really matters to the patient is not addressed, as there is no one who really takes time to understand the patient holistically, as a person. In orthopaedic surgery in some hospitals for instance, the specialists work in divisions called spine division, shoulder division, trauma division, ankle and foot division, hip and knee division and do almost exclusively spine, shoulder, trauma, ankle and foot, hip, or knee surgery, respectively. As our population ages and musculoskeletal problems become more common, the patient ends up seeing several different orthopaedic specialists just to have his musculoskeletal conditions managed. Similar fragmentation is evident in many other specialties.

The fragmentation of care in acute hospitals is compounded by the lack of depth in the primary care sector. It is not unusual to have a patient who could be taken care of by a good primary care physician being managed instead by a number of specialists in our acute tertiary care hospitals. This may be triggered by a single referral from primary care followed by several inter-specialist referrals even for conditions that could have been managed by the primary care physician. It has been regularly estimated that about a third of patients are wrongly sited in specialist clinics in acute care tertiary hospitals, when a good primary care doctor could provide as good or even better care by addressing these patients' needs holistically — including encouraging lifestyle changes and compliance with treatment.

The financing framework for care by specialists needs to be reviewed if we are to contain this worrying phenomenon. Sub-specialised care and holistic care should not each be seen as an end in itself or as opposing modes of treatment; rather as complementing good patient care. In a system or a hospital, when either sub-specialised care or holistic care exists without the other, healthcare is compromised.

2. Strengthening the Role of the Primary Care Practitioner

A healthcare system is only as strong as its weakest link. With the containment of infectious diseases, economic success, modern conveniences and increased life expectancy, lifestyle diseases have come to the fore. There is a need to manage chronic diseases better in the community setting. There is ample evidence that the burden of chronic disease can be contained by good primary care. We fall short here.

A significant factor contributing to the relative underdevelopment of the primary care sector is the prevailing business model for private sector primary care, which provides approximately 80% of primary care (by attendance) in Singapore. Because much of our private primary care is paid for out of pocket by the patient and most individuals can afford or are prepared to pay only relatively small sums, the private primary care model has remained underdeveloped and largely provides episodic care. The polyclinics serve as a high quality safety net for lower income Singaporeans, but the subsidy system distorts the primary care market such that even the more well-off are coming to the polyclinic especially for management of chronic disease, which requires lifelong care and is cumulatively expensive. Chronic disease management is increasingly being left to the state through its polyclinics and acute care hospital specialist outpatient clinics. Our polyclinics are staffed by about 300 doctors, whereas there are about 2000 general practitioners in the private sector. This leaves our polyclinics inundated by high patient volume every day, while the private sector remains relatively underdeveloped in managing chronic diseases. Some general practitioners have branched out into more lucrative areas of practice such as aesthetic medicine.

There is a need for greater investments in primary healthcare services. Family physicians should play an important role in the management of healthcare needs for seniors. Follow-up by a dedicated family physician in the neighbourhood or near the work place will ensure that our population's multiple needs will be comprehensively and holistically taken care of.

One option to increase the capability and capacity of our primary care sector is for the State to engage the Family Physicians in private practice and enable them through the provision of resources, to design and develop a viable (business) model for the management of patients with chronic conditions. As out-of-pocket payment alone will not sustain such a model, appropriate portable subsidies and other measures must make it attractive and nudge private primary care providers to develop the model. Appropriate training and practice opportunities would enable our family physicians and general practitioners to function at the peak of their capability, providing the more complex care necessary for managing patients with one or more chronic diseases. In this regard, the Community Healthcare Assist Scheme is a step in the right direction but much work remains to be done to transform the primary care sector.

Alternatively, similar to what the State has done for acute tertiary care, it will need to become a major player in the primary care sector. This will require more polyclinics to be built and more healthcare professionals to be recruited and retained in the public primary care sector. Recruiting and retaining a sufficient number of medical practitioners in the public primary care sector may be difficult. There may be a need to tap on other healthcare professionals, including nurse practitioners, to assist in the provision of care for some of the patients in the primary care sector.

There is also a need to grow inter-professional collaboration and to better integrate the primary care services as part of the Regional Health System. The funding framework, whether capitated or based on fee for service, needs to be structured to ensure accountability by providers and good outcomes.

3. Services for the Elderly

With the post-war baby boomers reaching the age of 65 from 2012 onwards, the proportion of elderly persons is set to increase sharply. We expect some 18% of the population (close to a million individuals) to be 65 years and older by 2030. It will be short-sighted to consider an aging society only as a dependent society, depleting the community's resources, as the elderly can remain socially and economically relevant with the appropriate interventions and support.

The State has had many committees appointed to advise on the issues of ageing and consequently has been working to implement many of their recommendations.[1,2] Some of the key recommendations include:

- The Government should systematically inform older persons of health promoting activities. For instance, the Government could publish an active lifestyle magazine to be made readily available to older persons.
- The Government should ensure that all public spaces in housing estates such as parks and sporting venues have facilities that cater to the whole family, including seniors, so as to make it convenient for seniors to engage in sports.
- The Health Promotion Board (HPB) should implement more programmes to inform seniors of the importance and benefits of healthy living and to increase public awareness of health issues.

- Sustain and grow strong family ties to ensure that the family continues to be the first line of support.
- Family physicians should play an important role in the management of healthcare needs for seniors.

One of the issues that needs to be addressed in the provision of services for the elderly is the long-term care for disabled elderly. It is not only a health problem, but it also has potentially significant social and economic impact as families become smaller and the dependency ratio worsens. Institutionalisation is a suboptimal choice as the elderly would usually prefer to live in familiar surroundings, but there may not be a choice if there are insufficient community support services or if these services are too costly. Even those who are relatively fit face challenges such as loneliness as their children leave home (empty nesters), or they are widowed and have to live alone.

In addition to living well, we need to help our population die well. Currently around 60% of deaths take place in acute hospitals,[3] although many patients prefer to die at home in familiar surroundings and the company of their loved ones. We need to build up our palliative care services and also extend such care beyond palliative care specialists, to include primary care providers.

Much is still unknown about ageing especially in the area of mental health and dementia. Filling these knowledge voids through research is vital to developing interventions to enable ageing with dignity and relieve caregiver burden.

The Business of Medicine

1. Managing International Demand for the Singapore Healthcare Brand — Singapore Medicine

Singapore Medicine began as a multi-agency government initiative to capitalise on Singapore's reputation as a preferred regional medical destination and to draw more foreign patients to Singapore by making Singapore's world-class healthcare services easily accessible to international patients. Many patients come not only because of the reputation of our medical services but because, through the years, Singapore has built a reputation for reliability and effectiveness. In 2006, the Political and Economic Risk Consultancy (based in Hong Kong) identified Singapore as having the government with the highest integrity in Asia. In 2007, the World Bank ranked Singapore as the world's easiest place to do business. For people searching for solutions to something as personal and critical as their health, this assurance of integrity and efficiency is important. The objective of Singapore Medicine was not just the health care dollars from patients, but also the dollars generated by the service industries used by the international medical tourist and their accompanying carers. Singapore Medicine was thus formally established at the beginning of the millennium.

In the early years, the Ministry of Health promoted this initiative and even set up a subsidiary, Temasia Health[4] in Indonesia. However, the Government recognised that this could work against the Ministry's social mission to serve our own citizens and the Ministry has recalibrated its involvement. However, some argue that a sizeable international patient load is useful to Singapore in more than one way. It allows for a minimum patient volume, larger than what our local population offers, that is needed to sustain the specialised training of our doctors and also the expensive technologies, all of which are important for our own population.

The challenge would be to sustain the Singapore Medicine initiative, welcoming international patients, yet maintaining a balance where Singapore Medicine serves Singaporeans best, without draining our resources. Until this balance can be achieved, it is best championed by the Singapore Tourist Promotion Board and private healthcare institutions.

2. Managing Inappropriate Utilisation

In a speech in 1980 Dr. Toh Chin Chye,[5] the then Minister of Health, spoke about how cost of medical care was rising and attributed the increase to some of the factors below, among others:

i. Third party payments such as through insurance and prepaid systems, which create the illusion that healthcare is "free." These generate demand not only for more healthcare, but also what might be viewed as "the best," or most expensive, healthcare.

ii. The supplier of medical care is also the main adviser to the consumer. This double role of the physician as adviser to the patient and as a profit oriented entrepreneur means that there is no interdependence between supply and demand as understood in the free market, because physicians as suppliers also create their own demand.

iii. The dominance of specialists in the healthcare system. This may lead to patients being treated with the most advanced current technology, whether these technologies are truly necessary or not, if specialists are restrained only by the state of the art of healing with little regard for cost-effectiveness or for other areas of healthcare needs. The intensity of treatment is regarded as an index of quality even though not all treatments contribute to patient recovery.

Although more than 30 years have passed, Dr. Toh's perceptive observations are still vaild, if not more so, today. The profit motive of healthcare companies and, increasingly, healthcare professionals, coupled with the ability to promote services through carefully crafted publicity materials that are in effect advertisements, have created demand for healthcare services that do not necessarily improve care outcomes. The social motives of wellbeing of the society which are the core values of healthcare professionals, that transcend individual characteristics of self-interest and profit, are being gradually eroded by the free market environment. As healthcare is traded on the stock exchange in Singapore some practitioners have begun to view healthcare services as no different from other commodities and that investors need to see profits. The public healthcare system is not immune from these pressures.

Medical advances have improved care outcomes, but have also increased healthcare demand. In the past there were many conditions for which there was no treatment. With better knowledge, medical equipment and pharmaceuticals, these conditions have become treatable. Reports of new treatment modalities have generated hope and supplier-induced demand. There may be a temptation to provide treatments that have as yet not been adequately evaluated or pressure to administer these treatments at a lower threshold of need than supported by evidence, especially when there is a willing payer as in terminal illness, when the treatment provided may neither be cost-effective nor change the patient's quality of life. Even for established procedures, the observed variations beg the question of the supplier's influence. The Caesarean section rate in 1965 was 1240 cases for 38,849 live births i.e. 3.2%.[6] In 2003, the rate in our public hospitals was about 25% and that in the private hospitals ranged from 30–40%[7]. In a more recent unpublished review, the rate in public hospitals exceeded 30% and that in private hospitals was close to 50% with some individual practitioners' rate exceeding 60%. While Caesarean section is critical to avoiding maternal and foetal complications, its dominance as the mode of delivery must certainly be reviewed.

With more people having health insurance or employee benefits which provide first dollar coverage, many now seek expensive investigations and treatment. Monitoring and regulations are important to contain abuses, but these are by nature reactive and applicable mainly to clear-cut transgressions. However there is a significant grey zone where the necessity of a particular treatment is debatable. While the provider may argue that this is the patient's choice, the provider is not a neutral party, but influences the choice by how the options are presented to the patient and family.

Another area where the government can play a key role in enabling the market to function for the benefit of Singaporeans is by ensuring transparent information about medical services and the outcomes in different healthcare facilities. Such information could be useful to influence behaviour of providers and healthcare choices by the population. Information should include bill sizes and intervention rates for the same conditions across institutions or clinics. This information would enable people to make more informed choices which could in turn influence supplier behaviour and pricing. At present, the Ministry of Health has been making such information available on their websites.

We need to also ensure that policies intended to improve the efficiency of care do not lead to unintended consequences. For example the Consultation Fee Scheme (CF Scheme) dramatically reduced waiting time for elective surgery, from months to within weeks and in many instances, within days. This may however, at the same time, result in unnecessary surgeries for conditions when rest with careful monitoring alone may have resulted in recovery. Taleb has aptly captured this dilemma:

In Praise of Procrastination — The Fabian Kind[8]:

> "There is an element of deceit associated with interventionism, accelerating in a professionalized society. It's much easier to sell "Look what I did for you" than "Look what I avoided for you." Of course a bonus system based on "performance" exacerbates the problem. I've looked in history for heroes who became heroes for what they did not do, but it is hard to observe nonaction; I could not easily find any. The doctor who refrains from operating on a back (a very expensive surgery), instead giving it a chance to heal itself, will not be rewarded and judged as favorably as the doctor who makes the surgery look indispensable, then brings relief to the patient while exposing him to operating risks, while accruing great financial rewards to himself."

The CF Scheme has recently been re-calibrated so that the ethics of practice are not diluted.

Resilient Healthcare System

1. Emergency Preparedness

Prosperity may provide a comfortable life, but it does not necessarily protect us against unforeseen events that cause significant loss of human life. In Singapore we have had our share of such crises, including an emerging infection like SARS or a civil disaster like the "Spyros disaster" or the Hotel New World collapse.

As a nation, especially with a small and open economy like ours, we have had to incorporate crisis management plans into our system. When the Emergency Unit was set up at the General Hospital in 1964, the unit was tasked to work out plans to handle a national emergency. We saw the first major post-independence crisis in 1978 when the "Spyros disaster" took place. An explosion in an oil tanker left 86 casualties with severe burns and 76 dead. Since then we have had other crises, such as SARS in 2003 and H1N1 in 2009. They have enabled us to improve our plans and to build redundancies into our system that can be called upon in case of emergencies. Yet we cannot be complacent as by its very nature, an emergency embodies the unexpected. We will need to be vigilant, constantly testing and renewing our readiness.

> *"I believe the answer lies not in convincing ourselves that the pandemic will not come, or in avoiding it should it come, but in being well prepared."[9]*

2. Improving Healthcare Productivity

Healthcare is a unique industry where innovations tend to increase costs, unlike industries such as information technology where computers become cheaper even as they become more powerful. Even if we assume that the State is able to meet the increased costs, ensuring sufficient manpower capacity and capability to meet the increased demand will always be a challenge. With the diverse needs of the nation, the local talent pool will need to be shared with other areas of growth and importance. To maintain the standards of healthcare for the nation, we will need to import talent, but we cannot assume that there will always be a ready pool that we can access and rely on.

We need to increase productivity in healthcare. Some headway has been made in areas such as telemedicine. For example, the introduction of teleradiology in Singapore has changed the way radiologists work. Once reporting was outsourced to external parties outside Singapore, some types of radiology reports in Singapore became almost immediate. Another example is information technology. The Electronic Medical Record (EMR) has made it possible for patients to have their records — which are physically located in one institution — seen by doctors in another institution when the patient moves between institutions. With advances like this, investigations do not need to be repeated and time for diagnosis and treatment is reduced, resulting in avoidance of additional costs, and more efficient and effective healthcare.

We must persist in improving productivity not just at the services, but also at the systems level through better models of care.

Conclusion

The leaders of the nation and healthcare professionals have worked diligently and have transformed healthcare services in the last half century. Singaporeans enjoy an unprecedented level of healthcare. The above challenges are not unique to Singapore and new challenges may arise from time to time requiring dynamic solutions. However we have benefitted from our predecessors and are in a stronger position compared with many other countries. With continued strong political and professional leadership, we are optimistic that every Singaporean can continue to have access to affordable and quality healthcare.

References

1. Ministry of Community Development. (1999) Report on the Inter-Ministerial Committee on Ageing Population. Singapore; ISBN 9971-88-718-5.
2. Committee on Ageing Issues. (2006) *Report on the Ageing Population*. Singapore.
3. Registrar-General of Births and Deaths. (2014) "Report on Registration Of Births and Deaths 2013." *Registry of Births and Deaths*, Immigration and Checkpoint Authority, Singapore.
4. Lim Meng-Kin. "Health Care Systems in Transition, Part I: An overview of health care systems in Singapore." *Journal of Public Health Medicine.* **20**(1): 16–22.
5. Toh Chin Chye. Some Causes of Spiraling Medical Care Costs; Health — A Crucial Concern; Excerpts from Ministerial Speeches on Health 1980/82 pp. 4–8. Singapore-Malaya Collection, National University of Singapore Medical Library
6. Singapore Ministry of Health Report 1965. Singapore-Malaya Collection, National University of Singapore Medical Library, p. 168.
7. Ganga Ganesan. (2004) *Deliveries in Singapore; Volume and Resources*. Ministry of Health information paper.
8. Nassim Nicholas Taleb. (2012) "Antifragile: Things That Gain from Disorder." *In Praise of Procrastination — the Fabian kind*. Random House, p. 121. ISBN 978-1-4000-6782-4.
9. "State of Health — Report of the Director of Medical Services 2003-2012." p. 95. ISBN 978-981-07-6828-7.

Index